Bob Weih

Modern Applied
Biostatistical Methods
Using S-Plus

MONOGRAPHS IN EPIDEMIOLOGY AND BIOSTATISTICS
Edited by Jennifer L. Kelsey, Michael G. Marmot,
Paul D. Stolley, Martin P. Vessey

2. CASE CONTROL STUDIES
Design, Conduct Analysis
James J. Schlesselman   1982

3. EPIDEMIOLOGY OF
MUSCULOSKELETAL
DISORDERS
Jennifer L. Kelsey   1982

6. THE LEUKEMIAS
Epidemiologic Aspects
Martha S. Linet   1984

8. CLINICAL TRIALS
Design, Conduct, and Analysis
Curtis L. Meinert   1986

12. STATISTICAL METHODS
IN EPIDEMIOLOGY
Harold A. Kahn and
Christopher T. Sempos   1989

13. RESEARCH METHODS
IN OCCUPATIONAL
EPIDEMIOLOGY
Harvey Checkoway, Neil E. Pearce,
Douglas J. Crawford-Brown   1989

14. CONCEPTION TO BIRTH
Epidemiology of Prenatal Development
Jennie Kline, Zena Stein,
Mervyn Susser   1989

15. NUTRITIONAL
EPIDEMIOLOGY
Walter Willet   1990

16. STATISTICAL MODELS
FOR LONGITUDINAL
STUDIES OF HEALTH
James H. Dwyer, Manning Feinleib,
Peter Lippert,
Hans Hoffmeister   1992

18. THE DRUG ETIOLOGY OF
AGRANULOCYTOSIS AND
APLASTIC ANEMIA
David W. Kaufman, Judith P. Kelly,
Micha Levy, Samuel Shapiro   1991

19. SCREENING IN CHRONIC
DISEASE, SECOND EDITION
Alan S. Morrison   1992

20. EPIDEMIOLOGY AND
CONTROL OF NEURAL TUBE
DEFECTS
J. Mark Elwood, Julian Little,
J. Harold Elwood   1992

21. PRINCIPLES OF EXPOSURE
MEASUREMENT IN
EPIDEMIOLOGY
Bruce K. Armstrong, Emily White,
Rodolfo Saracci   1992

22. FUNDAMENTALS OF
GENETIC EPIDEMIOLOGY
Muin J. Khoury, Terri H. Beaty,
Bernice H. Cohen   1993

23. AIDS EPIDEMIOLOGY:
A QUANTITATIVE APPROACH
Ron Brookmeyer and
Mitchell H. Gail   1994

24. META-ANALYSIS, DECISION
ANALYSIS, AND COST-
EFFECTIVENESS ANALYSIS
*Methods for Quantitative Synthesis in
Medicine*
Diana B. Petitti   1994

25. STATISTICAL ANALYSIS
OF EPIDEMIOLOGIC DATA,
SECOND EDITION
Steve Selvin   1996

26. METHODS IN
OBSERVATIONAL
EPIDEMIOLOGY,
SECOND EDITION
Jennifer L. Kelsey,
Alice S. Whittemore,
Alfred S. Evans,
W. Douglas Thompson   1996

27. DESIGN AND ANALYSIS OF
GROUP-RANDOMIZED TRIALS
David M. Murray   1998

28. MODERN APPLIED
BIOSTATISTICAL METHODS
USING S-PLUS
Steve Selvin   1998

Monographs in Epidemiology and Biostatistics
Volume 28

Modern Applied Biostatistical Methods
Using S-Plus

Steve Selvin, Ph.D.
University of California, Berkeley

New York   Oxford
Oxford University Press
1998

Oxford University Press

Oxford   New York
Athens   Auckland   Bangkok   Bogota
Bombay   Buenos Aires   Calcutta   Cape Town
Dar es Salaam   Delhi   Florence   Hong Kong   Istanbul
Karachi   Kuala Lumpur   Madras   Madrid
Melbourne   Mexico City   Nairobi   Paris
Singapore   Taipei   Tokyo   Toronto   Warsaw

and associated companies in
Berlin   Ibadan

Library of Congress Cataloging-in-Publication Data
Selvin S.
Modern applied biostatistical methods:
using S-Plus / Steve Selvin
p.   cm.
Includes bibliographical references and index.
ISBN 0-19-512025-6 (alk. paper)
1. Biometry.   2. Biology—Data processing.
3. S-Plus.
I. Title.
QH323.5.S448   1998   570'.1'5195—dc21   97-19777

987654321

Printed in the United States of America
on acid-free paper

For Nancy

Preface

Statistical texts are usually books that deal with theory or books that discuss applications or manuals that explain the details of an analytic computer language. Computer manuals typically omit explanations of statistical reasoning and theoretical or applied texts rarely make reference to issues of implementation. This text contains these related elements integrated into a single presentation. A statistical computer language called SPLUS is used in conjunction with a series of research data sets to describe fundamental and intermediate biostatistical methods. Explanations of the statistical logic (without elaborate mathematics), detailed applications, and descriptions of the accompanying computer/graphic analyses are the basic ingredients of the topics presented. Theory, data, implementation, graphics, and interpretation are combined to convey the entire biostatistical process.

Each section begins with a brief description of the reasoning underlying a particular statistical approach, followed by an analysis of a relevant data set. The SPLUS commands, S-functions, and computer code are used to produce numerical results along with the corresponding graphic output. Graphic analysis is a critical and sometimes neglected part of data analysis. Inferences and conclusions then complete the description of each statistical method.

The methods and examples covered in the text came from a one-semester course I have taught to first-year biostatistics and advanced epidemiology graduate students. The mathematical level is elementary, requiring a bit of first-year calculus and some matrix algebra (which can be omitted with only minor losses in continuity). Although it is not strictly necessary, the reader ideally should have access to SPLUS in either a UNIX or Windows computer environment. Clearly, it is important to verify the example analyses and to try other approaches (all data sets in the examples are complete). I have assumed that the exercises at the end of each chapter will be done with S-tools.

A large number of S-language examples are part of the text (not relegated to an appendix). These examples provide specific illustrations and, additionally, express in concrete terms the mechanics of the analytic process. Abstract symbols and mathematical manipulations are one way to communicate the concepts and issues underlying a statistical analysis. The purpose of the extensive number of S-language illustrations is to make the details of the statistical calculations readily accessible, providing another perspective on how and why statistical methods identify the properties of collected data. Of course, a by-product of studying the computer implementation is that one also learns the language of a modern statistical analysis system. The SPLUS language examples are intentionally made as simple as possible, at the expense of generality. By and large, the S-system contains general, "user-friendly" alternatives that perform the same or similar tasks.

A good question is: Why SPLUS? SPLUS is not a typical statistical analysis system. In fact, it is a computer language that facilitates statistical analysis. The language is made up of a large number of useful components. The distinct advantage of SPLUS is that the use is free to create a wide range of data-analysis schemes out of these components and is not restricted to the predetermined format typical of "batch" type analytic systems. The components can be linked together to create exactly the analysis desired. Furthermore, the creation of S-programs is done in an interactive environment. Results are continuously available and allow the user to modify or correct the S-program based on intermediate results. A particularly valuable tool in this interactive environment is the ability to create ongoing graphic displays. The S-graphic displays are easily and quickly produced. Yet another feature is the ability to generated random values with specific statistical properties. These random values are important in simulation and estimation procedures. The combination of a flexible computer language designed for statistical analysis, interactively applied with access to graphic displays and random numbers makes the S-system a powerful tool in the hands of individuals involved in data analysis.

The chapter-by-chapter topics that make up the text are:

Chapter 1 describes a selected set of S-language commands that are particularly useful for statistical applications. The S-commands discussed are only a small proportion of the commands available but consitute a "minimum" set, which is the basis of the statistical applications that follow. The S-tools are illustrated with numerous examples because, like the learning of most languages, imitation of existing patterns begins to provide an understanding of the language as a whole.

Chapter 2 combines two elements—descriptive statistics and S-graphics. Discussion of such descriptive techniques as histograms, stem-and-leaf displays, boxplots, qqplots, smoothing strategies, and cluster analyses is one purpose of the chapter. The interpretation of these descriptive techniques is considerably enhanced with graphic displays. Presentation of the S-tools to produce these graphic representations is the other major purpose of the chapter. For example, density estimation is one of the topics discussed, as well as the S-language necessary to produce the graphic displays of the estimated densities.

Chapter 3 is devoted to generating, testing, and applying random variables. Computer-simulated data with specified statistical features are an important part of exploring the properties of analytic techniques. Random values also play a fundamental role in estimation and statistical testing. The knowledge of both the statistical reasoning and the methods to produce random values is necessary to modern biostatistical analysis.

An extremely useful approach to identifying and understanding the relationship among multivariate measurements involves the application of linear models. Chapter 4 contains the logic, implementation, and interpretation of three commonly used analytic models—linear, logistic, and Poisson. Each model is applied to a research data set producing numerical results, again supplemented with graphic analysis. The logic of the approach and computer S-code are again included, giving a comprehensive picture of the application of linear models to explore the relationships within multivariable data.

Chapter 5 introduces three statistical estimation procedures—maximum likelihood, bootstrap, and both ordinary and nonlinear least squares techniques. Once again the logic, the S-code, the graphic displays, and a series of applications are presented. The study of these three basic estimation procedues, as before, produces insight into the entire analytic process with a focus on estimating summary values from sampled data.

Discrete data displayed in tables is certainly central to many data sets. Chapter 6 is an introductory discussion of the analysis of multivariate discrete data. The discussion of this broad topic begins with the analysis of 2×2 tables, continues with a discussion of $r \times c$ tables, and concludes with a presentation of using loglinear models to analyze discrete multivariate tabular data. Again, S-code and concrete data examples illustrate the concepts and implementation.

Chapter 7 is a collection of valuable statistical techniques (analysis of variance, model selection methods, principal components analysis, and canonical correlation analysis). For these four topics, the emphasis is on application and implementation.

Starting with rates and life tables and ending with Cox's proportional hazards model, Chapter 8 presents the logic, graphics, and analytic approaches to investigate a few basic issues that emerge from survival data. For example, leukemia follow-up data from a clinical trial are analyzed with S-tools, displayed with S-graphics, and the results interpreted from several points of view.

Berkeley, Cal.   S.S.
April 1997

Contents

1. S-language, 3

In the beginning, 3
Three data types—and some input conventions, 5
Reading values into SPLUS, 10
S-tools—a beginning set, 11
S-arithmetic, 19
More S-tools—intermediate set, 20
S-tools for statistics, 24
Statistical distributions in SPLUS, 29
Arrays and tables, 33
Matrix algebra tools, 39
Some additional S-tools, 43
Four S-code examples, 49
The .Data file, 57
Addendum: Built-in editors, 60
Problem set I, 61

2. Descriptive Techniques, 65

Description of descriptive statistics, 65
Basic statistical measures, 67
Histogram smoothing—density estimation, 72
Stem-and-leaf display, 76
Comparison of groups—t-test, 79
Comparison of groups—boxplots, 80
Comparison of data to a theoretical distribution—quantile plots, 84
Comparison of groups—qqplots, 89

xy-plot, 95
Three-dimensional plots—perspective plots, 98
Three-dimensional plots—contour plots, 101
Three-dimensional plots—rotation, 104
Smoothing, 109
Two-dimensional smoothing of spatial data, 113
Clusters as a description of data, 116
Additivity—"sweeping" an array, 126
Example—geographic calculations using S-functions, 133
Estimation of the center of a two-dimensional distribution, 135
Addendum: S-geometry, 136
Problem set II, 139

3. Simulation: Random Values, 141

Random uniform values, 142
An example, 152
Sampling without and with replacement, 155
Random sample from a discrete probability distribution—
    acceptance/rejection sampling, 156
Random sample from a discrete probability distribution—
    inverse transform method, 160
Binomial probability distribution, 162
Hypergeometric probability distribution, 165
Poisson probability distribution, 168
Geometric probability distribution, 172
Random samples from a continuous distribution, 174
Inverse transform method, 177
Simulating values from the normal distribution, 180
Four other statistical distributions, 183
Simulating minimum and maximum values, 185
Butler's method, 186
Random values over a complex region, 188
Multivariate normal variables, 190
Problem set III, 192

4. General Linear Models, 195

Simplest case—univariate linear regression, 195
Multivariable case, 199

Multivariable linear model, 199
A closer look at residual values, 217
Predict—pointwise confidence intervals, 221
Formulas for *glm( )*, 222
Polynomial regression, 223
Discriminant analysis, 227
Linear logistic model, 236
Categorical data—bivariate linear logistic model, 239
Multivariable data—linear logistic model, 243
Goodness-of-fit, 248
Poisson model, 250
Multivariable Poisson model, 257
Problem set IV, 263

5. Estimation, 266

Estimation: Maximum Likelihood, 266

Estimator properties, 266
Maximum likelihood estimator, 267
Scoring to find maximum likelihood estimates, 272
Multiparameter estimation, 277
Generalized scoring, 279

Estimation: Bootstrap, 283

Background, 283
General outline, 284
Sample mean from a normal population, 285
Confidence limits, 288
An example—relative risk, 289
Median, 290
Simple linear regression, 291
Jackknife estimation, 297
Bias estimation, 300
Two-sample test—bootstrap approach, 301
Two-sample test—randomization approach, 302

Estimation: Least Squares, 305

Least squares properties, 305
Non-linear least squares estimation, 309
Problem set V, 319

6. Analysis of Tabular Data, 323

   Two by two tables, 323
   Matched pairs—binary response, 328
   Two by k table, 330
   Measures of association—2×2 table, 334
   Measures of association—$r \times c$ table, 336
   Measures of association—table with ordinal variables, 338
   Loglinear model, 341
   Multidimensional—k-level variables, 348
   High dimensional tables, 354
   Problem set VI, 358

7. Analysis of Variance and Some Other S-Functions, 361

   Analysis of variance, 361
   One-way design, 361
   Nested design, 367
   Two-way classification with one observation per cell, 369
   Matched pairs—measured response, 378
   Two-way classification with more than one observation per cell, 381
   Leaps—a model selection technique, 384
   Principal components, 391
   Canonical correlations, 401
   Problem set VII, 407

8. Rates, Life Tables, and Survival, 410

   Rates, 410
   Life tables, 417
   Survival analysis—an introduction, 423
   Nonparametric estimation of a survival curve, 429
   Hazard rate—estimation, 430
   Mean/median survival time, 432
   Proportional hazards model, 437
   Problem set VIII, 450

Index, 453

Modern Applied
Biostatistical Methods
Using S-Plus

1

S-language

IN THE BEGINNING

To initiate the S-language, type the word *Splus* and press the enter-key. The computer reply looks something like:

```
SPLUS : Copyright (c) 1988, 1993 Statistical Sciences.
S : Copyright AT&T.
Version 3.2 Release 1 for Sun Sparc, SunOS 4.x : 1993
Working data will be in /h/name/.Data
>
```

The details of the response differ depending on the computer operating system, the particular version of SPLUS, and a variety of other generally inconsequential factors. The important part is the symbol ">". This prompt means that the S-program is in place and ready to respond to commands from the user. Anything typed at the terminal following the prompt is taken as a command and when the enter-key is pressed, the SPLUS program attempts to execute the command.

The second most important command after *Splus* is $q()$. This command ends an S-session and returns the computer to its operating system. The parentheses are an S-language convention that identifies input arguments, as will be seen. If only the command q is executed (no parentheses), SPLUS displays at the terminal the computer code invoked by the command and does not execute the command. This feature is a property of all S-functions.

A question immediately arises: what commands are available? The answer is not simple. There are hundreds of possibilities and only a subset is described in the following. To start, Table 1.1 lists symbols and functions that are likely useful for statistical analysis. To find out what these commands do and how they are used, the S-language provides "online" descriptions. These descriptions are invoked by typing *help*() where the specific command to be described is placed between the parentheses, such as any of the functions from Table 1.1. For example, *help*(q) produces on the terminal screen:

```
Quit From S-PLUS
```

Table 1.1. Partial list of S-functions and symbols (explained in detail by the S-help system)

!	all	df	kappa	phyper	replace
!=	anova	dgamma	kronecker	pi	resid
$	any	dgeom	kruskal.test	pie	residuals
%%	aperm	dget	labels	plnorm	rexp
%*%	apply	dhyper	lag	plogis	rf
%c%	approx	diag	lapply	plot	rgamma
%m%	array	diff	leaps	pnbinom	rgeom
%o%	arrows	dim	legend	pnorm	rhyper
&	asin	dimnames	length	pnrange	rlnorm
&&	asinh	discr	lgamma	points	rlogis
*	assign	dist	lines	poisson	rm
**	atan	dlnorm	list	poly	rnbinom
+	atanh	dlogis	lm	postscript	rnorm
-	attach	dnbinom	lo	ppois	round
->	attr	dnorm	loess	prcomp	row
:	audit.file	dotchart	log	pretty	rpois
<	axes	double	log10	prod	rt
<-	axis	dpois	logical	prompt	runif
<<-	backsolve	dput	loglin	pscript	rweibull
<=	barplot	drop	lowess	pt	rwilcox
==	binomial	dt	lpr	punif	sample
>	boxplot	dump	ls	pweibull	sapply
>=	break	dunif	lsfit	pwilcox	save
?	c	duplicated	mahalanobis	q	scale
AUDIT	cancor	dweibull	mantelhaen.test	qbeta	scan
BATCH	cat	dwilcox	match	qbinom	search
Beta	category	eigen	matpoints	qcauchy	segments
Binomial	cbind	else	matrix	qchisq	seq
Cauchy	ceiling	encode	max	qexp	show
Chisquare	chisq.test	end	mcnemar.test	qf	sign
Exponential	chol	exp	mean	qgamma	signif
F	coef	faces	median	qgeom	sin
For	col	factor	min	qhyper	single
GAMMA	compare	family	month	qlnorm	sinh
Gamma	contour	find	motif	qlogis	sink
Geometric	coplot	fix	na	qnbinom	smatrix
Hypergeometric	cor	floor	na.omit	qnorm	smooth
Logistic	cor.test	for	ncol	qpois	solve
Lognormal	cos	format	next	qqline	sort
NegBinomial	cosh	formula	nrow	qqnorm	source
Normal	coxreg	frequency	ns	quantile	spin
T	crossprod	friedman.test	null	qunif	spline
TRUNC_AUDIT	crt	function	order	qweibull	sqrt
Uniform	cstr	gaussian	outer	qwilcox	stars
Weibull	cumprod	get	pairs	random	stepwise
Wilcoxon	cumsum	glm	par	randomize	sum
X11	cut	hclust	paste	range	summary
abline	date	help	pattern	rank	sweep
abs	dbeta	hist	pbeta	rbeta	t
ace	dbinom	hist2d	pbinom	rbind	t.test
acf	dcauchy	history	pcauchy	rbinom	table
acos	dchisq	identify	pchisq	rcauchy	tabulate
acosh	density	if	persp	rchisq	tan
again	deriv	ifelse	pf	remove	tanh
aggregate	deviance	integer	pgamma	rep	tapply
alias	dexp	integrate	pgeom	repeat	terms

```
DESCRIPTION:
     Terminates the current S-PLUS session.
USAGE:
       q(n=0)
```

OPTIONAL ARGUMENTS:

```
n: integer value, to be used, modulo 256, as the
   exit status of the S-PLUS process. (In shell
   scripts, a non-zero exit status is conventionally
   an indication of an error.)
```

```
  SIDE EFFECTS:
     Causes termination of the S-PLUS session and
     returns to the operating system. If one or
     more graphics devices are active, a
     device-dependent wrap-up routine will be
     executed for each active device. The
     function or expression .Last, if it exists,
     will be called or evaluated before quitting.
```

$$\vdots$$

A quick way to invoke the help command is to type the function name preceded by a question mark. For example, *?q* produces the same response as *help(q)*. Also, an extensive online help-system using a menu approach is available. The S-command *help.start(gui="motif")* presents a menu that allows the user to choose among a number of categories and then among specific S-functions within these categories. For curiosity sake, "gui" stands for graphical user interface. To print an S-help "page," use the command *help(function.name,offline=T)* and the requested help "page" is sent directly to printer. Throughout the text the reader will be encouraged to use the "online" help system. It is an extremely useful S-tool. Several extensive manuals are available that completely describe the S-language from both a user's and a programmer's point of view ([1], [2], and [3]).

The quit command halts the SPLUS program but, on occasions, it is desirable to halt an executing command. To interrupt an S-command during execution, control/c-key (control and c-keys pressed simultaneously) stops the currently executing command and returns the system to the S-prompt, not to the operating system. Pressing the control key and the "back-slash" key simultaneously halts the executing SPLUS program and returns to the operating system.

THREE DATA TYPES—AND SOME INPUT CONVENTIONS

There are three primary data types in the S-language: a single value, a vector of values, and an array of values. All three types are referred to with a single symbol and SPLUS keeps track of the data type. A single value such as the number 10 can be labeled with a symbolic name such as x or

```
> x<- 10
```

The "arrow" means that the value 10 is assigned the symbolic name x. This same expression is also given by

```
> x_10
```

using an underscore to define x as 10. Both styles produce the same result and, for no particular reason, the "arrow" syntax is used in the following. The "arrow" convention does have the small advantage that assignments go both ways;

```
> 10 ->x
```

is an acceptable syntax but

```
> 10_x
```

is not. If a symbol alone is typed at the terminal followed by pressing the enter-key, the value of that symbol is displayed on the terminal screen. For example,

```
> x
[1] 10.
```

The S-labeling "[1]" will become clearer when more extensive variables are discussed. Variables can be manipulated to produce new values. For example,

```
> x+100
[1] 110
```

or

```
> x^2
[1] 100
```

where x^2 means the square of the value x (x^2).

Practically any combination of letters, numbers, and symbols is available to name a variable. A few choices conflict with function names that are already part of the S-language (e.g., *for*, *if*, *c*, and *t*—Table 1.1). When a variable name coincides with an established S-name, a warning or error message is issued. In some cases the user 's variable remains defined. However, it is best to avoid conflicting names altogether, which is easily done. Incidentally, variable names in SPLUS are case sensitive, which means that a distinction is made between upper and lower case letters in a variable name (e.g., x is different from X and fx is different from Fx).

A vector of values can also be labeled by a single symbol such as x. To define x as the vector containing values 10, 20, 30, and 40, an S-function $c()$ can be used ("c" for combine). The $c()$ command combines the series of values placed between the parentheses and separated with commas into a single variable representation, such as

```
> x<- c(10,20,30,40)
> x
[1] 10 20 30 40.
```

Like the single value variable, a vector variable can be manipulated to form new variables. Two examples are

```
> x+100
[1] 110 120 130 140
> x^2
[1]  100  400  900  1600.
```

Notice that the operator (e.g., + and ^) is applied to each element contained in the vector.

The c( ) command performs a variety of tasks. Two more examples are

```
> ctemp<- c(1,2,3,4,5,6,7,8,9)
> c(ctemp,ctemp,ctemp)
[1] 1 2 3 4 5 6 7 8 9 1 2 3 4 5 6 7 8 9 1 2
    3 4 5 6 7 8 9
> c(0,ctemp,10)
[1] 0 1 2 3 4 5 6 7 8 9 10.
```

Similar to a single value or vector value variable, an array of values can be assigned a single variable name. For two vectors, the commands

```
> c1<- c(10,20,30,40)
> c2<- c(5,10,15,20)
```

and the command *cbind*( ) ("cbind" for columns combined) form a two-dimensional array of values where

```
> x<- cbind(c1,c2)
> x
     c1 c2
[1,] 10  5
[2,] 20 10
[3,] 30 15
[4,] 40 20.
```

The *cbind*( ) command joins the vectors named as arguments (placed between the parentheses and separated with commas) so that they form the columns of an array. Like the previous two cases, this array can be manipulated using the single symbol x and, for example,

```
> x+100
      c1   c2
[1,] 110 105
[2,] 120 110
[3,] 130 115
[4,] 140 120
```

and

```
> x^2
       c1  c2
[1,]   100  25
[2,]   400 100
[3,]   900 225
[4,] 1600 400.
```

The *cbind()* command has a companion command *rbind()* ("rbind" for rows combined) that combines vectors into the rows of an array. For example,

```
> rbind(c1,c2)
    [,1] [,2] [,3] [,4]
c1    10   20   30   40
c2     5   10   15   20.
```

An increasing or decreasing sequence of integers is succinctly generated by the S-syntax *first value: last value* such as

```
> 0:10
 [1] 0 1 2 3 4 5 6 7 8 9 10
> temp<- 1:9
> temp
 [1] 1 2 3 4 5 6 7 8 9
> 20:8
 [1] 20 19 18 17 16 15 14 13 12 11 10 9 8
> c(1:5,5:1,1:5)
 [1] 1 2 3 4 5 5 4 3 2 1 1 2 3 4 5.
> rbind(1:6,11:16,111:116)
     [,1] [,2] [,3] [,4] [,5] [,6]
[1,]    1    2    3    4    5    6
[2,]   11   12   13   14   15   16
[3,]  111  112  113  114  115  116.
```

A two-dimensional array of values is also created with the S-function *matrix()* which has the general form

matrix(value or vector of values, number of rows, number of columns).

For example, an array labeled *darray* is created by

```
> darray<- matrix(1:12,3,4)
> darray
     [,1] [,2] [,3] [,4]
[1,]    1    4    7   10
[2,]    2    5    8   11
[3,]    3    6    9   12.
```

In some cases, the last argument is not needed. For example,

```
> array0<- matrix(1:12,6)
> array0
     [,1] [,2]
[1,]    1    7
[2,]    2    8
[3,]    3    9
[4,]    4   10
[5,]    5   11
[6,]    6   12
```

produces an array with six rows and, necessarily, two columns.

Specific values of an array are extracted using square brackets and the array name. The command *darray*[*i, j*] extracts a single value from the array named *darray* where *i* represents the row and *j* represents the column location of the value or, specifically,

```
> darray[2,2]
[1] 5.
```

An entire row or column can be extracted by leaving out the column or row specification. The expression *darray*[*i*,] extracts the ith row and the expression *darray*[*,j*] extracts the jth column of the array *darray*.

For example,

```
> darray[2,]
[1]   2   5   8 1
> darray[,3]
[1] 7 8 9.
```

Extracted values can be given a name and used in the same way as any S-variable. Therefore,

```
> cell12<- darray[1,2]
> cell12
[1] 4
> row2<- darray[2,]
> row2
[1]   2 5 8 11
> row2+10
[1] 12 15 18 21
> row2^2
[1]    4 25 64 121
> c(row2,row2^2,row2^3)
[1]   2   5   8   11   4   25   64   121   8   125   512   1331.
```

This "square-bracket" convention is additionally used to label the rows and the columns of an array (for example, *darray* in the above illustration). This convention provides a useful label and serves as a reminder of the syntax for extracting rows and columns. The ability to separate the elements of an array into components is an important property of the S-language and will be described in more detail.

A matrix of constants is easily created by *matrix(constant, nrows, ncols)*; to illustrate:

```
> matrix(1,3,5)
      [,1] [,2] [,3] [,4] [,5]
[1,]   1    1    1    1    1
[2,]   1    1    1    1    1
[3,]   1    1    1    1    1.
```

READING VALUES INTO SPLUS

A common method to bring data into SPLUS is by reading an exterior file. Say an exterior file called "test.file" has three lines and looks like

```
1 2 3 4
5 6 7
8 9
```

The S-language reads these values into the S-vector *data* with the command *scan( )* as follows:

```
> # read data from an exterior file named test.file
> data<- scan("test.file")
> data
[1] 1 2 3 4 5 6 7 8 9.
```

The symbol # identifies comments included in the S-code. Comment statements (words or symbols preceded by a #-sign) are used to add descriptive remarks to the S-code and are not executed. The quotes around a file name indicate that the file is exterior to SPLUS, a so-called system file. The S-function *scan( )* reads all numeric values encountered in the named exterior file (separated by any number of blanks) into a single vector. A number of other options exist for reading data with *scan( )* (see ?*scan*). For example, character data or data separated by other delimiters such as commas can be read with the *scan( )* command using special options.

Data entered directly from the keyboard are read also using the command *scan( )* where

```
> # data entered from the keyboard
> data<- scan()
> 1 # typed from the keyboard
> 2 # typed from the keyboard
> 3 # typed from the keyboard
> 4 # typed from the keyboard
> 5 # typed from the keyboard
> 6 # typed from the keyboard
> 7 # typed from the keyboard
> 8 # typed from the keyboard
> 9 # typed from the keyboard
> return # typed from the keyboard
> data
[1] 1 2 3 4 5 6 7 8 9
```

again produces the S-vector labeled *data*. Two consecutive S-functions that yield an S-array of values read from the exterior file labeled *test.file* are

```
> temp<- scan("test.file")
> d0<- matrix(temp,3,3)
> d0
      [,1] [,2] [,3]
[1,]    1    4    7
[2,]    2    5    8
[3,]    3    6    9.
```

This same result is achieved by nesting these two commands into a single command line producing the identical result, or

```
> d0<- matrix(scan("test.file"),3,3)
```

The nesting of S-functions is a general property of the S-language. Any number of commands can be nested into a single expression. The advantage is that the S-code is compact and brief. The disadvantage is that reading the code (by humans) is sometimes difficult and error prone.

Data values are automatically (by "default") formed into columns of an array by the S-function *matrix( )* or, if the user takes charge, then

```
> d0<- matrix(scan("test.file"),3,byrow=F)
> d0
     [,1] [,2] [,3]
[1,]   1    4    7
[2,]   2    5    8
[3,]   3    6    9.
```

To read the data in *test.file* and form the values into rows of an array, then

```
> d0<- matrix(scan("test.file"),3,byrow=T)
> d0
     [,1] [,2] [,3]
[1,]   1    2    3
[2,]   4    5    6
[3,]   7    8    9.
```

S-TOOLS—A BEGINNING SET

A good rule of thumb is—if you have to type more than a few repetitious values, there is probably an S-function that makes it possible for the computer to produce these values. The S-function *rep( )* ("rep" for repeat) is valuable in this context. This S-command produces a vector of repeating values using the general form

rep(value(s) to be repeated, number(s) of repetitions).

Some examples are

```
> rep(0,times=10)
[1] 0 0 0 0 0 0 0 0 0 0
> rep(0,10)
[1] 0 0 0 0 0 0 0 0 0 0
> rep(c(3,2,1),5)
[1] 3 2 1 3 2 1 3 2 1 3 2 1 3 2 1
> rep(c(3,2,1),c(1,2,3))
[1] 3 2 2 1 1 1
> rep(1:4,c(2,4,6,8))
[1] 1 1 2 2 2 2 3 3 3 3 3 3 4 4 4 4 4 4 4 4.
```

A related command produces a sequence of values and has the general form

$$seq(start, \ end, \ interval).$$

Some examples are

```
> 1:8
[1] 1 2 3 4 5 6 7 8
> seq(8)
[1] 1 2 3 4 5 6 7 8
> seq(1,8,1)
[1] 1 2 3 4 5 6 7 8
> seq(0,10,2)
[1]  0  2  4  6  8  10
>seq(from=0,to=1,by=0.1)
[1] 0.0 0.1 0.2 0.3 0.4 0.5 0.6 0.7 0.8 0.9 1.0
> seq(0,1,by=0.1)
[1] 0.0 0.1 0.2 0.3 0.4 0.5 0.6 0.7 0.8 0.9 1.0
> seq(0,1,0.1)
[1] 0.0 0.1 0.2 0.3 0.4 0.5 0.6 0.7 0.8 0.9 1.0
> seq(0,1,0.2)
[1] 0.0 0.2 0.4 0.6 0.8 1.0
> seq(0,1,length=5)
[1] 0.00 0.25 0.50 0.75 1.00
> seq(0,1,length=12)
[1] 0.00000000  0.09090909  0.18181818  0.27272727  0.36363636
[6] 0.45454545  0.54545455  0.63636364  0.72727273  0.81818182
[11] 0.90909091 1.00000000
> seq(20,2,-4)
[1] 20 16 12  8  4
> 20:8
[1] 20 19 18 17 16 15 14 13 12 11 10  9  8
> seq(20,8,-1)
[1] 20 19 18 17 16 15 14 13 12 11 10  9  8.
```

Note that 20:8 is equivalent to $seq(20, 8, -1)$ and, in general, for integers represented by a and b, $seq(b, a, -1)$ is equivalent to $b:a$ and $seq(a, b, 1)$ is equivalent to $a:b$ when $a < b$. If $a > b$, the S-language replies with an error message and does not execute the $seq()$ command.

A powerful command syntax that allows values within a vector to be extracted, rearranged, or deleted involves a process similar to the role of a subscript associated with a series of algebraic values. To select specific values from a vector, the vector name is followed by the locations (subscripts) of the values to be selected enclosed by square brackets. For example, z[c(1,3,5,7,9)] extracts the values z_1, z_3, z_5, z_7, and z_9 from $z_1, z_2, z_3, z_4, z_5, z_6, z_7, z_8, z_9, z_{10}$, and z_{11} or

```
> z<- c(1,2,3,4,5,6,5,4,3,2,1)
> z
[1] 1 2 3 4 5 6 5 4 3 2 1
> z[c(1,3,5,7,9)]
[1] 1 3 5 5 3.
```

Additional examples are

```
> z[7]
[1] 5
> z[c(2,4,6,8)]
[1] 2 4 6 4
> z[1:5]
[1] 1 2 3 4 5
> z[7:10]
[1] 5 4 3 2
> z[seq(1,10,2)]
[1] 1 3 5 5 3
> z[rep(9,6)]
[1] 3 3 3 3 3 3
> seq(1,10,length=4)
[1] 1 4 7 10
> z[seq(1,10,length=4)]
[1] 1 4 5 2.
```

Any ordering of the "subscript" has the same property, or, for example,

```
> z[c(3,9,1,7,5)]
[1] 3 3 1 5 5.
```

Unlike subscript, there can be more "subscript" than values in the vector, or

```
> rep(c(3,9,1,7,5),3)
 [1] 3 9 1 7 5 3 9 1 7 5 3 9 1 7 5
> z[rep(c(3,9,1,7,5),3)]
 [1] 3 3 1 5 5 3 3 1 5 5 3 3 1 5 5.
```

A last example is a bit different since it reorders rather than extracts the values contained in the vector z (a special type of selection—a permutation), or

```
> z<- z[c(1,3,5,7,9,2,4,6,8,11,10)]
> z
[1]  1 3 5 5 3 2 4 6 4 1 2.
```

The command $z[1, 2, 3]$ fails. The command $z[v]$ is valid only if the quantity between the square brackets v is a recognized S-vector, and the set of numbers 1, 2, 3 is not. A correct syntax $z[c(1, 2, 3)]$ extracts the first three elements of z.

The square-bracket syntax is also used to remove specified values from a vector. The "subscripts" listed between the square brackets preceded by a minus sign eliminate values from a vector. In general, the syntax $z[-v]$ removes the values indicated by the S-vector v. Some examples are

```
> z[-6]
[1] 1 2 3 4 5 5 4 3 2 1
> z[-c(2,4,6,8)]
[1] 1 3 5 5 3 2 1
> z[-seq(1,10,2)]
[1] 2 4 6 4 2 1.
 > z[c(-4,-7,-11,-1,-6)]
[1] 2 3 5 4 3 2.
```

Along the same lines, a logical condition can be placed between the square brackets and when that condition is true, the corresponding value or values are

extracted from the vector named. In general, the syntax is $z[S - condition]$.
Two examples are

```
> z[z<3]
[1] 1 2 2 1
> z[z<3 & z>=6]
[1] 1 2 6 2 1.
```

The S-language allows for logical input into the program structure. The major logical operators are

symbol	meaning
<	less than
<=	less than or equal to
>	greater than
>=	greater than or equal to
==	equals
!=	not equal

Logical expressions involving these symbols can be linked together by conjunctions—*and* (symbol = &) and *or* (symbol = |). An S-logical expression literally produces a series of values T and F, depending on whether the condition is "true" or "false." These character-values serve as input to other S-functions. Continuing the above example, T/F-sequences generated by logical conditions are

```
> z<3
[1] T T F F F F F F F T T
> z>=4
[1] F F F T T T T T F F F
> z<3 | z>4
[1] T T F F T T T F F T T
> z<3 | z<6
[1] T T T T T F T T T T T
> z<3 & z<6
[1] T T F F F F F F F T T
> (z<3 | z<6) | (z<3 & z<6)
[1] T T T T T F T T T T T.
```

Whenever the condition = T, the "square-bracket" convention causes the corresponding values to be extracted from the designated vector and these values can be given a new variable name for later use. For example,

```
> znew<- z[z<3]
> znew
[1] 1 2 2 1.
> znew+znew^2
[1] 2 6 6 2.
```

Further examples are:

```
> z
[1] 1 2 3 4 5 6 5 4 3 2 1
> z[z<3]
```

```
[1] 1 2 2 1
> (1:11)[z>=4]
[1] 4 5 6 7 8
> z[z<3 | z>4]
[1] 1 2 5 6 5 2 1
> z[z<3 | z<6]
[1] 1 2 3 4 5 5 4 3 2 1
> z[z<3 & z<6]
[1] 1 2 2 1
> z[(z<3 | z<6) | (z<3 & z<6)]
[1] 1 2 3 4 5 5 4 3 2 1
> z[(z<3 | z>4) & z!=2]
[1] 1 5 6 5 1.
```

The converse of a logical statement is caused with an explanation point or (!*condition*) which reverses the *T*'s and *F*'s generated by the condition. Note that,

```
> z==3
[1] F F T F F F F F T F F
> z[z==3]
[1] 3 3
> z!=3
[1] T T F T T T T T F T T
> z[z!=3]
[1] 1 2 4 5 6 5 4 2 1
> (!z==3)
[1] T T F T T T T T F T T
> z[!z==3]
[1] 1 2 4 5 6 5 4 2 1
> z==5
[1] F F F F T F T F F F F
> (z==3 | z==5)
[1] F F T F T F T F T F F
> z[(z==3 | z==5)]
[1] 3 5 5 3
> (!(z==3 | z==5))
[1] T T F T F T F T F T T
> z[!(z==3 | z==5)]
[1] 1 2 4 6 4 2 1.
```

A last application of "subscripting"—say it is desired to recode a series of integer values into a series of other values. When the integers to be recoded are placed between the square brackets applied to the vector holding the "new" values, the integers are correspondingly recoded. Specifically,

```
> # translates the values in a to values in b (recode)
> a<- c(4,1,3,2,4,3,2,1,1,2,3)
> b<- c(10,200,500,1000)
> b[a]
[1] 1000 10 500 200 1000 500 200 10 10 200 500.
```

The vector *a* contains the values to be recoded according the values contained in the vector *b*. As shown, this recoding is accomplished by the S-command *b*[*a*].

When a value is not available (e.g., the square root of a negative number, the logarithm of a value less than zero, or simply a missing data value), the position in an S-data structure is held by the letters "NA" ("Not Available").

For example, a sequence of values labeled s,

$$s = \{1, 2, 3, NA, 5, 6, 5, NA, 3, 2, 1\},$$

has two values that could not be computed. Frequently, it is necessary to remove NA-values. Without going into detail, this is best done with the S-command *is.na( )*. This logical command operates on the vector named between the parentheses generating a *T* for all NA-values and an *F* otherwise (answers the question: is the value NA?). The command *!is.na( )* generates an *F* for every NA-value and is used to eliminate the NA-values among the elements of the argument vector (the vector placed between the parentheses). For example, to extract the nine numeric values from s, eliminating the two NA-values,

```
> s<- c(1,2,3,NA,5,6,5,NA,3,2,1)
> is.na(s)
[1] F F F T F F F T F F F
> (!is.na(s))
[1] T T T F T T T F T T T
> s[!is.na(s)]
[1] 1 2 3 5 6 5 3 2 1.
```

The S-command *length( )* counts the number of elements in the vector named between the parentheses. For example,

```
> d<- 1:10
> length(d)
[1] 10
> length(seq(1,32,4))
[1] 8
> length(rep(1:7,1:7))
[1] 28.
```

Two commands illustrate the use of the *length()* function and generate an S-vector called *id* containing half zeros and half ones, or

```
> length(d)/2
[1] 5
> id<- c(rep(0,length(d)/2),rep(1,length(d)/2))
> id
[1] 0 0 0 0 0 1 1 1 1 1.
```

The *ifelse( )* command creates a vector of values according to two alternatives determined by a logical condition. The general form is

ifelse(logical condition(s), expression for true, expression for false)

where the conditions are generated using an S-logical expression. Employing the S-vectors *d* and *id* from above, some examples are

```
> id==0
[1] T T T T T F F F F F
> ifelse(id==0,2*d,d/2)
[1] 2.0 4.0 6.0 8.0 10.0 3.0 3.5 4.0 4.5 5.0
> d>=4
[1] F F F T T T T T T T
> ifelse(d>=4,1,0)
[1] 0 0 0 1 1 1 1 1 1 1
> d<=4
[1] T T T T F F F F F F
> ifelse(d<=4,d+1,0)
[1] 2 3 4 5 0 0 0 0 0 0
> (id==1 & d<7 | d>8)
[1] F F F F F T F F T T
> ifelse(id==1 & d<7 | d>8,1,0)
[1] 0 0 0 0 0 1 0 0 1 1.
```

Extra parentheses make the meaning of the last command clearer and

```
> ifelse((id==1 & d<7) | (d>8),1,0)
[1] 0 0 0 0 0 1 0 0 1 1.
```

Adding extra parentheses for clarity is always a good idea.

The S-language contains a variety of commonly used mathematical functions. Seven of these functions are:

S-symbol	symbol	function
$abs(x)$	$\lvert x \rvert$	absolute value (removes the sign)
$exp(x)$	e^x	the constant e raised to the value x
$log(x)$	$\log(x)$	logarithm of x, base e, $x > 0$
$log10(x)$	$\log_{10}(x)$	logarithm of x, base 10, $x > 0$
$sqrt(x)$	$\sqrt{x}$	square root of x, $x \geq 0$
$sign(x)$	$\text{sign}(x)$	-1 when $x < 0$, $+1$ when $x > 0$, and 0 when $x = 0$
$gamma(x)$	$\Gamma(x)$	gamma function evaluated at x, $x > 0$

Illustrations of these functions follow where values that cannot be evaluated are included:

```
> x<- c(-1,0,1,2,3,4)
> abs(x)
[1] 1 0 1 2 3 4
> exp(x)
[1] 0.3678794 1.0000000 2.7182818 7.3890561 20.0855369
    54.5981500
> log(x)
[1] NA -Inf 0.0000000 0.6931472 1.0986123 1.3862944
Warning messages:
  NAs generated in: log(x)
> log10(x)
[1] NA -Inf 0.0000000 0.3010300 0.4771213 0.6020600
Warning messages:
  NAs generated in: log(x)
> sqrt(x)
[1] NA 0.000000 1.000000 1.414214 1.732051 2.000000
Warning messages:
  (-1)^(0.5) DOMAIN error in: x in 0.5
```

```
> sign(x)
[1] -1 0 1 1 1 1
> gamma(x)
[1] NA NA 1 1 2 6
Warning messages:
  NAs generated in: gamma(x).
```

A gamma function is one way to produce factorials. When the function argument is an integer, $gamma(k + 1)$ yields $k! = k \times (k - 1) \times (k - 2) \times \cdots \times 1$; for example,

```
> gamma(5)
[1] 24
> gamma((1:9)+1)
[1] 1 2 6 24 120 720 5040 40320 362880.
```

Most trigonometric functions are part of the S-language. Twelve common S-trigonometric functions are:

trigonometric functions	$sin(x)$	$cos(x)$	$tan(x)$
inverse functions	$asin(x)$	$acos(x)$	$atan(x)$
hyperbolic functions	$sinh(x)$	$cosh(x)$	$tanh(x)$
inverse hyperbolic functions	$asinh(x)$	$acosh(x)$	$atanh(x)$

where arguments (single values, vectors, or arrays) are in radians.

Following the typical S-pattern, the trigonometric functions are applied to the elements of a vector or an array named as the argument.

Like all S-functions, these functions can be nested or take other S-functions as arguments. A few examples are:

```
> log(1:6)/log10(1:6)
[1] NA 2.302585 2.302585 2.302585 2.302585 2.302585
> exp(seq(0,1,0.2))
[1] 1.000000 1.221403 1.491825 1.822119 2.225541 2.718282
> sin(seq(0,2*pi,1))
[1] 0.0000000  0.8414710 0.9092974 0.1411200 -0.7568025
    -0.9589243 -0.2794155
> sqrt(exp(log(abs(x))))
[1] 1.000000 0.000000 1.000000 1.414214 1.732051 2.000000
> test<- c(0,pi/2,pi,3*pi/2)
> test
[1] 0.000000 1.570796 3.141593 4.712389
> sin(test)
[1] 0.000000e+00 1.000000e+00 1.224647e-16 -1.000000e+00
> asin(sin(test))
[1] 0.000000e+00 1.570796e+00 1.224647e-16 -1.570796e+00.
```

The constant $\pi = 3.14159$ (S-symbol $= pi$) is available as part of the S-language (type *help(pi)* to see an extremely accurate value of this universal constant).

S-ARITHMETIC

The SPLUS programming language accommodates any sort of arithmetic operation. Five symbols allow S-arithmetic—addition (+), subtraction (−), division (/), multiplication (*), and exponentiation (^ or **). Using these symbols, evaluations such as

```
> 7+4
[1] 11
```

or

```
> fact<- 12.4/3
> fact
[1] 4.133333
```

are easily executed. More complicated statements are the same in principle, for example,

```
> (1000-(7+4)/3*4)^2
[1] 970881.8.
```

Symbolic representations are equally available such as

```
> a<- 3
> b<- 12
> b/a
[1] 4
> 2*b-a^2+(b-a)^2
[1] 96
```

or

```
> x<- seq(-2,2,1)
> p<- (1+sqrt(1-exp(-2*x^2/pi)))/2
> p
[1] 0.9800112 0.8431189 0.5000000 0.8431189 0.9800112.
```

It is important to be aware of the rules SPLUS uses to make these computations. They are:

1. Quantities contained in a series of nested parentheses are evaluated starting with the expression contained between the innermost pair.
2. Within a set of parentheses or if no parentheses exist, the order of computation follows a strict hierarchy, which is
   (i) exponentiation first, (ii) multiplication and division second, and (iii) addition and subtraction third.
3. If the computation levels [(i), (ii), or (iii)] are equal within a set of parentheses or if no parentheses exist, the evaluation is done from left to right.

Rule 3 is unambiguous to the computer but sometimes causes problems for the human user. Algebraic S-statements are frequently made clear by explicitly using parentheses when confusion can arise. The expression *a/b*c* is evaluated as the ratio *a/b* multiplied by *c* where *(a/b)*c* clears up any ambiguity and is generally different from $a/(b*c)$. Another possibly ambiguous expression is $-x\char94 2$; does this mean $(-x)\char94 2$ or $-(x\char94 2)$? Including the parentheses makes the situation clear.

MORE S-TOOLS—INTERMEDIATE SET

Consider the test vector of 10 values labeled y where

```
> y<- c(0.234,1.561,5.320,0.053,3.333,7.688,2.116,5.72,
    9.321,0.844)
> y
[1] 0.234 1.561 5.320 0.053 3.333 7.688 2.116 5.720
    9.321 0.844.
```

The command *prod*( ) calculates the product of the values contained in the argument vector or $y_1 \times y_2 \times y_3 \times y_4 \times \cdots$ and

```
> prod(y)
[1] 251.2879.
```

The command *cumsum*( ) produces the cumulative sum of the values in the argument vector or $y_1, y_1 + y_2, y_1 + y_2 + y_3, y_1 + y_2 + y_3 + y_4, \cdots$ and

```
> cumsum(y)
 [1] 0.234 1.795 7.115 7.168 10.501 18.189 20.305 26.025
    35.346 36.190.
```

The command *diff*( ) produces a series of differences formed from the values in the argument vector or $y_2 - y_1$, $y_3 - y_2$, $y_4 - y_3$, $y_5 - y_4$, $\cdots$ and

```
> diff(y)
[1] 1.327 3.759 -5.267 3.280 4.355 -5.572 3.604
    3.601 -8.477.
```

The S-vector *diff(y)* contains one less value than y:

```
> length(diff(y))
[1] 9
> length(y)
[1] 10.
```

   Like all S-functions, these commands can be combined with other commands to perform specialized tasks. For example,

```
> prod(1:10)
[1] 3628800
> prod(1:10)/(prod(1:7)*prod(1:3))
[1] 120
> cumsum(y)/(1:length(y))
[1] 0.234000 0.897500 2.371667 1.792000 2.100200
[6] 3.031500 2.900714 3.253125 3.927333 3.619000
> prod(diff(y))
[1] -230054
> exp(cumsum(log(y)))
[1] 0.2340000 0.3652740 1.9432577 0.1029927
```

```
[5] 0.3432745 2.6390946 5.5843241 31.9423337
[9] 297.7344927 251.2879118
> cumprod(y)
[1] 0.2340000 0.3652740 1.9432577 0.1029927
[5] 0.3432745 2.6390946 5.5843241 31.9423337
[9] 297.7344927 251.2879118
> exp(diff(log(1:10)))
[1] 2.000000 1.500000 1.333333 1.250000 1.200000 1.166667
[7] 1.142857 1.125000 1.111111.
```

Numeric values from any S-expression can be rounded to a defined accuracy using the S-command *round( )* which has the general form

$$round(variable\ name,\ number\ of\ decimal\ places).$$

Continuing the example using the S-vector *y*,

```
> round(y)
[1] 0 2 5 0 3 8 2 6 9 1
> round(y,0)
[1] 0 2 5 0 3 8 2 6 9 1
> round(y,1)
[1] 0.2 1.6 5.3 0.1 3.3 7.7 2.1 5.7 9.3 0.8
> round(y,2)
[1] 0.23 1.56 5.32 0.05 3.33 7.69 2.12 5.72 9.32 0.84.
```

Two related commands are available where one function (*ceiling( )*) "rounds" all input values up to the next highest integer and the other function (*trunc( )*) "rounds" (truncates) all input values down to the next lowest integer. Examples are

```
> trunc(y)
[1] 0 1 5 0 3 7 2 5 9 0
> ceiling(y)
[1] 1 2 6 1 4 8 3 6 10 1
> # note: ceiling = trunc+1.
```

To sort a vector of values into ascending order, the command *sort( )* is used and to sort values into descending order *rev(sort( ))* ("rev" for reverse) is used. To illustrate:

```
> sort(y)
[1] 0.053 0.234 0.844 1.561 2.116 3.333 5.320 5.720
     7.688 9.321
> rev(sort(y))
[1] 9.321 7.688 5.720 5.320 3.333 2.116 1.561 0.844
     0.234 0.053.
```

The command *rev( )* reverses the ordering of any vector. For example,

```
> rev(1:12)
[1] 12 11 10 9 8 7 6 5 4 3 2 1.
```

The command *rev(x)* is equivalent to *x[length(x):1]*.

Frequently statistical analysis requires the ranking of a series of values. Ranking is done with the S-command *rank( )* or

```
> # smallest=rank 1, second smallest=rank 2, etc.
> rank(y)
[1] 2 4 7 1 6 9 5 8 10 3.
```

A related but a bit more complicated S-function is *order*( ). This command produces a vector of values so that its first value is the location of the smallest value in the argument vector, the second value is the location of the second ranking value in the argument vector, the third value is the location of the value ranked third in the argument vector, and so on until the last value in the resulting vector is the location of the largest value in the argument vector. In the language of computer science, the values generated by *order*( ) are called pointers, which "point out" the location of values with specific properties. An illustration makes this rather awkward description clearer:

```
> order(y)
[1] 4 1 10 2 7 5 3 8 6 9.
```

The first element is 4, indicating that the smallest element of y is located in position 4. That is, y[4] = 0.053 has rank = 1. The second element is 1, indicating that the next smallest element of y is located in position 1. That is, y[1] = 0.234 has rank = 2. And so forth, until the last element is 9, indicating that the largest element of y is located in position 9. That is, y[9] = 9.321 has rank = 10. This ordering process is related to sorting. Specifically,

```
> y[order(y)]
[1] 0.053 0.234 0.844 1.561 2.116 3.333 5.320 5.720 7.688 9.321
```

sorts the values in y. The command *order*( ) locates specific values in a vector without actually sorting the vector. For example, the smallest and the largest values in y are

```
> # the minimum
> sort(y)[1]
[1] 0.053
> order(y)[1]
[1] 4
> y[order(y)[1]]
[1] 0.053
> # the maximum
> sort(y)[10]
[1] 9.321
> order(y)[10]
[1] 9
> y[order(y)[10]]
[1] 9.321
> y[order(y)[length(y)]]
[1] 9.321.
```

Order can be used to find the k smallest or largest values within a vector or

```
> k<- 5
> yord<- order(y)
> # smallest k values (k = 5)
> yord[1:k]
```

```
[1]   4  1 10   2   7
> y[yord[1:k]]
[1] 0.053 0.234 0.844 1.561 2.116
> # largest k values
> m<- (length(y)-(k-1)):length(y)
> yord[m]
[1] 5 3 8 6 9
> y[yord[m]]
[1] 3.333 5.320 5.720 7.688 9.321.
```

An important use of the S-function *order*( ) is the sorting of the rows of an array according to a specific column. The process is illustrated by the following:

```
> # create a test array m0
> r1<- c(4,0,22)
> r2<- c(9,1,38)
> r3<- c(1,0,61)
> r4<- c(3,1,11)
> m0<- rbind(r1,r2,r3,r4)
> m0
     [,1] [,2] [,3]
r1    4    0    22
r2    9    1    38
r3    1    0    61
r4    3    1    11
> # order by column 1
> temp0<- order(m0[,1])
> temp0
[1] 3 4 1 2
> m0[temp0,]
     [,1] [,2] [,3]
r3    1    0    61
r4    3    1    11
r1    4    0    22
r2    9    1    38.
```

Another example of applying the S-function *order*( ) arises in a linear search to find a minimum (or maximum) of a function. For the function $x^3 - 8x - 20$,

```
> x<- seq(0,5,0.001)
> fx<- x^3-8*x-20
> m<- order(fx)
> m[1]
   [1] 1634
> fx[m[1]]
   [1] -28.7093
> x[m[1]]
   [1] 1.633
```

finds the approximate minimum value $f_{min} = -28.709$ that occurs at $x = 1.633$.

A valuable algebraic tool is a modulo operator. Despite the fancy name, a modulo operator or *mod*-function produces the value that remains after removing multiples of a fixed integer. Specifically, "9 modulo 4" is 1 since the largest multiple of 4 that does not exceed 9 equals 2×4 or 8 and is removed leaving 1. The S-operator that achieves this calculation is %% and, specifically, 9%%4. In general, the symbol $a\%\%b$ returns the value for a modulo b where a and b are integers. That is, the value computed is the remainder after the largest multiple of b that does not exceed a is subtracted from a. Some examples are:

```
> # mod = %%; test vector = g
> g<- 1:12
> g%%2
[1] 1 0 1 0 1 0 1 0 1 0 1 0
> g%%4
[1] 1 2 3 0 1 2 3 0 1 2 3 0
> # all values divisible by 4 in g
> g[g%%4==0]
[1] 4 8 12
> # all values not divisible by 4 in g
> g[g%%4!=0]
[1] 1 2 3 5 6 7 9 10 11.
```

The symbol $a\%\%b$ is equivalent to the S-code $a - b^* trunc(a/b)$ or, for example,

```
> g-4*trunc(g/4)
[1] 1 2 3 0 1 2 3 0 1 2 3 0
```

produces the same results as

```
> g%%4
[1] 1 2 3 0 1 2 3 0 1 2 3 0.
```

To test whether a number is odd or even illustrates:

```
> g%%2==0
[1] F T F T F T F T F T F T
> g[g%%2==0]
[1] 2 4 6 8 10 12
> g[g%%2!=0]
[1] 1 3 5 7 9 11
> ifelse(g%%2==0,0,1)
[1] 0 1 0 1 0 1 0 1 0 1 0 1.
```

The symbol "==" is used to test equality in a logical expression. A single equal sign "=" is used in other contexts but not in logical expressions.

S-TOOLS FOR STATISTICS

S-commands designed to execute specific statistical tasks follow the same style as the previous S-tools. Consider the S-vector x of numeric values where

```
> x<- c(14,1,8,3,4,4,5,5,5,6,7,2,1)
> x
[1] 14 1 8 3 4 4 5 5 5 6 7 2 1.
```

A basic necessity of many statistical operations is the sum $(\sum x_i)$ where $sum()$ is the S-function and

```
> sum(x)
[1] 65
> sum(x^2)
[1] 467.
```

Similarly the mean ($\bar{x} = \sum x_i/n$) and the median (the 0.5 quantile or 50th percentile) are fundamental summaries where the S-functions *mean*( ) and *median*( ) are used and

```
> mean(x)
[1] 5
> mean(x-5)
[1] 0
> median(x)
[1] 5.
```

The minimum and maximum values are found with *min*( ) and *max*( ) and

```
> min(x)
[1] 1
> max(x)
[1] 14.
```

A frequently important quantity is the estimated variance from a series of numeric values (*variance*$(x)= S_X^2 = \sum (x_i - \bar{x})^2/[n-1]$) where the S-function is *var*( ) and

```
> var(x)
[1] 11.83333
> # standard deviation
> S<- sqrt(var(x))
> S
[1] 3.439961.
```

The S-function is *range*( ) and

```
> r<- range(x)
> r
[1] 1 14
> r[2]-r[1]
[1] 13
> diff(range(x))
[1] 13.
```

These tools are readily combined, for example,

```
> (x-mean(x))/sqrt(var(x))
[1]   -1.1628038 -1.1628038 -0.8721028 -0.5814019
[5]   -0.2907009 -0.2907009 0.0000000 0.0000000
[9]    0.0000000 0.2907009 0.5814019 0.8721028
[13]   2.6163085
> sum((x-mean(x))/sqrt(var(x)))
[1] 0
> var((x-mean(x))/sqrt(var(x)))
[1] 1
> range((x-mean(x))/sqrt(var(x)))
[1] -1.162804 2.616309
> sum((x-mean(x))^2)/(length(x)-1)
[1] 11.83333
```

```
> var(x[x<=4])/var(x[x>4])
[1] 0.1813636.
```

Values that divide an ordered set of numbers such that a specific proportion is above and below that value (called a quantile) are frequently used to summarize data. The most common quantile is that value that divides the distribution in half (proportion = 0.5), producing the median. However, any specific proportion can be chosen. For example, if an exam score of 780 is the 0.90 quantile, then the proportion of scores exceeding 780 is 0.10. The S-function that produces quantiles from a set of numeric values is *quantile (vector, cut.points)* and

```
> quantile(x,0.5)
 50%
   5
> median(x)
[1] 5
> quantile(x,0.75)
 75%
   6
> quantile(x)
   0% 25% 50% 75% 100%
    1   3   5   6   14
> quantile(0:100,0.95)
 95%
  95
> quantile(0:1000,seq(0,1,0.1))
   0% 10% 20% 30% 40% 50% 60% 70% 80% 90% 100%
    0 100 200 300 400 500 600 700 800 900 1000.
```

A command that locates the 25th and 75th quantiles of the values in x is

```
> q<- quantile(x,c(0.25,0.75))
> q
 25% 75%
   3   6.
```

The inter-quartile range of x is then

```
> q[2]-q[1]
   3
> diff(q)
 75%
   3.
```

When the designated proportion is expressed as a percentage, a quantile is called a percentile.

A Pearson product-moment correlation coefficient reflecting the degree of linear association between two sets of numeric values is found with the S-function *cor(set1, set2)* and two examples are

```
> cor(x,1/x)
[1] -0.7168331
> cor(x,sqrt(x))
[1] 0.9757791.
```

The S-commands *var*( ) and *cor*( ) have a special property. When the S-function argument is an array of numeric values, the command *var*( ) calculates all possible variances and covariances among the columns of the array. That is,

```
> # create a test array xyz
> x0<- c(1,2,0,0,2,1)
> y0<- c(1,2,3,3,2,1)
> z0<- c(2,1,0,0,1,2)
> xyz<- cbind(x0,y0,z0)
> xyz
      x0 y0 z0
[1,]   1  1  2
[2,]   2  2  1
[3,]   0  3  0
[4,]   0  3  0
[5,]   2  2  1
[6,]   1  1  2
> var(xyz)
       x0    y0    z0
x0    0.8  -0.4   0.4
y0   -0.4   0.8  -0.8
z0    0.4  -0.8   0.8.
```

The variance of each column is 0.8 (diagonal elements) and the covariances are either 0.4, −0.4 or −0.8 (off-diagonal elements). A similar property is associated with the *cor*( ) command where all possible correlations are calculated among the columns of an argument array. To illustrate,

```
> cor(xyz)
      x0    y0    z0
x0   1.0  -0.5   0.5
y0  -0.5   1.0  -1.0
z0   0.5  -1.0   1.0.
```

Most statistical S-functions fail when NA-values occur in the input data. For example,

```
> xx<- c(1,1,2,4,NA,2,4,1,3)
> mean(xx)
[1] NA.
```

However, the following special case computes the mean from numeric values ignoring any NA-values:

```
> mean(xx,na.rm=T)
[1] 2.25.
```

The option *na.rm* = *T* ("rm" for remove NA-values) temporarily removes NA-values and allows the mean to be calculated based on the remaining numeric values. This option is not available in all situations; for example,

```
> var(xx,na.rm=T)
Error in call to var(): Argument na.rm= not matched
Dumped.
```

A more general approach employs the command *is.na()* to remove either permanently or temporarily the NA-values, such as

```
> mean(xx[!is.na(xx)])
[1] 2.25
> var(xx[!is.na(xx)])
[1] 1.642857.
```

In addition to a series of statistical functions, the S-language provides a number of commands that perform basic statistical tests. These functions are listed in Table 1.2.

Also a number of common multivariate methods are part of the S-language, listed in Table 1.3.

Further descriptions and applications of the functions given in Tables 1.2 and 1.3 are found in the following sections and chapters. As always, the help-system provides technical details.

Table 1.2. Simple statistical tests in SPLUS

Test	Function
binom.test(x, n, p=0.5, alternative="two.sided")	Exact test for binomial proportion
chisq.test(x, y=NULL, correct=T)	Chi-square test for independence of two factors in a contingency table
cor.test(x, y, alternative="two.sided", method="pearson")	Test of no linear association (correlation=0)
fisher.test(x, y=NULL)	Fisher's exact test for independece of two factors in a contingency table
friedman.test(y, groups, blocks)	Nonparametric test for no effect in a two-way classification
kruskal.test(y, groups)	Nonparametric test for no effect in a one-way classification
mantelhaen.test(x, y=NULL, correct=T)	Test of association within a series of 2 by 2 tables
mcnemar.test(x, y=NULL, correct=T)	Chi-square test for independence of two factors in a table of matched pairs
prop.test(x, n, p, alternative="two.sided", conf.level=0.95, correct=T)	Test for comparing a series of proportions
t.test(x, y=NULL, alternative="two.sided", mu=0, paired=F, var.equal=T, conf.level=0.95)	Student's test for the comparison of mean values from two independent groups
var.test(x, y, alternative="two.sided", conf.level=0.95)	Test of the equality of variances for two indepdendent groups
wilcox.test(x, y, alternative="two.sided", mu=0, paired=F, exact=T, correct=T)	Nonparametric test for the comparison of mean values from two independent groups

Table 1.3. Multivariate functions in SPLUS

Function	Action
cancor(x, y, · · ·)	Finds the correlation between two groups of multivariate data.
discr(x, k)	Finds the linear discriminant function in order to distinguish between a number of groups.
disct(x, metric="euclidean")	Finds the distance between all of the pairwise multivariate observations.
hclust(dist, method="compact", · · ·)	Performs hierarchical clustering on a distance or similarity array.
leaps(x, y, wt=, method="Cp", keep=, nbest=10, · · ·)	Attempts to find the "best" regression models using a subset of the explanatory variables.
plclust(tree, hang=0.1, unit=F, level=F, hmin=0, square=T, labels=, plot=T)	Creates a plot of a "tree" given a structure produced by hclust.

STATISTICAL DISTRIBUTIONS IN SPLUS

S-functions produce four important values calculated for 13 commonly encountered statistical distributions. They are:

1. a probability associated with a specific quantile (symbol p),
2. a quantile associated with a specific probability (symbol q),
3. a height (ordinate) of a statistical distribution (symbol d), and
4. a value selected at random from a given distribution (symbol r).

The commands are invoked by placing one of the four symbols (p, q, d, or r) on the front of an S-function root name associated with a specific distribution. The root names and the forms of the S-function are displayed in Table 1.4.

Application of the S-functions from Table 1.4 follows the same pattern and will be illustrated with the normal distribution; root name = *norm*. For a specific quantile, a statistical distribution associates a probability. In symbols, the quantile x is the value such that $P(random\ value \leq x) = probability$ or, more commonly denoted, $P(X \leq x) = F(x)$. The quantile x has associated probability $F(x)$, called a cumulative probability. The cumulative probability $F(x)$ from the standard normal distribution (mean = 0 and variance = 1) is generated by the S-function *pnorm*( ) ("p" for probability plus root name "norm" for normal). For example,

```
> # F(x) = p -- produces p
> x<- 1.0
> pnorm(x)
[1] 0.8413447
> pnorm(1.96)
[1] 0.9750021
```

Table 1.4. Statistical distributions in SPLUS

Distribution	Parameters
Beta distribution	dbeta(x, shape1, shape2)
	qbeta(p, shape1, shape2)
	pbeta(q, shape1, shape2)
	rbeta(n, shape1, shape2)
Binomial distribution	dbinom(x, size, probability)
	qbinom(p, size, probability)
	pbinom(q, size, probability)
	rbinom(n, size, probability)
Cauchy distribution	dcauchy(x, location=0, scale=1)
	qcauchy(p, location=0, scale=1)
	pcauchy(q, location=0, scale=1)
	rcauchy(n, location=0, scale=1)
Chi-square distribution	dchisq(x, df)
	qchisq(p, df)
	pchisq(q, df, ncp=0)
	rchisq(n, df)
Exponential distribution	dexp(x, rate=1)
	qexp(p, rate=1)
	pexp(q, rate=1)
	rexp(n, rate=1)
F-distribution	df(x, df1, df2)
	qf(p, df1, df2)
	pf(q, df1, df2, ncp=0)
	rf(n, df1, df2)
Gamma distribution	dgamma(x, shape)
	qgamma(p, shape)
	pgamma(q, shape)
	rgamma(n, shape)
Lognormal distribution	dlnorm(x, meanlog=0, sdlog=1)
	qlnorm(p, meanlog=0, sdlog=1)
	plnorm(q, meanlog=0, sdlog=1)
	rlnorm(n, meanlog=0, sdlog=1)
Logistic distribution	dlogis(x, location=0, scale=1)
	qlogis(p, location=0, scale=1)
	plogis(q, location=0, scale=1)
	rlogis(n, location=0, scale=1)
Normal (Gaussian) distribution	dnorm(x, mean=0, sd=1)
	qnorm(p, mean=0, sd=1)
	pnorm(q, mean=0, sd=1)
	rnorm(n, mean=0, sd=1)
Poisson distribution	dpois(x, lambda)
	qpois(p, lambda)
	ppois(q, lambda)
	rpois(q, lambda)
Student's t-distribution	dt(y, df)
	qt(p, df)
	pt(q, df)
	rt(n, df)
Uniform distribution	dunif(x, min=0, max=1)
	qunif(p, min=0, max=1)
	punif(q, min=0, max=1)
	runif(n, min=0, max=1)

```
> pnorm(1.644854)
[1] 0.95
> pnorm(c(-0.5,0.5))
[1] 0.3085375 0.6914625
> pnorm(seq(-2,2,1))
[1] 0.02275013 0.15865525 0.50000000 0.84134475 0.97724987.
```

Geometrically, *pnorm(x)* is the area of the probability density function (Chapter 3) to the left of the value *x* under the curve describing the standard normal probability distribution.

These probabilities can be calculated for any normal distribution. That is, for a normal distribution with mean represented by *m* and standard deviation by *s*, then *pnorm(x, m, s)* or

```
> pnorm(2,0,2)
[1] 0.8413447
> pnorm(c(-3,5,13),5,4)
[1] 0.02275013 0.50000000 0.97724987
> pnorm(1:5,3,1.5)
[1] 0.09121122 0.25249254 0.50000000 0.74750746 0.90878878
> z<- (1:5-3)/1.5
> pnorm(z)
[1] 0.09121122 0.25249254 0.50000000 0.74750746 0.90878878.
```

Quantiles associated with a probability are generated with the command *qnorm( )* ("q" for quantile). Technically, *qnorm( )* is the inverse function $F^{-1}(p)$ for the standard normal distribution where $F(x) = p$. Quantiles for the standard normal distribution for specific input probabilities are

```
> # F(x) = p -- produces x
> p<- 0.8
> qnorm(p)
[1] 0.8416212
> qnorm(0.9750021)
[1] 1.96
> qnorm(0.95)
[1] 1.644854
> qnorm(c(0.3,0.7))
[1] -0.5244005 0.5244005
> qnorm(c(0.9,0.95,0.975,0.99))
[1] 1.281552 1.644854 1.959964 2.326348.
```

Geometrically, *qnorm(p)* is the value *x* associated with the area size *p* from a standard normal distribution. To illustrate that *qnorm( )* is the inverse function of *pnorm( )*, note that

```
> pnorm(qnorm(c(0.9,0.95,0.975,0.99)))
[1] 0.900 0.950 0.975 0.990,
```

demonstrating that $F[F^{-1}(p)] = p$.

The height of the standard normal probability distribution is given by *dnorm( )* ("d" for density) where, for example,

```
> dnorm(0)
[1] 0.3989423
```

```
> dnorm(c(-2,-1,0,1,2))
[1] 0.05399097 0.24197072 0.39894228 0.24197072 0.05399097
> dnorm(qnorm(c(0.05,0.95)))
[1] 0.1031356 0.1031356.
> dnorm(c(-2,-1,0,1,2),2,2)
[1] 0.02699548 0.06475880 0.12098536 0.17603266 0.19947114.
```

A powerful feature of the S-language is the ability to generate randomly selected values from a specified probability distribution. Values selected at random from a standard normal distribution are generated using *rnorm( )* ("r" for random). A sample of 10 random values is generated by

```
> rnorm(10)
[1] 0.9640383 -0.5154206 -1.3833759 0.1764667 0.4535188
[7] 1.1371895 -1.3334224 1.3967793 1.6329620 1.4855619.
```

The input argument is the number of desired random values. A sample of n random normal values from any normal distribution is generated by *rnorm(n, mean, standard deviation)* with a specified mean and a standard deviation. For example, $n = 10$ random values are

```
> rnorm(10,12,3)
[1] 7.555013 10.065110 8.901517 15.948688 12.899141
    14.450648 14.218464 13.883906 8.587446 14.214624
```

where the mean value is 12 and the standard deviation is 3 of the normal population generating the 10 sampled values. If the mean and standard deviation are not specified, the value mean = 0 and standard deviation = 1 are assumed, producing a random selection from the standard normal distribution. As all S-functions, these functions can be nested or serve as arguments to other S-functions. Some examples are:

```
> mean(rnorm(1000))
[1] 0.01110404
> median(rnorm(1000))
[1] 0.05197204
> range(rnorm(1000))
[1] -3.040432 2.990719
> var(rnorm(1000))
[1] 1.000899
> quantile(rnorm(1000),c(0.05,0.1,0.5,0.90,0.95))
        5%       10%       50%      90%      95%
-1.700898 -1.301734 -0.001976516 1.295501 1.617297
> qnorm(c(0.05,0.1,0.5,0.90,0.95))
[1] -1.644854 -1.281552 0.000000 1.281552 1.644854.
```

Another important statistical distribution is the uniform distribution invoked by the S-root *unif*. Following the same pattern used to generate random normal values gives

```
> runif(12)
[1] 0.11964098 0.26525373 0.28375461 0.94273316 0.17228740
    0.08763699 0.15057526 0.86111738 0.80631937 0.28082356
    0.60405288 0.40858894,
```

which are 12 uniformly distributed values between 0 and 1 selected at random. To generate 12 random values between 0 and 10, then

```
> 10*runif(12)
[1] 1.887413 3.110879 3.438027 1.958919 7.396346 5.205491
    8.076091 5.563600 9.197182 7.017570 5.807942 4.392242.
```

Random uniform values between any two values are generated using *runif*(*n*, *a*, *b*) where *n* is the number of values desired, *a* is the left-hand bound (minimum) and *b* is the right-hand bound (maximum). To illustrate, $n = 12$ uniformly distributed random values between 0 and 10 are

```
> runif(12,0,10)
[1] 3.760145 6.528759 9.747343 6.175687 1.553015 0.866855
    6.148760 9.818910 9.315106 8.925914 3.968154 4.849827.
```

To generate 12 random (equally likely) integers between 1 and 10, then

```
> ceiling(10*runif(12))
[1] 10 10  1  8  8  6 10  9  6  5  4  3
> ceiling(runif(12,0,10))
[1] 10  1  9  2  1  1  6  9  5  6  4  7.
```

An application of *runif*( ) might be to simulate flipping a coin where

```
> # flip a fair (p=0.5) coin n=100 times and count the heads
> sum(ifelse(runif(100)<0.5,1,0))
[1] 49
> # flip an unfair (p=0.6) coin n=100 times and count the heads
> sum(ifelse(runif(100)<0.6,1,0))
[1] 64.
```

The same S-syntax generates probabilities, quantiles, heights, or random values for any of the statistical distributions (continuous or discrete) listed in Table 1.4, using the root name and the prefix letters *p*, *q*, *d*, or *r*.

ARRAYS AND TABLES

An important S-function that provides the capability of making calculations from an array of values is *apply*( ). This command applies an S-function to the rows or columns of a two-dimensional array and to the rows, columns, or levels of a three-dimensional array. The general form is

$$apply(array,\ indicator, S\text{-}function)$$

where the indicator is 1 for rows, 2 for columns and denotes specific rows, columns, or levels for a three-dimensional array. Since arrays are a primary data form in SPLUS, this S-function is an important tool. Some examples are:

```
> # create an array to illustrate the command apply
> a<- rbind(c(1,2,3),c(2,3,2),c(3,2,1))
> # a = test array
```

```
> a
     [,1]  [,2]   [,3]
[1,]    1    2      3
[2,]    2    3      2
[3,]    3    2      1
> # sum of the rows
> apply(a,1,sum)
[1] 6 7 6
> # mean of the columns
> apply(a,2,mean)
[1] 2.000000 2.333333 2.000000
> # variance of the columns
> apply(a,2,var)
[1] 1.0000000 0.3333333 1.0000000
> # product of the rows
> apply(a,1,prod)
[1]    6 12   6
> # sum of squares for each row
> apply(a,1,function(x){sum((x-mean(x))^2)})
[1] 2.0000000 0.6666667 2.0000000
> # geometric mean of the columns
> apply(a,2,function(x){prod(x)^(1/length(x))})
[1] 1.817121 2.289428 1.817121.
```

The S-language allows the user to create specialized functions (such as the last two examples) that are not part of the S-language. These "homemade" functions then can be applied to the elements of an array with *apply*(). The creation of these specialized functions will be discussed in detail.

Data are tabulated with two S-functions—*table*() and *cut*(). The arguments employed in the S-function *table*() are the variable names of the data to be tabulated:

$$table(variable1, variable2, variable3, \cdots).$$

These input variables consist of vectors of integers indicating categorical classifications. For example, one-dimensional tabulations are created by

```
> data<- ceiling(10*runif(100))
> table(data)
  1  2 3 4 5  6  7 8 9 10
 10 17 9 9 8 10 14 8 9  6
> table(ifelse(runif(300)<0.6,1,0))
   0   1
 108 192.
```

The first row of output contains the S-supplied labels of the tabulated counts that are displayed in the second row.

Similarly, a two-dimensional tabulation is illustrated by

```
> x<- c(rep(0,3),rep(1,4),rep(2,4),rep(3,6),rep(4,3))
> x
[1] 0 0 0 1 1 1 1 2 2 2 2 3 3 3 3 3 3 4 4 4
> y<- rep(c(1,0),10)
> y
[1] 1 0 1 0 1 0 1 0 1 0 1 0 1 0 1 0 1 0 1 0
> tab<- table(y,x)
```

```
> tab
  0 1 2 3 4
0 1 2 2 3 2
1 2 2 2 3 1.
```

A table such as those illustrated can be further manipulated with S-functions where the input argument is the named table. For example,

```
> sum(tab)
[1] 20
> prod(tab)
[1] 576
> length(tab)
[1] 10
> tab*tab
  0 1 2 3 4
0 1 4 4 9 4
1 4 4 4 9 1.
```

Continuing the example, a single element can be extracted by

```
> tab[2,3]
[1] 2
```

or a column by

```
> tab[,3]
  0 1
  2 2.
```

New tables that are a function of the tabulated values can be created, such as

```
> tab/2
    0 1 2   3   4
0 0.5 1 1 1.5 1.0
1 1.0 1 1 1.5 0.5
```

or

```
> (tab-4)/2
     0  1  2    3    4
0 -1.5 -1 -1 -0.5 -1.0
1 -1.0 -1 -1 -0.5 -1.5.
```

The *apply*( ) command can be used in conjunction with tabulated data or

```
> apply(tab,1,sum)
  0  1
 10 10
> apply(tab,2,sum)
 0 1 2 3 4
 3 4 4 6 3
> apply(tab,1,mean)
  0 1
  2 2.
> apply(tab,2,mean)
    0 1 2 3   4
  1.5 2 2 3 1.5.
```

In short, a table created by *table*( ) is treated by SPLUS as any S-vector or S-array of values.

To tabulate continuous values, first they must be classified into a series of defined categories. To place numeric values into a series of categories, the command *cut*( ) is used. The general form of the command is

$$cut(data, \ category.limits).$$

The result of applying this S-function is a set of integer category classification values and a corresponding set of category labels for the limits specified. The data classified according to these categories can then be tabulated with *table*( ). Consider $n = 100$ random values from a standard normal distribution:

```
> x<- rnorm(100)
> cut(x,c(-9,-2,-1,0,1,2,9))
 [1]  2 5 4 5 4 4 4 4 3 2 4 4 4 3 2 4 4 3 4 2 2 3 4 4 3
[26]  4 3 4 3 3 4 3 4 4 4 3 3 2 3 5 2 2 2 5 4 3 4 5 3 4
[51]  4 4 3 5 2 4 5 3 3 3 6 5 1 5 4 3 3 1 3 2 3 4 3 4 3
[76]  4 3 3 4 3 3 4 3 5 3 4 2 4 2 4 2 4 2 3 3 4 4 3 4 4 4
attr(, "levels"):
[1] "-9+ thru -2" "-2+ thru -1" "-1+ thru  0"
    " 0+ thru  1" " 1+ thru  2" " 2+ thru  9"

        > table(cut(x,c(-9,-2,-1,0,1,2,9)))
        -9+ thru -2 -2+ thru -1 -1+ thru  0
                  2          15          32
         0+ thru  1  1+ thru  2  2+ thru  9
                 40          10           1.
```

The S-function *cut*( ) also divides values into a predetermined number of categories. For example, say 10 categories are desired, then

```
> u<- runif(100)
> cut(u,10)
 [1] 5 10 10 7 4 9 8 4 8 8 5 2 9 7 4 1 5 2 9 6 8 7 6 1 9
[26] 5 3 5 6 7 6 9 9 3 5 4 4 1 4 10 1 5 7 5 7 3 9 6 3 8
[51] 2 1 2 6 7 3 6 10 5 1 4 3 2 5 10 8 9 7 10 5 10 5 1 9 10
[76] 4 2 6 7 2 3 6 2 3 8 9 5 4 7 7 3 2 2 10 4 4 9 4 4 1
attr(, "levels"):
[1] "0.02920983+ thru 0.1268125" "0.12681252+ thru 0.2244152"
[3] "0.22441522+ thru 0.3220179" "0.32201791+ thru 0.4196206"
[5] "0.41962060+ thru 0.5172233" "0.51722330+ thru 0.6148260"
[7] "0.61482599+ thru 0.7124287" "0.71242869+ thru 0.8100314"
[9] "0.81003138+ thru 0.9076341" "0.90763407+ thru 1.0052368"

> table(cut(u,10))
0.02920983+ thru 0.1268125 0.12681252+ thru 0.2244152
                         8                         10
0.22441522+ thru 0.3220179 0.32201791+ thru 0.4196206
                         9                         13
0.41962060+ thru 0.5172233 0.51722330+ thru 0.6148260
                        13                          9
0.61482599+ thru 0.7124287 0.71242869+ thru 0.8100314
                        11                          7
0.81003138+ thru 0.9076341 0.90763407+ thru 1.0052368
                        11                          9.
```

Labels that are not as cumbersome as the S-supplied values are frequently introduced. Continuing the example,

```
> # user defined category labels
> deciles<- c("1st","2nd","3rd"','"4th","5th","6th","7th"
  ,"8th","9th","10th")
> table(cut(u,10,label=deciles))
 1st 2nd 3rd 4th 5th 6th 7th 8th 9th 10th
   8  10   9  13  13   9  11   7  11    9.
```

In the same way, higher dimensional tables can be created. The *cut*( ) command establishes the categories and the *table*( ) command produces the table. Using the *x*-values from above and

```
> y<- x+rnorm(100)
> table(cut(x,c(-9,-2,-1,0,1,2,9)),cut(y,c(-9,-1,0,1,9)))
            -9+ thru -1 -1+ thru  0  0+ thru  1  1+ thru 9
-9+ thru -2      2            0           0           0
-2+ thru -1      7            6           2           0
-1+ thru  0     14           12           3           3
 0+ thru  1      8            7          18           7
 1+ thru  2      0            0           3           7
 2+ thru  9      0            0           0           1.
```

A command *tapply*( ) ("tapply" for table apply) allows summary values to be calculated based on the values contained in each cell of a table. In other words, the S-function *tapply*( ) applies a specified function to calculate summary values within each of a series of categories. In general,

$$tapply(data, categories, function)$$

applies the named *function* to calculate summary values for values contained in *data* (a vector or an array) defined by *categories*. For example,

```
> n<- 100
> u<- runif(n)
> cc<- cut(u,seq(0,1,length=4),
    label=c("low","medium","high"))
> table(cc)
  low  medium high
   29      33   38
> tapply(u,cc,length)
  low  medium high
   29      33   38
> tapply(u,cc,mean)
       low      medium        high
 0.1622614   0.4986871   0.8351344
> tapply(u,cc,var)
        low      medium        high
 0.01035142  0.007466902  0.008681872.
```

The *tapply*( ) command applies S-functions to data classified into any size table. The categories are identified by a *list* option. For example, if one categorical variable classifies numbers divisible evenly by 2 or not and another categorical variable classifies numbers divisible evenly by 9 or not, then these two binary variables define the following table:

```
> x<- 0:999
> # divisible by 2 categories
```

```
> f1<- ifelse(x%%2,1,0)
> # divisible by 9 categories
> f2<- ifelse(x%%9,1,0)
> table(f1,f2)
   0   1
0 56 444
1 56 444
> tapply(x,list(f1,f2),length)
   0   1
0 56 444
1 56 444
> tapply(x,list(f1,f2),mean)
>      0         1
0    495   499.5045
1    504   499.4955
> tapply(x,list(f1,f2),median)
   0   1
0 495 499
1 504 500
> sqrt(tapply(x,list(f1,f2),var))
          0         1
0 293.5711 288.7092
1 293.5711 288.7092.
```

The variables used to form the table (classification vectors named in the list option) have the same length as the vector of values to be classified.

An S-function that produces an array of any size from a vector is *array*( ). The general form is

$$array(vector, \ c(rows, \ columns, \ levels, \cdots), \cdots)$$

and, specifically,

```
> # array(vector, dimensions)
> array(c(1:10,101:110,1001:1010),c(2,5,3))

, , 1
     [,1] [,2] [,3]  [,4] [,5]
[1,]    1    3    5     7    9
[2,]    2    4    6     8   10

, , 2
     [,1] [,2] [,3] [,4] [,5]
[1,]  101  103  105  107  109
[2,]  102  104  106  108  110

, , 3
     [,1] [,2] [,3]  [,4] [,5]
[1,] 1001 1003 1005 1007 1009
[2,] 1002 1004 1006 1008 1010.
```

This S-function is a generalization of the previously described *matrix*( ) command but produces arrays with any number of dimensions. Therefore,

```
> array(1:24,c(3,8))
     [,1] [,2] [,3] [,4] [,5] [,6] [,7] [,8]
[1,]    1    4    7   10   13   16   19   22
[2,]    2    5    8   11   14   17   20   23
[3,]    3    6    9   12   15   18   21   24
```

```
> matrix(1:24,3,8)
      [,1] [,2] [,3] [,4] [,5] [,6] [,7] [,8]
[1,]    1    4    7   10   13   16   19   22
[2,]    2    5    8   11   14   17   20   23
[3,]    3    6    9   12   15   18   21   24
```

are equivalent S-functions. The converse is also achieved by the command *array( )*. If the only argument is an array, then this S-function *array( )* makes a vector out of the array values. For example,

```
> mtemp<- matrix(1:24,3,8)
> mtemp
      [,1] [,2] [,3] [,4] [,5] [,6] [,7] [,8]
[1,]    1    4    7   10   13   16   19   22
[2,]    2    5    8   11   14   17   20   23
[3,]    3    6    9   12   15   18   21   24
> array(mtemp)
 [1]  [2]  [3]  [4]  [5]  [6]  [7]  [8]  [9] [10] [11] [12] [13]
   1    2    3    4    5    6    7    8    9   10   11   12   13
[14] [15] [16] [17] [18] [19] [20] [21] [22] [23] [24]
  14   15   16   17   18   19   20   21   22   23   24.
```

MATRIX ALGEBRA TOOLS

Matrix algebra is another method to manipulate numeric values contained in an array. The S-language provides matrix algebra tools implemented as S-functions. A brief discussion of some of the most useful of these S-tools is worthwhile.

The number of rows, columns, and dimensions of an array are found with the S-functions *nrow( )*, *ncol( )*, and *dim( )* where the argument is a matrix. For example,

```
> # matrix functions: m = test matrix
> m<- matrix(1:36,9,4)
> m
      [,1] [,2] [,3] [,4]
[1,]    1   10   19   28
[2,]    2   11   20   29
[3,]    3   12   21   30
[4,]    4   13   22   31
[5,]    5   14   23   32
[6,]    6   15   24   33
[7,]    7   16   25   34
[8,]    8   17   26   35
[9,]    9   18   27   36
> nrow(m)
[1] 9
> ncol(m)
[1] 4
> dim(m)
[1] 9 4
> # dimensionality
> length(dim(m))
[1] 2.
```

The command *diag()* extracts the elements on the diagonal of an array (e.g., elements $= m_{ii}$). For example,

```
> diag(m)
[1] 1   11 21 31.
```

Also, for a $k \times k$ diagonal matrix, then

```
> k<- 6
> diag(k)
      [,1] [,2] [,3] [,4] [,5] [,6]
[1,]    1    0    0    0    0    0
[2,]    0    1    0    0    0    0
[3,]    0    0    1    0    0    0
[4,]    0    0    0    1    0    0
[5,]    0    0    0    0    1    0
[6,]    0    0    0    0    0    1
> diag(1:3)
      [,1] [,2] [,3]
[1,]    1    0    0
[2,]    0    2    0
[3,]    0    0    3
```

when the input argument is an single value or a S-vector. Exactly as before, the elements of a matrix can be extracted by employing the square-bracket syntax (S-subscript). For example,

```
> m[2,3]
[1] 20
> m[,3]
[1] 19 20 21 22 23 24 25 26 27
> m[3,]
[1]  3 12 21 30
> m[,-3]
      [,1] [,2] [,3]
[1,]    1   10   28
[2,]    2   11   29
[3,]    3   12   30
[4,]    4   13   31
[5,]    5   14   32
[6,]    6   15   33
[7,]    7   16   34
[8,]    8   17   35
[9,]    9   18   36.
```

Subsets of a matrix can also be selected with square brackets. Using the matrix *m*, two examples are

```
> # select rows 3-8 and columns 2-4
> m[3:8,2:4]
      [,1] [,2] [,3]
[1,]   12   21   30
[2,]   13   22   31
[3,]   14   23   32
[4,]   15   24   33
[5,]   16   25   34
[6,]   17   26   35
```

```
> # eliminate rows 3-8 and select columns 2-4
> m[-(3:8),2:4]
     [,1] [,2] [,3]
[1,]   10   19   28
[2,]   11   20   29
[3,]   18   27   36.
```

The S-function $t()$ transposes a matrix (array elements m_{ij} become elements m_{ji} and an $r \times c$ matrix becomes an $c \times r$ matrix); that is,

```
> t(m[3:8,2:4])
     [,1] [,2] [,3] [,4] [,5] [,6]
[1,]   12   13   14   15   16   17
[2,]   21   22   23   24   25   26
[3,]   30   31   32   33   34   35.
```

The S-language allows multiplication of vectors and matrices but it is a bit tricky since two types of multiplication exist. One type produces an element by element product and the other produces the product expected from linear algebra rules. The difference between these two types of multiplication is identified by the multiplication sign – the operator "$*$" multiplies the elements of two vectors or arrays and the operator "$\%*\%$" performs linear algebra vector or matrix multiplication. In symbols, if x and y are vectors, then the product z is either $z = \{x_1 y_1, x_2 y_2, x_3 y_3, \cdots\}$ (symbol = "$*$"and $x*y$) or $z = \sum x_i y_i$ (symbol = "$\%*\%$" and $x\%*\%y$). If x and y are arrays, then the elements of the product array are either $z_{ij} = x_{ij} y_{ij}$ (symbol = "$*$"and $x*y$) or $z_{ij} = \sum x_{ik} y_{kj}$ (symbol = "$\%*\%$" and $x\%*\%y$). The following contrasts these two possibilities:

```
> # x and y are test vectors
> x<- c(1,2,3)
> y<- c(3,0,1)
> x*y
[1] 3 0 3
> x%*%y
     [,1]
[1,]    6
> # crossprod(x,y) = x%*%y
> crossprod(x,y)
     [,1]
[1,]    6
> # a = test array
> a<- rbind(c(1,2,3),c(2,3,2),c(3,2,1))
> a
     [,1] [,2] [,3]
[1,]    1    2    3
[2,]    2    3    2
[3,]    3    2    1
> a*a
     [,1] [,2] [,3]
[1,]    1    4    9
[2,]    4    9    4
[3,]    9    4    1
> a%*%a
```

```
        [,1] [,2] [,3]
[1,]    14    14    10
[2,]    14    17    14
[3,]    10    14    14
> a/a
     [,1] [,2] [,3]
[1,]    1     1     1
[2,]    1     1     1
[3,]    1     1     1
> a*x
     [,1] [,2] [,3]
[1,]   1     2     3
[2,]   4     6     4
[3,]   9     6     3
> a%*%x
       [,1]
[1,]    14
[2,]    14
[3,]    10.
```

The S-function *solve( )* produces the inverse of a matrix, illustrated by

```
> solve(a)
         [,1] [,2]     [,3]
[1,]    0.125 -0.5    0.625
[2,]   -0.500  1.0   -0.500
[3,]    0.625 -0.5    0.125.
```

To verify that *solve( )* indeed produces the inverse of array *a*,

```
> round(solve(a)%*%a,2)
       [,1]  [,2] [,3]
[1,]     1    0    0
[2,]     0    1    0
[3,]     0    0    1.
```

The command *solve(a, y)* finds the solution to a set of k linear equations where a is a $k \times k$ matrix of coefficients and y is a vector with k elements. For example, if

$$z_1 + 2z_2 + 3z_3 = 3$$

$$2z_1 + 3z_2 + 2z_3 = 0$$

$$3z_1 + 2z_2 + z_3 = 1$$

then the solution $z = \{z_1, z_2, z_3\}$ is

```
> # a%*%z=y, find the solution vector z
> # input values
> a
[,1] [,2] [,3]
[1,]    1    2    3
[2,]    2    3    2
[3,]    3    2    1
> y
[1] 3 0 1
> # solution
> z<- solve(a,y)
> z
```

```
[1]   1 -2   2
> # verify solution
> z%*%a
        [,1] [,2] [,3]
[1,]    3    0    1.
```

A special S-function to manipulate vectors to produce a matrix is *outer*() ("outer" for outer-product). The general form of the *outer*() command is

$$outer(vector1, vector2, function)$$

and evaluates the named S-function at all possible pairs of values contained in the two input vectors. The vectors, one with m elements and one with n elements, form an $m \times n$ array of results. For example, the product of all possible pairs of values from x and values from y (i.e., $x_i y_j$ for all possible pairs i and j) is, continuing the above example,

```
> x
[1] 1 2 3
> y
[1] 3 0 3
> # outer(x,y,"*") = outer(x,y)
> outer(x,y)
        [,1]  [,2]  [,3]
[1,]    3     0     1
[2,]    6     0     2
[3,]    9     0     3.
```

Additional examples are

```
> # x+y for all possible pairs
> outer(x,y,"+")
        [,1]  [,2]  [,3]
[1,]    4     1     2
[2,]    5     2     3
[3,]    6     3     4
> # x^y for all possible pairs
> outer(x,y,"^")
        [,1]  [,2]  [,3]
[1,]    1     1     1
[2,]    8     1     2
[3,]    27    1     3
> # (1+x^2)/(1+y^2) for all possible pairs
> outer(x,y,function(x,y){(1+x^2)/(1+y^2)})
        [,1] [,2] [,3]
[1,]    0.2   2   1.0
[2,]    0.5   5   2.5
[3,]    1.0  10   5.0.
```

SOME ADDITIONAL S-TOOLS

The S-command *for*() is used to execute repeatedly the same set of commands, sometimes called a loop. These *for*-loops are slow executing and, if possible, should be avoided in creating S-code. However, situations arise where a *for*-loop is needed to generate the required values when no good alternative exists. The general form of a *for*-loop is

$$for(index\ in\ range)\{command(s)\ to\ be\ executed\}.$$

The value *index* takes on each value found in the vector labeled *range*. The command(s) in the brackets{} are executed once for each value of the *index*. An example is

```
> # illustration of a for-loop
> counts<- c(0,0,0,0)
> n<- c(2,4,6,4)
> for(i in 1:length(n)){
      counts<- c(counts,rep(i,n[i]))
    }
> counts
[1] 0 0 0 0 1 1 2 2 2 2 3 3 3 3 3 3 4 4 4 4.
```

To avoid the loop syntax:

```
> counts<- rep(0:4,c(4,2,4,6,4))
> counts
[1] 0 0 0 0 1 1 2 2 2 2 3 3 3 3 3 3 4 4 4 4.
```

The following *for*-loop calculates the terms of a Fibonacci series $(f_{i+2} = f_{i+1} + f_i)$ and, additionally, computes the ratio of consecutive pairs of terms (i.e, $r_i = f_{i+1}/f_i$) with and without a *for*-loop:

```
> n<- 15
> f<- NULL
> r<- NULL
> f[1]<- 1
> f[2]<- 2
> for(i in 1:(n-2)) {f[i+2]<- f[i+1]+f[i]}
> f
[1]    1    2    3    5    8   13   21   34   55   89  144  233  377  610  987
> # ratio with a for-loop
> for(i in 1:(n-1)) {r[i]<- f[i+1]/f[i]}
> round(r,3)
[1] 2.000 1.500 1.667 1.600 1.625 1.615 1.619 1.618 1.618 1.618
[11] 1.618 1.618 1.618 1.618
> # ratio without a for-loop
> r<- exp(diff(log(f)))
> round(r,3)
[1] 2.000 1.500 1.667 1.600 1.625 1.615 1.619 1.618 1.618 1.618
[11] 1.618 1.618 1.618 1.618.
```

The expressions *f<– NULL* and *r<– NULL* predefine the vectors *f* and *r* created in the loop, which is required by the S-language when a vector or an array is generated inside a *for*-loop.

Another example is

```
# illustration of a for-loop
> y<- NULL
> k<- 0
> x<- c(1,0,2,0,3,0,4,0,5,0,6,-1,0,6,0,5,0,4,0,3,0,2,0,1)
```

```
> for(i in 1:length(x)) {
  if(x[i]==0) next
  if(x[i]<0) break
  k<- k+1
  y[k]<- 1/x[i]
  }
> y
[1] 1.00000 0.50000 0.33333 0.25000 0.20000 0.16667.
```

The command *if*(*condition*) *next* skips the following commands and goes to the next value of the index when the condition is "true." The *if*(*condition*) *break* command causes the program to leave the *for*-loop and execute the first statement after the end bracket when the condition is "true." In general, the S-command *if*(*condition*) *expression* executes the expression if the condition is true and goes to the following statement if the condition is false.

A last example—to create k sums of n random normal values (mean = 10 and variance = 4) with a *for*-loop:

```
> s<- NULL
> for (i in 1:k) {s[i]<- sum(rnorm(n,10,2))}
```

and to avoid the *for*-loop:

```
> s < -apply(matrix(rnorm(n*k,10,2),n,k),2,sum)
```

When n and k are large numbers, the second S-command executes considerably faster.

The S-language not only provides a large number of system functions but also allows the user to create specialized functions that become part of the S-language either permanently or temporarily. The general form is

function.name <– function(arguments){code to be executed}

Then,

function.name(*arguments*)

executes the code contained between the brackets {} for the given arguments. These "homemade" functions can be nested within other S-commands, called by S-functions such as *apply*(), *tapply*(), or *outer*() and, in general, used in exactly the same way as all S-functions. For example, say it is necessary to evaluate the function $f(x) = x^3 + x^2 + x + 10$ for a number of x-values, then

```
> # homemade function
> f<- function(x){x^3+x^2+x+10}
> x<- 1:6
> f(x)
[1]   13   24   49   94  165  268
> f(2*x)
[1]   24   94  268  594 1120 1894
> f(x/2)
[1] 10.875 13.000 17.125 24.000 34.375 49.000.
```

Continuing the example, the approximate derivative of the function f is

```
> devf<- function(x){(f(x+0.001)-f(x))/0.001}
> devf(2.5)
[1] 24.7585
> devf(c(10,1.8,5,13))
[1] 321.0310   14.3264   86.0160 534.0400
> round(devf(x),3)
[1]    6.004   17.007   34.010   57.013   86.016 121.019
> round(3*x^2+2*x+1,3)
[1]    6   17   34   57   86 121.
```

Another example of a "homemade" S-function that computes the covariance between two sets of values is

```
> cov<- function(x,y){sqrt(var(x)*var(y))*cor(x,y)}
> x0<- c(1,2,0,0,2,1)
> y0<- c(1,2,3,3,2,1)
> cov(x0,y0)
[1] -0.4
> cov(x0,x0)
[1] 0.8
> cov(x0+5,y0/10)
[1] -0.04
> cov(x0^2,y0^2)
[1] -2.533333.
```

An S-function created to generate binomial coefficients is

```
> bcoef<- function(n){
  gamma(n+1)/(gamma(0:n+1)*rev(gamma(0:n+1)))
  }
> bcoef(2)
[1] 1 2 1
> bcoef(6)
[1]   1   6 15 20 15 6 1
> bcoef(10)
[1]    1   10 45 120 210 252 210 120 45 10 1.
```

Factorials can also be generated with the S-function $prod(1:k)$ which produces the value $k!$ (e.g., $prod(1:10) = 3,628,800$).

Most S-code can be incorporated into a function. A bit more complex example occurs when the three probabilities $p_1 = pm + dp^2$, $p_2 = dpq$, and $p_3 = qm + dq^2$ are calculated from the input values $p = 1 - q$ and $d = 1 - m$:

```
> probs<- function(p,d){
    m<- 1-d
    q<- 1-p
    p1<- m*p+d*p^2
    p2<- 2*p*q*d
    p3<- m*q+d*q^2
    c(p1,p2,p3)
  }
> probs(0.5,0.5)
[1] 0.375 0.250 0.375
> probs(0.5,0.8)
[1] 0.3 0.4 0.3
> probs(0.2,0.2)
```

```
[1] 0.168 0.064 0.768
> p<- 0.2
> d<- 0.2
> probs(p,d)
[1] 0.168 0.064 0.768
> sum(probs(p,d))
[1] 1.
```

The last statement in the function code defines the values returned (results of the function calculation) and is characterized by the absence of an "arrow." An additional example—when it is necessary to produce the squared sums among all possible combinations of two sets of values x and y (i.e., $f(x,y) = x^2 + y^2$), then

```
sqdist<- function(x,y){
n1<- length(x)
n2<- length(y)
xy<- matrix(0,n1,n2)
for(i in 1:n1){
for(j in 1:n2){
xy[i,j]<- x[i]^2+y[j]^2
}}
xy
}
> sqdist(1:10,1:10)
       [,1] [,2] [,3] [,4] [,5] [,6] [,7] [,8] [,9] [,10]
 [1,]    2    5   10   17   26   37   50   65   82   101
 [2,]    5    8   13   20   29   40   53   68   85   104
 [3,]   10   13   18   25   34   45   58   73   90   109
 [4,]   17   20   25   32   41   52   65   80   97   116
 [5,]   26   29   34   41   50   61   74   89  106   125
 [6,]   37   40   45   52   61   72   85  100  117   136
 [7,]   50   53   58   65   74   85   98  113  130   149
 [8,]   65   68   73   80   89  100  113  128  145   164
 [9,]   82   85   90   97  106  117  130  145  162   181
[10,]  101  104  109  116  125  136  149  164  181   200
> sqdist(1:4,1:6)
      [,1] [,2] [,3] [,4] [,5] [,6]
 [1,]    2    5   10   17   26   37
 [2,]    5    8   13   20   29   40
 [3,]   10   13   18   25   34   45
 [4,]   17   20   25   32   41   52.
```

The command *outer*() achieves the same results and again executes considerably faster, especially when a large number of calculations is involved. That is,

```
> outer(1:4,1:6,function(x,y){x^2+y^2})
      [,1] [,2] [,3] [,4] [,5] [,6]
 [1,]    2    5   10   17   26   37
 [2,]    5    8   13   20   29   40
 [3,]   10   13   18   25   34   45
 [4,]   17   20   25   32   41   52
```

or

```
> distance2<- function(x,y){x^2+y^2}
> outer(1:4,1:6,distance2)
```

```
      [,1] [,2] [,3] [,4] [,5] [,6]
[1,]     2    5   10   17   26   37
[2,]     5    8   13   20   29   40
[3,]    10   13   18   25   34   45
[4,]    17   20   25   32   41   52.
```

An odds ratio measures association in a 2×2 table (Chapter 6). An S-function that calculates the odds ratio and an approximate 95% confidence interval provides a last illustration of constructing an S-function. The S-function labeled *or.ci*() is

```
or.ci<- function(tab){
or<- tab[1,1]*tab[2,2]/(tab[1,2]*tab[2,1])
logor<- log(or)
v<- 1/tab[1,1]+1/tab[2,1]+1/tab[1,2]+1/tab[2,2]
bounds<- c(logor-1.96*sqrt(v),logor+1.96*sqrt(v))
cat("odds ratio =",round(or,3)," 95% confidence bounds: ",
        round(exp(bounds),3),"\n")
}
```

The output value calculated by this S-function is the estimated odds ratio plus the upper and lower bounds for an approximate 95% confidence interval where a 2×2 table is the input argument (*tab*, in the example). For example,

```
> # odds ratio + 95% confidence interval
> f.tab<- matrix(c(178,79,1411,1486),2,2)
> f.tab
       [,1] [,2]
[1,]   178 1411
[2,]    79 1486
> or.ci(f.tab)
 odds ratio = 2.373 95% confidence bounds: 1.803 3.123.
```

The S-function *cat*() ("cat" for concatenate) allows output (numeric) to be displayed along with alphabetic characters (enclosed in quotes). The S-function

$$cat(\text{``character expression(s)''}, \text{S-output variable(s)}, \cdots, \text{``} \setminus n\text{''})$$

combines labels and numeric results in any order for output. The somewhat obscure expression just before the last parenthesis "\n" is the S-language symbol for "start a new line."

Except for the specifically designated values, all values created by an S-function are local to that function (not communicated to other S-functions or the calling program). To make an S-function variable "globally" available a double arrow convention is used. For example, to make the variable *xvalue*, generated within an S-function, available in general, the syntax

$$xvalue <<- \{expression\} \text{ is used instead of } xvalue <- \{expression\}.$$

FOUR S-CODE EXAMPLES

Example 1

To illustrate an S-language program, the chi-square test for independence based on data classified by two categorical variables follows; specifically, seven levels of one variable (x) and two levels of the other variable (y). A 2×7 table of observed frequencies collected to compare the distribution of bone traumas found in Neanderthal man with those of the modern cowboy is

	foot	leg	pelvis	head	arm	trunk	head	total
Neanderthals	24	24	16	16	25	15	40	160
Cowboys	10	8	8	6	25	10	30	97

A chi-square analysis to examine the relationship between these two sets of observations is

```
> #chi-square example
> row1<- c(24,24,16,16,25,15,40)
> row2<- c(10,8,8,6,25,10,30)
> data<- rbind(row1,row2)
> data
     [,1] [,2] [,3] [,4] [,5] [,6] [,7]
row1   24   24   16   16   25   15   40
row2   10    8    8    6   25   10   30
> rsum<- apply(data,1,sum)
> csum<- apply(data,2,sum)
> n<- sum(data)
> # expected values
> ex<- outer(rsum,csum)/n
> round(ex,2)
      [,1]  [,2]  [,3] [,4]  [,5]  [,6]  [,7]
row1 21.17 19.92 14.94 13.7 31.13 15.56 43.58
row2 12.83 12.08 9.06  8.3 18.87  9.44 26.42
> x2<- sum((data-ex)^2/ex)
> df<- (nrow(data)-1)*(ncol(data)-1)
> pvalue<- 1-pchisq(x2,df)
> round(cbind(x2,df,pvalue),3)
        x2 df pvalue
[1,] 8.471  6  0.206.
```

The S-function *chisq.test*() performs the same test and

```
> chisq.test(data)

Pearson's chi-square test without Yates'
  continuity correction

data: tdata
X-squared = 8.4708, df = 6, p-value = 0.2056
```

gives the same results. No evidence exists of a difference (p-value = 0.206) in the distribution of the bone traumas (types of injuries) sustained by

Neanderthal man and the modern cowboy—both groups appear to lead similar violent and dangerous lives.

Example 2

The data contained in Table 1.5 are cholesterol levels recorded for two behavior types (where type-A is a time conscious, hard driving individual and type-
B is a more relaxed, less competitive person) for $n = 40$ men who weigh more
than 225 pounds. The following S-code performs a Student t-test and a
Wilcoxon two-sample test. The S-code and output are

```
> # t-test example
> # read data from exterior file ab.data
> temp<- scan("ab.data")
> data<- matrix(temp,2)
> # separate the A/B-type individuals
> d<- data[1,]
> id<- data[2,]
> d1<- d[id==1]
> d1
[1] 233 291 312 250 246 197 268 224 239 239 254 276
      234 181 248 252 202 218 212 325
> d2<- d[id==0]
> d2
[1] 344 185 263 246 224 212 188 250 148 169 226 175
      242 252 153 183 137 202 194 213
> # calculate the mean difference in cholesterol levels
> mdiff<- mean(d1)-mean(d2)
> mdiff
[1] 34.75
> n<- length(d1)
> m<- length(d2)
> N<- n+m
> # estimated pooled variance
> vp<- ((n-1)*var(d1)+(m-1)*var(d2))/(N-2)
> vp
[1] 1839.557
> # t-statistic
> tstat<- mdiff/sqrt(vp*(1/n+1/m))
```

Table 1.5. Cholesterol (mg/100 ml) and behavior type A (coded 1) and B (coded 0) for
heavy men (>225 lbs.)

	chol	A/B		chol	A/B		chol	A/B		chol	A/B		chol	A/B
1	344	0	9	246	0	17	224	1	25	242	0	33	252	1
2	233	1	10	224	0	18	239	1	26	252	0	34	202	1
3	291	1	11	212	0	19	239	1	27	153	0	35	218	1
4	312	1	12	188	0	20	254	1	28	183	0	36	202	0
5	185	0	13	250	0	21	169	0	29	234	1	37	212	1
6	250	1	14	197	1	22	226	0	30	137	0	38	325	1
7	263	0	15	148	0	23	175	0	31	181	1	39	194	0
8	246	1	16	268	1	24	276	1	32	248	1	40	213	0

```
> pvalue<- 2*(1-pt(abs(tstat),N-2))
> round(cbind(tstat,pvalue),3)
        tstat pvalue
 [1,]   2.562  0.014

> # S-version of a t-test
> t.test(d1,d2)

      Standard Two-Sample t-test

data: d1 and d2
t = 2.5621, df = 38, p-value = 0.0145
alternative hypothesis: true difference in means
 is not equal to 0
95 percent confidence interval:
  7.293091 62.206909
sample estimates:
 mean of x mean of y
    245.05    210.3

> t.test(d1,d2,var.equal=F)

      Welch Modified Two-Sample t-Test

data:   d1 and d2
t = 2.5621, df = 35.413, p-value = 0.0148
alternative hypothesis: true difference in means is
  not equal to 0
95 percent confidence interval:
  7.227071 62.272929
sample estimates:
 mean of x mean of y
    245.05    210.3

> # Wilcoxon test --- behavior type and cholesterol
> w<- sum(rank(c(d1,d2))[1:m])
> ew<- n*(N+1)/2
> v<- m*n*(N+1)/12
> # z = approximate normal test statistic
> z<- (w-ew-0.5)/sqrt(v)
> pvalue<- 2*(1-pnorm(abs(z)))
> round(cbind(z,pvalue),3)
          z pvalue
[1,]   2.502  0.012

> # S-version of the Wilcoxon test
> wilcox.test(d1,d2,exact=F)

      Wilcoxon rank-sum test

data: d1 and d2
rank-sum normal statistic with correction
      Z = 2.5029, p-value = 0.0123
alternative hypothesis: true mu is not equal to 0.
```

Example 3

A central feature of the S-language is the ability to create a large number of useful summary results with a single command. These results are stored under a single name and are individually accessed to fit particular needs. To illustrate, simulated data ($n = 12$ observations) are created based on the linear regression model $y_i = 10 + 3x_{1i} - 0.5x_{2i} + error_i$, and

```
> # random data
> # generates x1, x2 and y=a+b1*x1+b2*x2+error
> x1<- rep(c(1:4),3)
> x2<- rep(c(1,2,3),rep(4,3))
> a<- 10
> b1<- 3
> b2<- -0.5
> y<- a+b1*x1+b2*x2+rnorm(length(x1))
> # data
> cbind(x1,x2,y)
        x1 x2          y
  [1,]  1  1  11.93879
  [2,]  2  1  15.47869
  [3,]  3  1  18.61216
  [4,]  4  1  21.48232
  [5,]  1  2  12.80333
  [6,]  2  2  15.65158
  [7,]  3  2  17.99809
  [8,]  4  2  22.35833
  [9,]  1  3  11.86457
 [10,]  2  3  12.98607
 [11,]  3  3  20.07852
 [12,]  4  3  22.14333.
```

An S-function *lsfit*() ("lsfit" for least squares fit) calculates a variety of useful summary results generated by a least squares analysis based on a linear model. The first argument is a vector or an array of independent variables (x), the second argument is a vector of dependent variables (y). The function *lsfit*(x,y) produces the elements of a least squares regression analysis (discussed in detail in Chapters 4 and 5). Using the generated "data," these elements are (identified by $name:$)

```
> # regression analysis of simulated data
> lsfit(cbind(x1,x2),y)

$coef:

Intercept        x1            x2
 8.667485 3.35681 -0.05493098

$residuals:
[1] -0.03057686   0.15251090 -0.07082644 -0.55747987
     0.88889519   0.38034090 -0.62995880  0.37346722
     0.00506804 -2.23023815  1.50539877  0.21339900

$intercept:
[1] T

$qr:
$qr$qt:
[1] -58.71530494   13.00087048  -0.15536828
     -0.46886587    0.84611244   0.37861483
     -0.59062828    0.45385437  -0.04594156
     -2.24019112    1.53650244   0.28555936

$qr$qr:
```

```
            Intercept          x1           x2
 [1,]  -3.4641016  -8.66025404  -6.928203e+00
 [2,]   0.2886751   3.87298335  -1.554312e-15
 [3,]   0.2886751  -0.21585785   2.828427e+00
 [4,]   0.2886751  -0.47405674   3.991304e-01
 [5,]   0.2886751   0.30053993  -1.583042e-01
 [6,]   0.2886751   0.04234104  -9.034379e-02
 [7,]   0.2886751  -0.21585785  -2.238337e-02
 [8,]   0.2886751  -0.47405674   4.557706e-02
 [9,]   0.2886751   0.30053993  -5.118576e-01
[10,]   0.2886751   0.04234104  -4.438972e-01
[11,]   0.2886751  -0.21585785  -3.759368e-01
[12,]   0.2886751  -0.47405674  -3.079763e-01

$qr$qraux:
[1] 1.288675 1.042341 1.331170
$qr$rank:
[1] 3
$qr$pivot:
[1] 1 2 3
$qr$tol:
[1] 1e-07.
```

It is not necessary to list these values and generally only some of the estimates or summaries are needed (see *help(lsfit)* for a complete description). The command *otemp* <– *lsfit(x, y)* stores all results and is referred to by the variable name *otemp*, called an "object" or "S-object." The name *otemp* ("otemp" for temporary object) is completely arbitrary and most any label can be used to designate an S-object. Continuing the illustration,

```
> otemp<- lsfit(cbind(x1,x2),y)
```

creates an S-object containing the elements of the least squares analysis of the simulated data (shown explicitly above). A summary of the available elements continued in the S-object generated by *lsfit()* is obtained with the command *summary(object.name)* where the name of the S-object is placed between the parenthesis. From the example,

```
> # available summaries from the lsfit results
> summary(otemp)
              Length      Mode
      coef       3        numeric
 residuals      12        numeric
 intercept       1        logical
        qr       6        list.
```

Various elements of the S-object (*object.name*) are retrieved by using the syntax *object.name$element.name* where *element.name* identifies the particular element within the object to be extracted (i.e., listed by the *summary()* function). For the least squares example,

```
> otemp$coef
 Intercept       x1          x2
  8.667485 3.35681 -0.05493098
> b<- otemp$coef
> b[2]
     x1
  3.35681
```

```
> b
[1]   8.66748500   3.35681000  -0.05493098
> x1<- c(1,1,4,4)
> x2<- c(1,4,1,4)
> b[1]+b[2]*x1+b[3]*x2
[1] 11.96936 11.80457 22.03979 21.87500
> otemp$intercept
[1] T
> otemp$residuals
[1] -0.03057686   0.15251090  -0.07082644  -0.55747987
     0.8889519    0.38034090  -0.62995880   0.37346722
     0.00506804  -2.23023815   1.50539877   0.21339900
> sum(otemp$residuals^2)
[1] 9.096867.
```

An additional series of summary values from a least squares analysis can be created using the S-function *ls.diag(object.name)* ("ls.diag" for least squares diagnostics). The output from *ls.diag()* is also an S-object created from the input of another S-object. Executing the S-command, for example, *summary(ls.diag(otemp))* lists all available elements based on the results contained in the S-object *otemp*. The elements contained in *ls.diag()* are again extracted using the general S-convention where *ls.diag(object.name)$ element.name* produces the summary values of the specific element named. These elements frequently play an important role in regression analyses (Chapter 4).

Example 4

Hotelling's T^2-test for comparing multivariate mean values from two groups illustrates a more advanced application of SPLUS programming making use of the matrix algebra features. The data in Table 1.6 show the heights (inches), weights (pounds), and ages (years) of $n = 63$ individuals with coronary heart disease. These individuals are classified into two groups based on personality assessments, type-A and type-B. The multivariate T^2-test provides an evaluation of the differences between two sets of multivariate mean values when the data are sampled from multivariate normal distributions. Two vectors of k mean values are compared where $\bar{\mathbf{x}}_1 = \{\bar{x}_{11}, \bar{x}_{12}, \bar{x}_{13}, \cdots, \bar{x}_{1k}\}$ and $\bar{\mathbf{x}}_2 = \{\bar{x}_{21}, \bar{x}_{22}, \bar{x}_{23}, \cdots, \bar{x}_{2k}\}$. For the example data, $\bar{\mathbf{x}}_1 = \{\overline{ht}_1, \overline{wt}_1, \overline{age}_1\} = \{70.280, 174.400, 47.120\}$ for type-A individuals and $\bar{\mathbf{x}}_2 = \{\overline{ht}_2, \overline{wt}_2, \overline{age}_2\} = \{69.763, 177.447, 49.947\}$ for type-B individuals $(k = 3)$. Bold-face symbols denote vectors and arrays.

The question is: are the differences observed between these two vectors of three mean values due to chance variation? A necessary part of assessing differences between two vectors of mean values is the pooled variance/covariance array estimated by

Table 1.6. Height, weight, and age measured on type-A and type-B coronary heart disease patients

Type-B			Type-A		
Height	Weight	Age	Height	Weight	Age
65	150	54	73	165	54
67	173	49	70	175	59
68	173	45	67	157	44
74	185	41	70	168	40
69	167	44	68	180	59
76	265	53	70	165	39
70	160	52	70	200	40
70	172	58	68	175	46
69	165	59	72	178	47
63	155	57	70	170	46
68	164	51	69	167	49
69	190	43	71	145	41
70	160	52	74	172	48
72	200	59	68	162	43
72	176	58	77	210	49
70	180	55	70	170	48
72	160	59	71	180	44
71	168	54	71	170	39
63	137	48	68	153	52
70	175	52	74	226	57
68	185	49	70	180	39
71	228	40	71	174	53
72	180	48	68	178	43
74	200	52	70	140	45
72	191	44	67	200	54
68	178	40			
72	190	52			
66	160	39			
69	165	49			
70	165	52			
69	145	52			
69	168	40			
74	205	51			
69	185	59			
68	182	49			
70	188	51			
72	188	41			
70	165	47			

$$V = \frac{(n_1 - 1)\mathbf{v}_1 + (n_2 - 1)\mathbf{v}_2}{n_1 + n_2 - 2}$$

where n_1 and n_2 are the number of observations in each group. The values $\mathbf{v}_1$ and $\mathbf{v}_2$ represent two $k \times k$ variance/covariance arrays estimated from within each group. The test-statistic

$$F = \frac{(n_1 + n_2 - k - 1)T^2}{(n_1 + n_2 - 2)k}$$

where

$$T^2 = \frac{n_1 n_2 (\bar{\mathbf{x}}_1 - \bar{\mathbf{x}}_2)' \mathbf{V}^{-1} (\bar{\mathbf{x}}_1 - \bar{\mathbf{x}}_2)}{n_1 + n_2}$$

has an F-distribution with k and $n_1 + n_2 - (k + 1)$ degrees of freedom when the data are sampled from the same multivariate normal distribution and only random differences exist between the two vectors of mean values. Example S-code applied to the A/B-data (Table 1.6) is

```
> # multivariate t-test (Hotelling's t-squared test)
> # reads the 63 by 3 array of data -- ttest.data
> temp<- scan("ttest.data")
> dtemp<- t(matrix(temp,3))
> # dtemp -- rows 1-25 = type-A, rows 26-63 = type-B
> d1<- dtemp[1:25,]
> # d1 = 25 by 3; type-A
> d2<- dtemp[26:63,]
> # d2 = 38 by 3; type-B
> n1<- nrow(d1)
> n2<- nrow(d2)
> k<- ncol(dtemp)
> xbar1<- apply(d1,2,mean)
> xbar2<- apply(d2,2,mean)
> dbar<- xbar2-xbar1
> round(cbind(xbar1,xbar2,dbar),3)
       xbar1    xbar2    dbar
[1,]   70.28   69.763  -0.517
[2,]  174.40  177.447   3.047
[3,]   47.12   49.947   2.827
> # pooled variance/covariance array
> v<- ((n1-1)*var(d1)+(n2-1)*var(d2))/(n1+n2-2)
> round(v,3)
        [,1]     [,2]     [,3]
[1,]   6.917   33.414   1.224
[2,]  33.414  457.597   6.372
[3,]   1.224    6.372  37.484
> t2<- n1*n2*dbar%*%solve(v)%*%dbar/(n1+n2)
> f<- (n1+n2-k-1)*t2/((n1+n2-2)*k)
> pvalue<- 1-pf(f,ncol(dtemp),n1+n2-k-1)
> cbind(f,pvalue)
             f        pvalue
[1,]  1.797264     0.1575505.
```

The F-statistic indicates that little evidence exists of a systematic difference in the measured characteristics between the type-A and type-B coronary patients.

When $k = 1$ measurement per variable, Hotelling's T^2-test is identical to the previous Student's two-sample t-test.

THE .DATA FILE

All commands, all variables, all functions, and all responses to S-commands are recorded by the SPLUS program. The input and output from an S-session are recorded in a directory called ".Data." The dot preceding a directory name is a UNIX convention and means that the directory is not listed unless the UNIX command *ls -al* is used. When SPLUS is executed with an operating system other than UNIX, the name of the directory and the details of this record keeping feature differ but the process is essentially the same. When a variable or function is defined, it is stored in the directory ".Data" and remains there until removed. Therefore, data, variables, and functions created in previous S-sessions continue to be available for subsequent S-sessions. The names of the stored variables and functions are viewed with the command *ls()*. To delete any of these quantities the command *remove("variable.name")* is used where the variable to be removed is placed between the quotes. For example, the command *remove("temp3")* removes from the directory ".Data" the S-variable named "temp3." The combined commands *remove(ls())* removes all variables and functions contained in the .Data-directory.

A special file is created and maintained in the .Data-directory labeled .Audit. The .Audit-file contains all input commands and a record of the SPLUS responses. It is a complete history of an S-session. An example of part of a .Audit-file is

```
#~New session: Version: S Wed Oct 21 14:16:16 PDT 1995,
     Time: Mon Oct 31 10:25:40 1995
#~get "/home/machine/Splus/Splus/.Datasets/.Copyright" 719540429...
#~get "/home/machine/Splus/Splus/.Datasets/version" 719540430 ...
#~
temp <- scan("temp.data")
#~put "/export/home/sigma/staff/user/.Data/temp" 783627967 ...
#~
d <- matrix(temp, 3, length(temp)/3)
#~get "/export/home/sigma/staff/user/.Data/temp" 783627967 ...
#~put "/export/home/sigma/staff/user/.Data/d" 783627982 ...
#~
d
#~get "/export/home/sigma/staff/user/.Data/d" 783627982 ...
#~
t(d)
#~get "/export/home/sigma/staff/user/.Data/d" 783627982 ...
#~put "/export/home/sigma/staff/user/.Data/.Last.value" 783627987...
#~
ctemp <- cbind(d[, 1], d[2, ], d[3, ])
```

```
#˜error: No. of observations in time, status, and x must match
#˜put "/export/home/sigma/staff/user/.Data/last.dump" 783628088 ...
#˜
time <- d[, 1]
#˜get "/export/home/sigma/staff/user/.Data/d" 783627982 ...
#˜put "/export/home/sigma/staff/user/.Data/time" 783628105 ...
#˜
status <- d[2, ]
#˜get "/export/home/sigma/staff/user/.Data/d" 783627982 ...
#˜put "/export/home/sigma/staff/user/.Data/status" 783628111 ...
#˜
g <- d[3, ]
#˜get "/export/home/sigma/staff/user/.Data/d" 783627982 ...
#˜put "/export/home/sigma/staff/user/.Data/g" 783628119 ...
#˜
cbind(time, status.g)
#˜error: Object "status.g" not found
#˜
.
.
.
```

The .Audit-file accumulates commands until it becomes extremely large. At a given size limit a warning message is issued indicating that the records will be truncated from the .Audit-file as new commands are entered and executed. The .Audit-file can be manipulated with the usual system commands (e.g., the UNIX command *rm* ˜/.*Data*/.*Audit* deletes the file) or specialized S-functions exist for managing the .Audit-file. For example, to remove the entire contents of the .Audit-file, the command *Splus* TRUNC_AUDIT 0 does the job.

The .Audit-file can be edited to recover the commands entered at the terminal during an interactive session since all lines beginning with #˜ are produced by SPLUS in response to a command. Lines without this "prefix" are a record of the S-commands entered from the terminal. From the example fragment, deleting all lines starting with the two characters "#˜ " gives

```
temp <- scan("temp.data")
d <- matrix(temp, 3, length(temp)/3)
d
t(d)
ctemp <- cbind(d[, 1], d[2, ],  d[3, ])
time <- d[, 1]
status <- d[2, ]
g <- d[3, ]
cbind(time, status.g)
.
.
.
```

There are several ways to recover the S-commands in the .Audit-file. Perhaps the most direct way is to use a text editor. The recovered input commands can be then edited (e.g., remove the error in the last line— *status.g* should be *status, g*) and saved with a file name such as *read.s*. Such script files containing S-commands can be run again in three ways. The

S-function *source("input.code")* executes the code in the named file from within SPLUS. For example, the command *source("read.s")* reads the data from the exterior file "temp.data" and defines the variables *time, status,* and *g,* making them available for subsequent use (i.e., stored in ".Data"). More usually, S-script files are run with the syntax *Splus <input.code >output.file* where this command is issued at the system prompt. The code found in *input.code* is run and any generated output is placed in the second file, *output.file.* For example, the command *Splus < read.s > temp.out* executes the code within *read.s* and places the resulting output in the file *temp.out.* If an output file name is not included in the command, the output is displayed on the terminal screen as it is being created ("real time"). Again, the variables *time, status,* and *g* are stored in the directory .Data. Alternatively, the command *Splus BATCH input.code output.file* executes the S-script found in file *input.code* and places the output in file *output.file.* Additionally, the commands from the input code are included as part of the output file. This "batch" command runs the S-script in the "background" so that the computer is free for other tasks while the S-program is executing.

System commands can be executed without leaving SPLUS. If a command issued during an S-session is preceded by an exclamation point (!), the command is interpreted as a system command (temporarily ignoring the SPLUS program). The exclamation point is an "escape" character. For example, during an S-session, the UNIX command *!ls* lists the files contained in the present working directory and then returns to the current S-session. This feature allows a variety of tasks to be executed without interrupting the flow of the S-commands. Escape characters occur in a variety of contexts and are a valuable computer tool.

Occasionally, a UNIX command is needed as part of an S-program. The S-function *unix("command")* allows UNIX commands to be executed as part of an S-code program. For example, *unix(ls)* is the same as the command *!ls.* To count the number of files in the current directory as part of an S-program

```
> temp<- length(unix("ls")).
```

Or, a bit more complicated example follows:

```
> temp<- unix("wc -l <input.dat")
> temp
[1] "9"
> numlines<- as.numeric(temp)
> numlines
[1] 9
> data<- matrix(scan("input.dat"),numlines,byrow=T)
```

and gives the number of lines in the file labeled "input.dat" where the UNIX word count command "wc" is used. The S-function *as.numeric*( ) turns character representations of numbers into numeric S-values.

ADDENDUM: BUILT-IN EDITORS

The initial S-command *Splus* followed by −*e* ("e" for editor) can invoke one of two UNIX editors, called *vi* and *emacs*. These editors become part of the S-system by setting specific environmental variables (see [4]). The "-*e*" option makes commands from these editors available to modify interactively S-command lines. The process will be illustrated using the *vi*-editor.

As described, SPLUS keeps a history of previously executed commands. To recall a command from this history, press the *Esc*-key and use the *k*-key to scroll up through previous commands or the *j*-key to scroll down though this list. To re-submit a command, press the *enter*-key at any time and the current command line will be executed. Previous commands containing a specific string of characters can be located in the history list by typing "?" followed by the string of characters to be located. For example, *?pnorm* finds the last command containing the character string *pnorm*.

To change a previous command or to edit a current command, the process again starts with pressing the *Esc*-key making the current command line available for editing or allowing a previous command to be recalled and made current. To move horizontally on the current command line a number of options are available. To move the cursor to the left, the *h*-key is used and to move to the right the *l*-key is used. The cursor moves one character each time the key is pressed. To move to the right from word to word the *w*-key is used and to move to the left from word to word the *b*-key is used. To move to the end of the line, type $ and to move to the beginning of the line, type 0.

Once the cursor is in position, the command line can be edited. To add to the command line, the *i*-key ("i" for insert) and the *a*-key ("a" for append) are the most useful. If the *i*-key is pressed, the next character or characters typed are inserted before the position of the cursor. Any number of characters or words can be inserted. Pressing the *Esc*-key returns the system to the editor mode. The same process is achieved with the *a*-key but the characters or words typed are added after the cursor position. Pressing the *x*-key deletes the character under the cursor and pressing the *r*-key ("r" for replace) replaces the character under the cursor with the next character typed. When the pair of letters *x* and *p* are typed, the letter under the cursor and the following letter are transposed. Typing *dw* ("dw" for delete word) deletes the entire word located by the cursor and to change a word, type *cw* ("cw" for change word) followed by the new word or words that replace the old word. As before, to re-submit an edited command press the *enter*-key and SPLUS then executes the newly edited command line.

To summarize:

key	function
Esc	invokes or terminates the editor
recall commands	
k	moves up through the S-history
k	moves up through the S-history
j	moves down through the S-history
?<*string*>	locates <*string*> in the S-history
cursor movement	
h	moves the cursor one character to the left
l	moves the cursor one character to the right
w	moves the cursor one word to the right
b	moves the cursor one word to the left
$	moves the cursor to the end of the line
0	moves the cursor to the beginning of the line
editing	
i	inserts characters to the left of the cursor
a	adds characters starting with the cursor position
x	deletes the character under the cursor
r	replaces the character under the cursor
xp	transposes two characters
dw	deletes the word located by the cursor
cw	changes the word located by the cursor

Problem set I

1. Write and test a command that creates absolute values; other than *abs*().

2. Write and test a command that evaluates the standard error of the mean associated with a vector of n values labeled x without using *var*(x) where

$$\text{standard error} = \sqrt{\frac{\sum (x_i - \bar{x})^2}{n(n-1)}}.$$

3. Write and test a set of commands that calculates the square root of T using the relationship $x_{i+1} = (x_i + T/x_i)/2$.

4. Compare the S-function *pnorm*() to the approximation $P(x)$ where

$$P(x) = \frac{1 + \sqrt{1 - e^{-2x^2/\pi}}}{2}$$

when x is between 0 and ∞.

Find the maximum difference between these two functions and the value at which the maximum difference occurs.

5. Pascal's triangle is

row 1	1
row 2	1 1
row 3	1 2 1
row 4	1 3 3 1
row 5	1 4 6 4 1

.
.
.

Write and test an S-function that generates the kth row. Verify that the rows sum to 2^k.

6. The estimated standard deviation is

$$S = \sqrt{\frac{\sum(x_i - \bar{x})^2}{n - 1}}.$$

A correction for the bias of this estimate is

$$\alpha_n = \sqrt{\frac{2}{n}} \frac{\Gamma(n/2)}{\Gamma([n-1]/2)}$$

where $\Gamma(x)$ represents a gamma function evaluated at x. Calculate α_n for $n = 2, 3, 4, \cdots,$ 50. An approximation is $\alpha'_n = 1 - 0.75/(n - 1)$. Compare this approximation to α_n.

Show that

$$\alpha_n = \frac{3.5n - 3.62}{3.5n - 1}$$

is a better approximation.

7. Write and test S-commands that create the following two patterns of numbers:

1 2 3 4 5 1 2 3 4 5 1 2 3 4 5 1 2 3 4 5 1 2 3 4 5
1 1 1 1 1 2 2 2 2 2 3 3 3 3 3 4 4 4 4 4 5 5 5 5 5

Write and test S-commands that will generate this pattern in general; that is, for any chosen integer.

8. Create an S-vector with 1000 values set to 1. Then add one to every second value, then add one to every third value, then add one to every fourth value, and so on 1000 times. Which values are odd and which are even? Justify the observed pattern.

9. Write and test an S-function that accepts two vectors of observations x and y as input and returns the Spearman rank correlation (the correlation coefficient calculated using ranks of the observations).

Verify the S-code using $cor.test(x, y, method = spearman)$.

10. A perfect shuffle of a deck of 52 playing cards occurs when the deck is split perfectly into halves (26/26) and the cards are exactly alternated. If the top card remains on the top after each perfect shuffle, the shuffle is called a perfect outside shuffle. If the deck is ordered before the first shuffle, how many perfect outside shuffles are necessary to restore the original order? If the top card becomes the second card on

each shuffle, the shuffle is called a perfect inside shuffle. If the deck is ordered before the first shuffle, how many perfect inside shuffles are necessary to restore the original order?

11. Generate a vector (denoted *ybar*) containing $k = 20$ mean values each composed of $n = 50$ random observations from a normal distribution with mean $= 2$ and standard deviation $= 2$.

Generate *ybar* using a "*for*-loop."

Generate *ybar* without using a "*for*-loop."

Increase k and n and note the difference in execution times.

12. Evaluate

$$f(x, y) = \frac{sin(x)}{\sqrt{1 + cos^2(y)}}$$

over the ranges $-2\pi < x < 2\pi$ and $-2\pi < y < 2\pi$.

Construct and test S-code using and not using a "*for*-loop." Note the difference in execution times.

13. Construct a three-column array where column $1 = rnorm(100, 2, 2)$, column $2 = rnorm(100, 4, 4)$, and column $3 = rnorm(100, 0, 1)$. Use S-code to produce an array so that each column has exactly mean $= 0$ and exactly variance $= 1$.

Use the command $scale(cbind(x1, x2, x3), center = T)$ which does the same thing to verify your results.

Verify that $cor(cbind(x1, x2, x3)) = var(scale(cbind(x1, x2, x3)))$

14. An approximation for $n!$ is

$$n! \approx \sqrt{2n\pi}(n/e)^n.$$

Write an S-code program to show that the difference between this approximation and $n!$ increases with increasing n but the relative error (i.e., (*absolute difference*)/n) decreases.

15. For the 100 observations in the following table, write an S-command that produces a vector labeled *test* with 100 observations with the same distribution of values (e.g, 1, 1, 1, $\cdots$,5, 5, 5, 5):

	1	2	3	4	5
count	20	35	25	10	10

To check: *table(test)* will reproduce the above table.

16. In a random matching of two equivalent decks of k cards the probability P_m of exactly m matches is

$$P_m = \frac{1}{m!}\left\{1 - 1 + \frac{1}{2!} - \frac{1}{3!} + \frac{1}{4!} - \cdots \pm \frac{1}{(n - m)!}\right\}$$

where $m = 0, 1, 2, 3, \cdots, n - 1$.

Write an S-code function to calculate P_m for a given value of $m < n$.

Show that for $m > 9$, $P_m \approx \frac{1}{m!}e^{-1}$.

REFERENCES

1. Chambers, M. J. and Hastie, T. J., (eds), *Statistical Models in S*. Wadsworth & Brooks/Cole Advanced Books, Pacific Grove, CA, 1992.
2. Becker, R. A., Chambers, M. J., and Wilks, A. R., *The New S Language*. Wadsworth & Brooks/Cole Advanced Books, Pacific Grove, CA, 1988.
3. Spector, P., *An Introduction to S and S-Plus*. Duxbury Press, Belmont, CA, 1994.
4. Venables, W. N. and Ripley, B. D., *Modern Applied Statistics with S-Plus*. Springer-Verlag, New York, NY, 1994.

2

Descriptive Techniques

DESCRIPTION OF DESCRIPTIVE STATISTICS

Descriptive statistics are at the heart of organizing and summarizing numerical values. Data are not particularly interesting until they are reduced to a few summary values indicating general properties of the entire sample. Five general properties of a sample of numerical observations are:

location—the central or most typical value,

variability—the dispersion or spread of the observations,

distribution—the concentrations (or gaps) within a sample of observations,

extreme values—the locations of the large and small values, and

outlier values—observations with patterns that differ from most other collected values.

Without summarization, the assessment of these properties is not easy or even possible. Additionally, the first step of a statistical analysis is typically a description of each of the variables under investigation. For example, Table 2.1 contains 750 birth weights (grams) of first born children. Without some sort of summary technique, these values do not convey much meaning. It is necessary to translate the large number of birth weights into a few descriptive values and create graphic representations of the data so that a picture of the entire distribution can be grasped. Such tools as

summary statistics: averages, variances, ranges, quantiles, tables,

visual displays: histograms, stem-and-leaf plots, density plots, univariate plots, quantile-plots, bivariate plots

display methods: smoothing techniques, cluster analyses, and tabular approaches

help make sense out of the collected values. Descriptive statistics produce summary values or display the observations "visually" so that the general properties of the structure underlying the sampled data emerge. The S-language provides computer tools to implement these descriptive statistics.

Table 2.1. Birth weights (grams) of 750 newborn infants

3500	3050	2920	3050	2620	3380	620	4240	4160	3010	3360	3800	3460	4260	4500
4190	3220	3920	3700	3400	3340	3500	3560	4100	3100	3870	3520	2920	3480	4400
2210	4100	3580	3500	3550	3500	3200	3250	3380	3900	3400	4600	3100	3940	3485
4000	3760	3420	3420	3040	3880	1170	2340	3760	3860	2160	3510	3480	3150	3560
4240	3920	3620	3410	3400	4280	2920	3360	3920	2800	3180	3320	3700	4860	4020
3440	2380	2400	3120	4040	3110	4180	4280	3090	3980	3520	1880	3340	3760	3940
2360	3050	3080	3500	3860	3260	3100	4300	2840	1210	3600	3960	3540	3890	890
4320	3500	3290	3900	4040	2680	3590	3020	4030	3140	3000	3620	3150	3950	3180
3970	3520	2780	3300	4000	3220	3800	3890	2380	2740	3400	3900	3120	3070	3790
3820	3300	1800	1600	3400	3100	3720	4215	3180	3740	3700	3660	3110	3200	1570
4490	3500	3620	340	1030	3700	2900	4150	3560	1170	3980	3160	3760	2380	4120
3880	2750	3880	4120	1080	790	3390	910	3540	3540	3320	3980	1050	4060	4480
2430	3780	3580	3700	1640	3720	3900	4130	3350	4480	4140	4100	3000	3380	3300
3260	3580	3840	3150	4040	3500	3260	3900	2900	2860	3240	3780	2260	3700	4520
2760	1000	4020	4190	3140	3840	4120	3830	3100	3470	3300	3380	990	3500	3340
4440	3860	3100	3240	3540	3340	3280	3215	3620	4080	3780	3580	4280	3220	4480
3240	4260	4100	3600	3480	3860	680	3520	3000	3720	3030	3560	3340	4350	2960
2930	4080	3300	1700	3480	3580	3730	3590	3300	3380	3500	4180	4030	3640	3660
3960	3060	3690	3990	3900	3530	3400	3320	2790	3900	3160	3520	1980	4520	3620
3388	4280	4040	3750	3500	3990	2150	1330	4060	3400	3900	3540	4480	3480	2320
3440	2495	3020	3340	3340	3460	3920	3720	3100	1820	2860	3020	2610	3540	3740
3480	4100	3240	2920	3880	3800	3380	2370	3540	3180	3150	3930	4080	3275	3675
3400	3880	2930	4140	2020	3960	3660	3080	3700	2540	3480	3680	4200	3640	3600
3680	3840	4180	3340	3840	3640	4130	1790	3460	3200	3450	4100	3520	4360	3580
3180	3950	1060	3710	3120	3460	3980	3560	1960	3120	3370	3480	3700	3770	3280
4240	3680	3460	2960	4240	3920	3100	3540	3100	760	4420	3260	4200	4010	4180
4060	2550	3420	2920	3530	2490	3400	3160	3360	3720	3640	4320	4000	2550	2920
4800	3420	3120	3910	3700	4000	3160	3130	3265	3940	3960	2220	2740	4140	2510
1270	635	2680	4060	3440	3140	3320	3900	3820	3050	790	2860	2960	3200	3500
3800	3160	3680	2420	3600	3550	2520	3600	4440	3580	2180	3500	3320	3680	3660
2700	3220	4350	3640	3280	3660	3180	4720	4130	3650	3720	2830	3700	2440	2970
4300	3400	2350	2800	4220	4170	3820	4140	3540	3400	3100	4260	3540	3160	3585
3540	4280	3000	3780	3120	2900	2960	4080	2840	2525	3175	4120	2100	3800	2380
3660	3880	4200	4100	3570	3600	4320	4120	3900	4040	3125	3990	3600	3740	3140
3530	3750	3990	3840	3450	3180	3970	3440	3420	3300	3100	3460	2960	3670	3530
3360	3560	3450	4400	3420	3240	3420	3660	3160	2760	3370	2520	4290	3040	2960
3500	4100	820	3320	3940	3380	3370	1060	3715	2750	3760	2980	3620	3520	2660
3860	3380	3540	2900	3560	3330	3470	3240	3700	4400	2700	3380	3740	3600	3890
3820	3550	3220	3040	3330	3420	4120	4050	3540	2920	3460	4180	3460	4060	3120
3460	3160	3020	3840	1070	3440	3430	3820	4240	4280	3180	2030	3740	3240	2980
4480	3900	2900	3800	2980	3920	3280	3750	3640	3820	3380	3200	3880	3220	4460
3700	3480	3540	3360	3740	3360	3220	3460	3820	3740	3460	3240	3260	3360	4260
3880	2800	3040	3230	3180	4040	2730	3125	3880	3660	3940	2980	2540	3540	3200
4920	3900	3240	3040	3100	2790	3280	3840	4040	3620	3240	4350	3460	3000	3980
3740	2700	3280	3280	3400	4000	3420	3810	3940	3615	3300	2260	3700	3320	4280
3850	3310	3760	3110	3550	3760	3680	3700	3580	3660	3040	3580	3320	4180	3600
3220	2550	3760	3260	3280	3200	3960	4330	4115	3100	3860	3190	4430	5020	3580
3025	3600	4260	3930	2910	3220	3660	2820	4150	3750	3520	3500	3660	3200	3420
3820	3010	4060	3950	3050	3260	4000	3440	3480	3940	2980	4300	3650	3190	3060
3220	4080	3780	3230	3200	2960	4000	3240	3090	4420	4800	3220	4260	3840	4310

BASIC STATISTICAL MEASURES

Nine elementary statistical summaries associated with a collection of numeric values are:

sample size	mean	median
variance	standard deviation	standard error
minimum	maximum	range.

Of course, there are other possibilities but these measures serve as a start and can be calculated with an S-function. For example,

```
describe<- function(x){
n<- length(x)
xbar<- mean(x)
md<- median(x)
s2<- var(x)
s<- sqrt(s2)
se<- s/sqrt(n)
xmin<- min(x)
xmax<- max(x)
rng<- xmax-xmin
cbind(n,xbar,md,s2,s,se,xmin,xmax,rng)
}
```

The argument vector x contains input data consisting of measurements made on a single variable, such as the birth weights in Table 2.1. Using the $n = 750$ birth weight observations (labeled *bwt*), the S-function *describe*( ) produces

```
> describe(bwt)
       n     xbar    md      s2       s     se xmin xmax   rng
[1,] 750 3421.484 3500 475861.4 689.83 25.19  340 5020 4680.
```

A similar S-command *summary*( ) applied to the birth weight data gives

```
> summary(bwt)
 Min. 1st Qu. Median Mean 3rd Qu.  Max.
 340    3160   3500   3421  3860   5020.
```

Sample size is a necessary description of any data set. The mean and the median are different averages indicating the location of the distribution of observations. Once the location is established, variability becomes an important description. The variance or standard deviation (square root of the variance) provide measures of variability. The standard error of the mean is also a description of variability but refers to the variability associated with an estimated mean and not the observations themselves. In symbols, the estimated variance of n numeric values is represented as S^2 and the square root is then the estimated standard deviation S, making the estimated standard error of the mean $S/\sqrt{n}$. These two quantities are sometimes confused in the description of a specific variable. The standard deviation refers to the variability of a single observation while the standard error reflects the variability of an estimated mean value, based on n observations. Other measures of dispersion are the minimum and the maximum values as well as the range (the maximum minus the minimum value).

The nine summary statistics calculated by *describe( )* begin to describe specific properties of the data but it is also valuable to view the distribution of the observations as a whole. A simple one-way frequency tabulation created by the S-function *table( )* yields a summary table and for the birth weight data

```
> ints<- seq(0,6000,500)
> table(cut(bwt,ints))
   0+ thru   500   500+ thru 1000 1000+ thru 1500 1500+ thru 2000
                1               11              11              10
2000+ thru 2500 2500+ thru 3000 3000+ thru 3500 3500+ thru 4000
               25              69             255             249
4000+ thru 4500 4500+ thru 5000 5000+ thru 5500 5500+ thru 6000
              110                8               1               0
```

displays the general features of the 750 observations.

Several kinds of visual displays of a one-way table exist and provide important ways to describe sampled values. A popular display is a histogram. To construct a histogram, each observation is represented by the area of a rectangle. Within the limits of a series of intervals, these rectangles are accumulated (summed) so that the total area is proportional to the number of observations occurring in the interval (*area = interval width × total height*). These summary rectangles are placed side by side producing a picture of the distribution corresponding to a one-way tabulation of the data. The total area is proportional to the sample size (n).

Figure 2.1 is a histogram of the birth weight data organized into 12 intervals of 500 gram widths corresponding to the tabulation of the 750 infant birth weights. The small number of intervals leads to a histogram lacking detail. Increasing the number of intervals to 50 produces a histogram (Figure 2.2) where the concentrations and gaps in the birth weight distribution are clearly seen but, more importantly, the general shape of the distribution becomes apparent. For birth weights, the distribution is skewed toward the left (negative skewness) showing more extremely light weight infants than heavy infants. The birth weight distribution above 2500 grams is more or less symmetric.

A histogram is generated with the S-function *hist( )* and the S-function that generated Figure 2.2 is

```
> hist(bwt,nclass=50,main="n = 750 birth weight (parity = 1)")
```

The 750 birth weights contained in the input vector *bwt* are classified into 50 intervals (option = *nclass*; where *nclass*=50) and the counts of birth weights in each of these 50 intervals determine the heights of the histogram rectangles. The S-option *main = "n = 750 birth weight (parity = 1)"* labels the top of the

n = 750 birthweight (parity = 1)

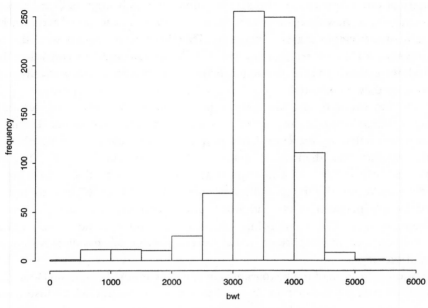

Figure 2.1

n = 750 birthweight (parity = 1)

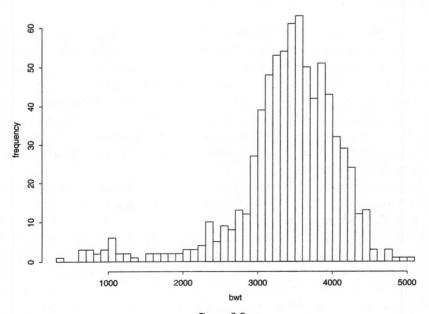

Figure 2.2

plot with the words or symbols placed between the quotation marks. A large variety of other options are available to "fine-tune" a histogram (see *?hist*).

One way to view this plot or other graphic output on a terminal screen is by means of a separate graphics window. This window is created with the S-command $X11()$ or *motif()* for the UNIX system and *win.graph* for the Windows system. Executed graphic S-functions are then automatically displayed as they are created.

The key property of a histogram relates to area. The area to the left of a given interval point is proportional to the count of observations less than that point, reflecting the cumulative frequency. For example, the number of birth weights less than 2500 grams is 58 or 58 out of 750. That is, $100 \times 58/750 = 7.7\%$ of a histogram area is to the left of the 2500 gram birth weight on the horizontal axis. Similarly, 504 or 67.2% of infant weights are between 3000 and 4000 grams and are also depicted as a histogram area. The relationship between area and specific values makes as a histogram an important visual representation of the distribution of the observations.

Another version of the histogram is produced with the S-function *density()*. Application of the S-function *density()* generates an outline of the histogram such as the one shown in Figure 2.3. Figure 2.3 is an outline of a histogram of birth weights (Figure 2.2) created with the specific S-function

```
> plot(density(bwt),type="l",
    main="n = 750 birth weight (parity = 1)")
```

where the option *type* = *"l"* produces a line plot ("l" for line). The option *type* = *"b"* would produce both points and lines ("b" for both) and if no *type* option is specified only points are plotted. The heights (vertical axis) are adjusted so that the total area enclosed by the curve equals 1.0.

These two representations of a single distribution of observations (histogram or density plot) differ primarily in esthetics but, as will be seen, the density representation has a more extensive interpretation. The S-function *density()* employs a general process used to estimate density functions under a variety of circumstances.

A plot resembling a histogram is a barplot. The fundamental difference between these two graphic representations is that the "x-axis" on a barplot has no particular ordering. The "x-axis" is a series of categories and the area enclosed by the barplot rectangles generally has no useful interpretation. A barplot represents frequency by the height of the bar (not area). For example, the counts of four races from a data set are: white = 815, Hispanic = 319, black = 123, and Asian = 171. A barplot with bar heights equal to these counts is created by the S-function *barplot(data, names = c(< list >), · · ·)*. Specifically,

n = 750 birthweight (parity = 1)

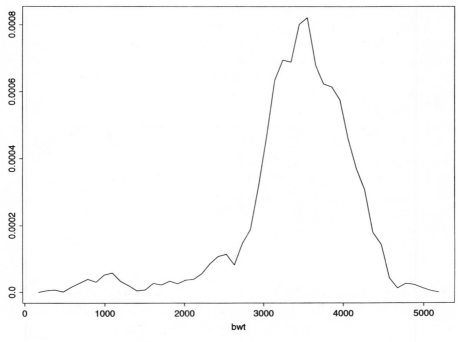

Figure 2.3

```
> count<- c(815,319,123,171)
> barplot(count,names=c("white","hispanic","black","asian"),
  angle=c(45,30,15,0),xlab="race/ethnic group",
  main="Barplot")
```

plots Figure 2.4 (left side). The options *main* and *xlab* label the figure (top) and x-axis (bottom) with any symbols or words placed between the quotes. The option *angle* produces the type of fill for the rectangles representing each count with lines at the given angles. In the example, the angles are 45°, 30°, 15°, and 0, respectively. When the *angle* option is omitted, the rectangles are given the same solid fill. The S-vector *names* provides a label for each bar plotted.

A pie chart is not much different in principle from a bar plot. A pie chart can be created with the S-function *pie(data, names = c(< list >), ⋯)* and for the race/ethnicity counts

```
> percent<- 100*count/sum(count)
> round(percent,1)
[1] 57.1 22.3  8.6 12.0
> pie(percent,names=c("white","Hispanic","black","Asian"),
  density=0,xlab="race/ethnic group",main="Pie chart")
```

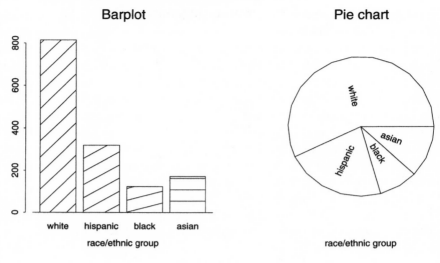

Figure 2.4

plots Figure 2.4 (right side). The option *density* =< *value* > determines the density of the fill (*density* = 0 yields no fill). Both a barplot and a pie chart, like *hist*( ), can be "fine-tuned" with various S-options (see *?barplot* or *?pie*).

HISTOGRAM SMOOTHING—DENSITY ESTIMATION

A histogram depicts a distribution of sampled values as rectangles with areas proportional to the frequency of the observations occurring in each of a series of predefined intervals. The nature of a histogram is such that discontinuous jumps in frequency counts occur between intervals where frequently the underlying data varies smoothly across the horizontal axis. Nevertheless, the area of a histogram, as mentioned, relates to the distribution associated with the observed data, making a histogram a rough estimate of the underlying probability function.

If the values that form the bases for constructing a histogram are a sample from a continuous distribution and if enough data are available, then a "smooth" histogram can be created using small interval widths. This smoother version more plausibly reflects the underlying sampled population. A density estimation approach produces a smooth representation of a continuous variable that does not require a large number of observations to estimate the underlying probability distribution.

To produce such an estimate, each observation is replaced by a normal distribution (other distributions are used) with mean value equal to the value of the replaced observation. This distribution is called the kernel function. There is one kernel function for each observation. The standard deviation of the normally distributed kernel functions, in this context, is called a smoothing parameter or bandwidth. Each "data value" is now a function (not a single discrete observation) that continuously varies across the entire range of the data set with the most concentration at the value of the replaced observation. The degree of concentration is determined by the bandwidth. A small bandwidth completely locates an "observation" at the mean and a large bandwidth spreads the "observation" more or less uniformly over the range of the data. An intermediate bandwidth is a compromise so that each observation contributes a balance between location and spread.

The height of an estimated probability function or density function is the sum of the heights of the the kernel functions and can be constructed at any point. That is, the heights of the kernel functions, for all sampled observations, are added together producing a summary height at any point in the range of the sampled variable. The process is analogous to constructing a histogram but based on heights constructed at a continuous series of points rather than at a set of discrete intervals. These heights smoothly vary with changes in the variable plotted producing a continuous estimate of the distribution that generated the sampled data. Again, the area to the left of a point x_0 estimates the probability that a random observation X is observed less than or equal to x_0 (i.e., estimates $P[X \leq x_0]$).

Fifteen observations (Figure 2.5) are:

$$x = \{2.3, 0.8, 2.0, 1.2, 1.3, 0.9, 3.8, 2.2, 5.5, 1.0, 3.4, 5.3, 1.1, 0.7, 2.7\}.$$

To estimate the distribution from which the sample was selected each value is replaced by a normal distribution with mean = x_i and bandwidth = standard deviation = 0.2 (dotted lines). The heights of these 15 kernel functions added together at a series of points between 0 and 6 form a smooth representation of the distribution of the observed data (solid line). A histogram employs rectangles to reflect the frequency of a series of observations while a density estimate uses sums of a less severe geometric form (such as a normal distribution) to spread the frequency over the entire range.

The following example S-code is a simple density estimation algorithm for plotting the data contained in the S-vector x (kernel = normal distribution, bandwidth = standard deviation = h = 1.0):

```
> # x contains the observed values
> x<- c(2.3,0.8,2.0,1.2,1.3,0.9,3.8,2.2,5.5,1.0,3.4,5.3,1.1,
       0.7,2.7)
> n<- length(x)
> dx<- 2
> z<- seq(min(x)-dx,max(x)+dx,0.1)
> y<- matrix(0,n,length(z))
> # smoothing parameter = bandwidth = h
```

Illustration of a density plot

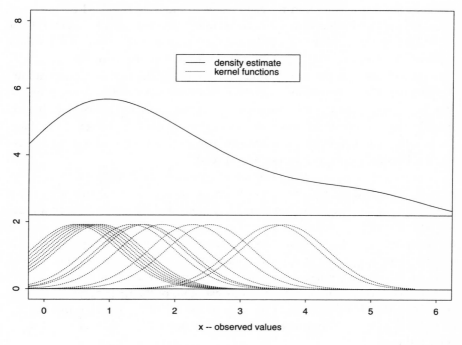

Figure 2.5

```
> h<- 1.0
> for(i in 1:n) {y[i,]<- dnorm(z,x[i],h)}
> zfreq<- apply(y,2,sum)
> plot(z,zfreq,xlab="x -- observed values",
  xlim=c(0,6),ylim=c(0,4),type="l")
```

The plot options *xlab* = "label for x axis" and *ylab* = "labels for y axis" allow the axes to be labeled with the letters or symbols placed between the quotes. If this option is omitted, the names of the x-argument and y-argument in the plot command are used.

The plot limits are defined by a two-value S-vector (e.g., $c(a, b)$ defines the limits as a and b) or by the *range*( ) command. The options *xlim* = $c(a, a')$ and *ylim* = $c(b, b')$ define the limits of the plot field to a and a' in the x-direction and b to b' in the y-direction. When values a and b are not known, *xlim* = *range*(x) and *ylim* = *range*(y) define limits based on the ranges of the vectors x and y. When no limits are specified (*xlim* and *ylim* are not included in the plot command) the plot ranges are determined based on the input vectors containing the coordinate points.

A sophisticated and "user-friendly" S-function to plot estimated probability distributions,

$$density(input.vector, window = < kernel\ function >, width = h, \cdots),$$

is available with several choices for the kernel function ("cosine," "gaussian," "rectangular," or "triangular") and with an option for setting the bandwidth $width = h$). The S-command

```
> plot(density(x,width=3.5),xlab="x -- sampled values",
    xlim=c(0,6),ylim=c(0,0.3),ylab="frequency",type="l")
```

produces essentially the same density plot displayed in Figure 2.5 (using a different scale).

The smoothness of the plot is influenced by the choice of the kernel function but is primarily controlled by the bandwidth. Small values of the bandwidth parameter make the estimated density into a series of spikes located at each observed value. As the value of the bandwidth parameter increases, a smoother estimate of the sampled distribution emerges. Like most smoothing techniques, a trade-off occurs between the loss of detail and the visibility of broad characteristics. Figure 2.6 shows the same set of values sampled from a normal distribution plotted with increasing bandwidth parameter (h) using a normal kernel function.

The bandwidth option $width$ depends on the scale of the data. One suggestion for selecting a bandwidth (value of h) is to use a multiple of the interquartile range (i.e., the distance between the third and first quartile). S-commands setting a bandwidth at two times the interquartile range are

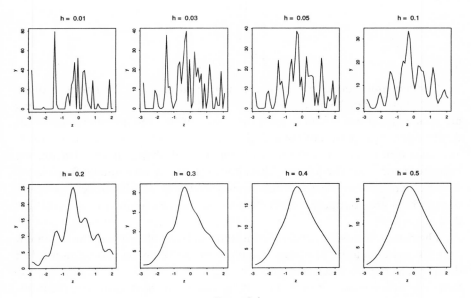

Figure 2.6

```
> h<- 2.0*(quantile(x,0.75) - quantile(x,0.25))
```

and often creates a smooth but not too smooth plot based on the data contained in the S-vector x. However, no hard and fast rule exists for setting the bandwidth.

STEM-AND-LEAF DISPLAY

A cross between a table and a histogram is a description of sampled data called a stem-and-leaf display. Like a histogram, the stem-and-leaf display is used to organize and summarize numeric values producing a compact picture of the properties of a data set without elaborate theory. A stem-and-leaf plot is constructed from the digits of the values to be displayed. These values are split into high order digits (stems) and lower order digits (leaves). Then, a separate row (stem) is allocated for each high order digit and the lower order digits are accumulated within their associated rows in increasing order (leaves). The process is easier to illustrate than describe. A small sample of 26 recent California lottery numbers follows:

$$3, 6, 46, 33, 23, 34, 15, 16, 12, 9, 33, 44, 48, 39, 31, 22, 38, 22, 11, 19, 27, 43, 45, 40, 21, \text{ and } 18.$$

For the lottery values, the stem-and-leaf display is

$$
\begin{aligned}
&0 : 369 \\
&1 : 125689 \\
&2 : 12237 \\
&3 : 133489 \\
&4 : 034568
\end{aligned}
$$

Each lottery number is split into tens digits and ones digits. The tens digits {0, 1, 2, 3 and 4} make up the five stems and the associated ordered ones digits are attached to these stems to form the leaves. When the 26 lottery values are displayed, the properties of the group are easily determined (e.g., ranks, median, maximum, and minimum) and the general shape of the distribution becomes apparent. The lottery values appear more or less equally frequent.

Another stem-and-leaf example comes from $n = 187$ birth weights where the mothers are young, less than 20 years old, and classified by race (Table 2.2).

The S-function *stem*( ) constructs a stem-and-leaf plot, where the argument vector is the data to be displayed. It produces the following two stem-and-leaf displays for the Moffitt Hospital data. Input data are an S-vector *bwtw* <– *bwt[race==1]* containing $n_1 = 111$ white infant birth weights and *bwtb* <– *bwt[race==2]* containing $n_2 = 76$ black infant birth weights.

Table 2.2. Infant birth weights (grams) classified by race (white = 1 and black = 2) where the maternal age is less than 20 years (University of California, Moffitt Hospital, 1980–90)

bwt	race	bwt	race	bwt	race	bwt	race	bwt	race	bwt	race	bwt	race	bwt	race
3500	1	2980	1	3080	1	3680	1	3140	1	3570	1	3580	2	3320	2
3800	1	3370	1	4000	1	4000	1	3080	1	3155	2	3965	2	2300	2
4420	1	4800	1	4200	1	4520	1	460	1	2205	2	3650	2	2240	2
3500	1	3940	1	4180	1	3760	1	4700	1	3160	2	1940	2	3400	2
3940	1	3690	1	3800	1	3820	1	3000	1	3350	2	3050	2	3755	2
4220	1	3840	1	3230	1	4320	1	3977	1	3280	2	3520	2	3080	2
2420	1	3700	1	4200	1	3380	1	3590	1	3480	2	4420	2	3500	2
3980	1	3540	1	2960	1	3900	1	680	1	3030	2	2560	2	2580	2
3760	1	4750	1	5150	1	3530	1	4060	1	3020	2	3500	2	3990	2
3290	1	3800	1	3210	1	3700	1	820	1	300	2	4300	2	960	2
3700	1	3420	1	4100	1	3800	1	3550	1	3040	2	3060	2	3450	2
3730	1	3500	1	4310	1	2830	1	2650	1	3940	2	3460	2	3870	2
3510	1	3880	1	4360	1	4150	1	3870	1	3500	2	3420	2	3300	2
4520	1	3740	1	3640	1	410	1	3815	1	4400	2	3700	2	4260	2
3970	1	3940	1	4300	1	4420	1	1930	1	4240	2	3100	2	2940	2
2320	1	5070	1	4620	1	3320	1	4150	2	3980	2	3120	2	3007	2
4120	1	3040	1	3860	1	2780	1	3820	2	2760	2	3100	2	2220	2
3400	1	3860	1	780	1	4000	1	1240	2	3320	2	3060	2	3625	2
1700	1	3550	1	3950	1	4255	1	4170	2	3460	2	2580	2	3845	2
3955	1	3470	1	3820	1	4180	1	3260	2	3285	2	2780	2		
3520	1	3000	1	4920	1	3500	1	2740	2	4190	2	3020	2		
3620	1	3650	1	2920	1	3870	1	3510	2	3080	2	3730	2		
4480	1	3840	1	4250	1	2540	1	3160	2	2400	2	2905	2		
3380	1	3440	1	3810	1	3140	1	3020	2	3340	2	3100	2		

For the white infants,

```
> stem(bwtw)
```

```
            N = 111 Median = 3760
            Quartiles = 3370, 4000

            Decimal point is 2 places to the right of the colon

            Low:    410    460    680    780    820   1700   1930

    23 : 2
    24 : 2
    25 : 4
    26 : 5
    27 : 8
    28 : 3
    29 : 268
    30 : 00488
    31 : 44
    32 : 139
    33 : 2788
    34 : 0247
    35 : 00001234559
    36 : 24589
    37 : 0003466
    38 : 000011224466778
    39 : 044455788
    40 : 0006
    41 : 02588
```

```
42 : 00255
43 : 0126
44 : 228
46 : 2
47 : 05
48 : 0
49 : 2
50 : 7
51 : 5
```

Extreme values ("outliers") are listed separately (top—labeled "Low") as part of the general description of the data.

For the black infants,

```
> stem(bwtb)
          N = 76 Median = 3292.5
          Quartiles = 3020, 3637.5

          Decimal point is 2 places to the right of the colon

          Low:     300    960   1240

   19 : 4
   20 :
   21 :
   22 : 024
   23 : 0
   24 : 0
   25 : 688
   26 :
   27 : 468
   28 :
   29 : 04
   30 : 12223456688
   31 : 0002566
   32 : 688
   33 : 02245
   34 : 025668
   35 : 0001278
   36 : 25
   37 : 035
   38 : 247
   39 : 4689
   40 :
   41 : 579
   42 : 46
   43 : 0
   44 : 02
```

The least significant digits are not used in the birth weight stem-and-leaf displays. That is, 19 : 4 (first line of the black infant's stem-and-leaf display) represents the observed birth weight 1940 grams, the fourth line 22 : 024 represents birth weights 2205, 2220, and 2240 grams, and so forth.

A comparison of a stem-and-leaf display with a histogram shows no substantial difference except the stem-and-leaf display allows a more detailed assessment of the location (ranks) of the observations. Both approaches display the prominent features of the distribution of the collected data classified by race (e.g., location, symmetry, variability, concentrations, gaps, and extreme values).

COMPARISON OF GROUPS—*t*-TEST

Data are commonly collected to make comparisons among several groups. These comparisons take a variety of forms. For example, a series of descriptive statistics for each group can be calculated and compared. Again using the birth weight data (Table 2.2),

```
> # entire birth weight data set
> round(describe(bwt),4)
      n    xbar    md        s2      s    se xmin xmax   rng
[1,] 187 3434.0 3520.0 703171.6 838.6 61.3  300 5150 4850
> # restricted to whites
> round(describe(bwtw),4)
      n    xbar    md        s2      s    se xmin xmax rng
[1,] 111 3579.7 3760.0 767267.9 875.9 83.1  410 5150 4740
> # restricted to blacks
> round(describe(bwtb),4)
      n    xbar     md        s2      s    se xmin xmax  rng
[1,]  76 3221.3 3292.5 541284.6 735.7 84.4  300 4420 4120
```

where *bwt* is a vector containing all observed birth weights and, as before, *bwtw* and *bwtb* contain the birth weights for each of the two racial groups.

Frequently a two-sample *t*-test provides a valuable comparison of the mean values from two groups, such as:

```
> t.test(bwtw,bwtb)

        Standard Two-Sample t-Test

data: bwtw and bwtb
t = 2.9284, df = 185, p-value = 0.0038
alternative hypothesis: true difference
    in means is not equal to 0
95 percent confidence interval:
  116.9393 599.8234
sample estimates:
mean of x mean of y
  3579.658  3221.276.
```

The white birth weight mean (3579.7 grams) is significantly (p-value = 0.004) higher than the black birth weight mean (3221.3 grams).

Throughout, the term p-value is frequently used instead of the more formal but equivalent term, significance probability. A p-value is defined as the probability of observing a more extreme result than the one observed under the hypothesis that the observed differences are due entirely to chance variation. In less precise language, a significance probability is a numeric guide to deciding whether an observed difference is likely due to non-random influences.

Since a t-test is based on the assumption that the variances associated with the sampled populations are equal, a test of variance is a relevant description, and

```
> var.test (bwtw,bwtb)
              F test for variance equality
data: bwtw and bwtb
F = 1.4175, num df = 110, denom df = 75, p-value = 0.1079
alternative hypothesis: true ratio of variances
    is not equal to 1
95 percent confidence interval:
    0.9256439 2.1347387
sample estimates:
variance of x      variance of y
     767267.9           541284.6.
```

Statistical tests certainly reflect specific aspects of a comparison between samples of data but fail to describe completely the overall distributions associated with two or more sets of observations. For example, two distributions can have the same mean and variance but differ substantially in "shape." Furthermore, many analytic techniques, like the t-test and the test of equal variances, require the sampled data to have at least an approximate normal distribution. Statistical techniques to compare distributions under all conditions (normal or not) also play an important role in describing data. Such techniques are called distribution-free, "exploratory," "sturdy," "resistant," and "robust." Examples are boxplots and quantile plots which are the topics of the next three sections.

COMPARISON OF GROUPS—BOXPLOTS

One effective approach to compare visually samples of data involves the construction of a set of boxplots. A boxplot is constructed from five summary numbers computed from a sample. These values are derived from a general concept called depth [1]. The depth of the median, for example, is $depth = (n+1)/2$ where n is the number of observations. The median (denoted F_m) is the value x_{depth} when the sample size n is odd and, by convention, $x_{depth-\frac{1}{2}} + x_{depth+\frac{1}{2}})/2$ when the sample size n is even where x represents a value from n ordered observations, $\{x_1 \leq x_2 \leq x_3 \leq \cdots \leq x_n\}$. As the term suggests, depth is a measure of the extent inward in a series of ordered values.

Another special case is called depth of a fourth, defined by

$$depth \ of \ a \ fourth = \frac{[depth \ of \ the \ median] + 1}{2}$$

where the symbol $[z]$ stands for the largest integer not exceeding z (S-function $trunc(z)$ produces $[z]$). The lower fourth observation (F_l) is found by counting up to the *depth of a fourth* value and the upper fourth (F_u) is found by counting down the number of observations equal to the *depth of a fourth* where again the observations are ordered from low to high. Each fourth is close to halfway between the median and the corresponding extreme value. When the fourth is not an integer, the same convention of averaging the two adjacent values is used that is employed to find the median when n is even. For technical reasons these two values F_l and F_u) sometimes differ from the 25th and 75th quantiles but are essentially the same, particularly in large samples of data. Two other important values computed from a sample are the "outlier cut-offs" defined as

$$lower\ cut\text{-}off = F_l^* = F_l - 1.5(F_u - F_l)\ \text{and}$$

$$upper\ cut\text{-}off = F_u^* = F_u + 1.5(F_u - F_l).$$

The difference $F_u - F_l$ is called the fourth-spread and is similar to the inter-quartile range. To summarize, the five summary values are: F_l^* (lower cut-off), F_l (lower fourth), F_m (median), F_u (upper fourth), and F_u^* (upper cut-off). These five values are computed by the S-function *five( )*:

```
five<- function(data){
x<- sort(data)
n<- length(x)
m<- (n+1)/2
fm<- 0.5*(x[ceiling(m)]+x[trunc(m)])
m<- (trunc(m)+1)/2
fl<- 0.5*(x[ceiling(m)]+x[trunc(m)])
m<- n+1-m
fu<- 0.5*(x[ceiling(m)]+x[trunc(m)])
upper<- fu+1.5*(fu-fl)
lower<- fl-1.5*(fu-fl)
cbind(lower,fl,fm,fu,upper)
}
```

A small sample of industrial hygiene data measuring exposure of refinery workers processing gasoline at a marine loading facility illustrates. Fifteen measured levels of benzene exposure (ppm) are

$$data = \{0.51, 0.01, 0.08, 0.09, 0.14, 0.20, 0.01, 0.09, 0.06, 0.05, 0.01, 0.03,$$
$$0.05, 0.22, 0.68\}$$

and

```
> data<- c(0.51,0.01,0.08,0.09,0.14,0.20,0.01,0.09,0.06,
  0.05,0.01,0.03,0.05,0.22,0.68)
> five(data)
      lower     fl     fm     fu     upper
[1,] -0.155   0.04   0.08   0.17   0.365
> quantile(data)
   0%   25%   50%   75% 100%
  0.01 0.04 0.08 0.17 0.68.
```

The benzene data produce $F_l^* = -0.155$, $F_l = 0.04$, $F_m = 0.08$, $F_u = 0.17$, and $F_u^* = 0.365$.

A boxplot is constructed by placing these five values on a scale that ranges beyond the minimum and maximum observed values as follows:

1. a symbol is placed at the median F_m,
2. a box is drawn with end points at F_l and F_u (length = fourth-spread),
3. two lines are extended from the end of the box to the most remote observation that does not exceed F_l^* and F_u^* (not an "outlier"), and
4. all observations outside these limits are marked on the plot ("outliers").

Figure 2.7 shows a boxplot of the benzene exposure data constructed with the S-function *boxplot*( ), or specifically

```
> boxplot(data,main="Benzene exposure data")
```

The median is indicated on the S-boxplot by solid line within the box.

Using the birth weight data in Table 2.3 and the S-function *boxplot*( ), then

```
> boxplot(bwtw,bwtb,names=c("whites","blacks"),
    ylab="birth weight", main="Birth weight
    distributions -- whites versus blacks")
```

produces two boxplots (Figure 2.8) comparing white and black birth weight distributions. The plot option *ylab* produces a label for the *y*-axis and the option *names* labels each of the boxplots on the *x*-axis (the order of the data sets and the order of the labels must be the same). A comparison of the

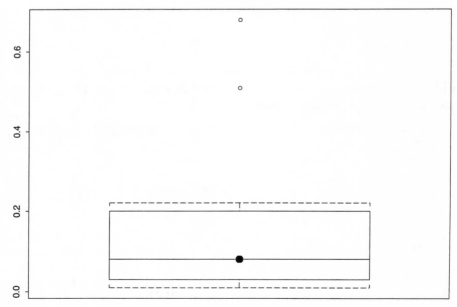

Figure 2.7

Birth weight distributions -- whites and blacks

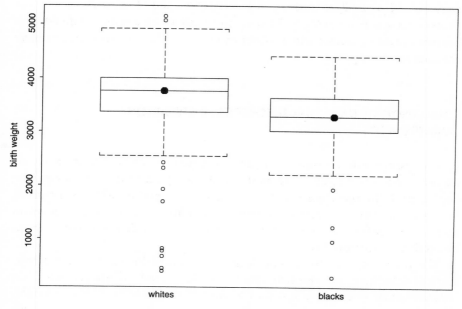

Figure 2.8

boxplots shows that white infants appear to have a higher median birth weight than black infants with similar fourth-spreads (difference between the F_l and F_u). Additionally, the white birth weight distribution contains a larger proportion of very light weight infants ("outlier observations"—whites = 11/111 = 0.099 versus blacks = 4/76 = 0.053).

The fundamental properties of a boxplot are: (1) it is valid for any distribution of values (distribution-free), (2) it is essentially unaffected by extreme values (robust), and (3) it defines rigorously but somewhat arbitrarily the term outlier.

The interval given by *mean value* $\pm z_{1-\alpha/2} \times$ *standard deviation* contains $(1 - \alpha)\%$ of the values of a normal distribution where $z_{1-\alpha/2}$ is the $(1 - \alpha/2)^{th}$ quantile from a standard normal distribution. When a sample of data comes from a normal distribution, such limits can define a likely "outlier" observation based on small values of α. However, most data are not normally distributed and in many cases data are not even approximately normally distributed. In the non-normal case, a boxplot remains an effective statistical tool. Nevertheless, it is interesting to compare these two approaches. For a normal distribution with mean μ and standard deviation σ, the lower fourth is $F_l = \mu - 0.674\sigma$ (*qnorm*(0.25) returns 0.674) and the upper fourth is

$F_u = \mu + 0.674\sigma$, making the fourth-spread 1.348σ. The cut-off values are then $F_l^* = F_l - 2.022\sigma$ and $F_u^* = F_u + 2.022\sigma$ and $P(observation < F_l^*) = P(observation > F_u^*) = 0.0035$. That is, an "outlier" observation defined by a boxplot occurs by chance with probability of 0.007 when the data are normally distributed.

COMPARISON OF DATA TO A THEORETICAL DISTRIBUTION— QUANTILE PLOTS

It is frequently interesting to compare a distribution derived from collected observations to a theoretical distribution. A histogram or density plot can be compared to the corresponding theoretical curve. Another useful comparison that is visually easy to assess contrasts two cumulative probability distributions, one constructed entirely from the data and the other constructed from theoretical considerations.

When a theoretical probability distribution is described in terms of cumulative probabilities, these probabilities are the likelihood a random observation is less than or equal to a specified value—$P(X \le x) = F(x)$. For example, standard normal distribution (mean = 0 and standard deviation = 1) cumulative probabilities are generated by $pnorm(x)$ for a specific value x, as noted. If $x = 0.771$, then $P(X \le 0.771) = F(0.771) = 0.780$ ($pnorm(0.771)$ returns 0.780) or, in other words, 78% of the normal distribution from which x was selected is less than or equal to the value 0.771. In general, the constructed S-function $p + root.name(\ )$ (Table 1.4) produces cumulative probabilities.

An empirical cumulative probability distribution developed directly from the sampled data, completely independent of theoretical considerations, is

$$\hat{P}(X \le x) = \hat{F}(x) = \frac{\text{the number of values less than or equal to } x}{\text{total number of values observed}}.$$

The symbol $\hat{F}(x)$ simply represents the observed proportion of the sampled values less than or equal to x. The empirical cumulative distribution is not a smooth continuous sequence of values but increases in discrete jumps at each observed value x. Such a function is referred to as a step-function and each step has height $1/n$ when n observations are sampled. For example, consider the $n = 20$ values given in Table 2.3 (first column) where the values are transformed to have mean $= \bar{x} = 0$ and variance $= S^2 = 1$. When these values are ordered (low to high), the empirical cumulative probability associated with the ith ranked value is $\hat{F}(x_i) = i/n = i/20$.

For example, the value $x_{17} = 0.771$ is the 17th ranked value so an estimate of the cumulative probability at that point is $\hat{F}(x_{17}) = \hat{F}(0.771) = 17/20 = 0.85$. That is, 85% of the values of the distribution from which x_{17} was selected

Table 2.3. Two cumulative probability distributions—one based on the data $\hat{F}(x)$ and one based on the theoretical standard normal distribution $F(x)$

obs	x	$\hat{F}(x)$	$F(x)$
1	-2.293	0.05	0.011
2	-1.349	0.10	0.089
3	-1.005	0.15	0.158
4	-0.683	0.20	0.247
5	-0.434	0.25	0.332
6	-0.235	0.30	0.407
7	-0.204	0.35	0.419
8	-0.193	0.40	0.423
9	-0.117	0.45	0.453
10	-0.102	0.50	0.460
11	-0.010	0.55	0.496
12	0.013	0.60	0.505
13	0.128	0.65	0.551
14	0.235	0.70	0.593
15	0.250	0.75	0.599
16	0.254	0.80	0.600
17	0.771	0.85	0.780
18	0.832	0.90	0.797
19	1.932	0.95	0.973
20	2.209	1.00	0.986

are estimated to be less than or equal to 0.771. The empirical cumulative distribution function estimated from the 20 values given in Table 2.3 (third column) is displayed in Figure 2.9 (solid line).

To compare the empirical values $\hat{F}(x)$ to a standard normal distribution, the theoretical cumulative probabilities $F(x)$ are also found for each observed value in the data set. These values are given in Table 2.3 (fourth column) and the theoretically derived cumulative standard normal probability distribution is also plotted (Figure 2.9—dotted line). If the observed distribution closely corresponds to the theoretical distribution, these two sets of probabilities are similar. A formal comparison of the difference $|F(x) - \hat{F}(x)|$ is accomplished with the Kolmogorov procedure (Chapter 3). A good way to compare informally the degree of similarity is to plot the two sets of values, one against the other. The plot will be close to a straight line where the distributions are similar and where they are not similar, the plot will deviate from a straight line. Such a plot is created by SPLUS with the S-function *qqnorm( )* and is illustrated in Figure 2.10 where *qqnorm(sort(x), type="l")* is used to plot the probabilities associated with x from Table 2.3 (theoretical normal versus empirical cumulative distribution functions). The argument vector contains the values to be compared to a standard normal distribution. A comparison line is constructed with the S-function *qqline( )*. The S-function *qqnorm( )* does not directly plot the values $\hat{F}(x)$ and $F(x)$ but rather the quantiles associated

Cumulative distributions

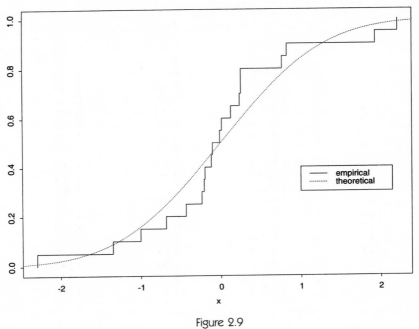

Figure 2.9

S-qqnorm

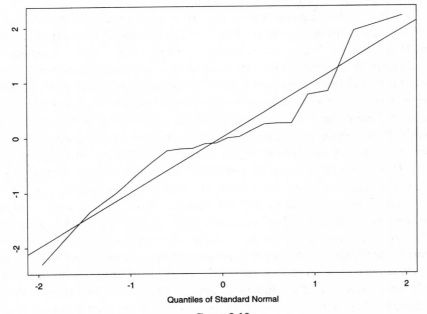

Figure 2.10

with both these probabilities. The result is a change in scale, which does not affect the interpretation of the plot.

The essence of the S-function *qqnorm*( ) is captured in a few lines of example S-code where

```
> # rdata = vector of rdata -- mean = 0 and variance = 1
> n<- length(rdata)
> y0<- sort(rdata)
> x0<- qnorm(((1:n)-1/3)/(n+1/3))
> # quantile plot
> plot(x0,y0,type="l")
```

Or, alternatively,

```
> y1<- pnorm(sort(rdata))
> x1<- ((1:n)-1/3)/(n+1/3)
> # cumulative probability plot
> plot(x1,y1,type="l")
```

The vector $y0$ contains the sorted data standardized to have mean = 0 and variance = 1. The vector $x0$ contains the corresponding expected quantile values based on applying the inverse normal S-function *qnorm*( ) to the empirical cumulative distribution function. Using the correction factor 1/3 improves the accuracy of the estimate. When the data are normally distributed, a plot of these pairs (either $x0$ against $y0$ or $x1$ against $y1$) deviates from a straight line only because of random variation.

Figure 2.11 shows the qqnorm plot for the 750 birth weights (Table 2.1) where

```
> z<- sort((bwt-mean(bwt))/sqrt(var(bwt)))
> qqnorm(z,type="l",main="n = 750 birthweight (parity = 1)")
> qqline(z)
```

creates the plot. The asymmetry seen in the previous histogram and density plots is clearly displayed in the comparison of the empirical cumulative distribution to the normal cumulative distribution. The major contribution to the asymmetry comes from the low birth weight infants. To further explore the distribution of newborn birth weights, the data restricted to "normal" weight infants (i.e., birth weights > 2500 grams) produce

```
> nbwt<- bwt[bwt>2500]
> describe(nbwt)
        n   xbar    md      s2      s    se xmin xmax   rng
[1,] 692 3568.1 3540 202653.5 450.2 17.1 2510 5020 2510.
```

The qqnorm-plot of these "normal" weight infants shows a remarkably close fit between the observed and theoretical cumulative probability distributions (Figure 2.12). Three graphic descriptions of the birth weight distribution *hist*( ), *density*( ), and *qqplot*( ) S-functions) are summarized in Figure 2.13.

n = 750 birthweight (parity = 1)

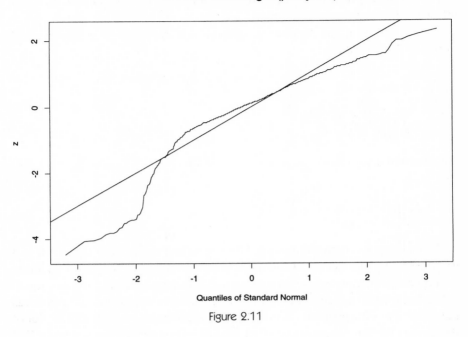

Quantiles of Standard Normal

Figure 2.11

n = 692 birthweight (bwt >2500g and parity = 1)

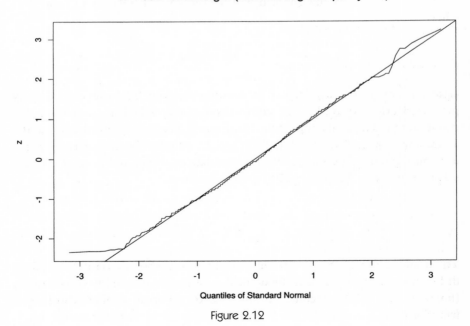

Quantiles of Standard Normal

Figure 2.12

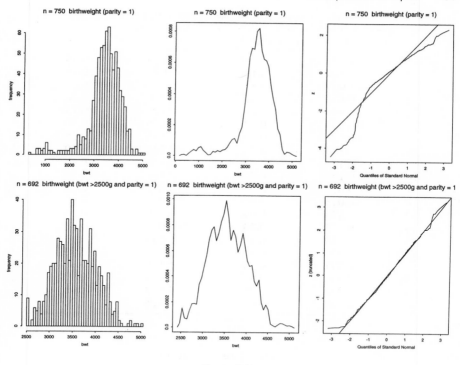

Figure 2.13

COMPARISON OF GROUPS—QQPLOTS

Another effective visual comparison of groups of observations is achieved by contrasting their estimated cumulative distribution functions. Identical to the previous empirical cumulative probability distribution function, the cumulative probabilities $\hat{F}_k(x)$ are estimated for each group and compared. The subscript k indicates different cumulative probability functions, one from each of a series of collected samples (i.e., $\hat{F}_1(x)$, $\hat{F}_2(x)$, $\hat{F}_3(x)$, $\cdots$). For the 20 observations in Table 2.4, the estimated cumulative probabilities are given in column 3 (group 1) and column 5 (group 2) where $\hat{F}_k(x_i) = i/n_k$ for sample sizes $n_1 = 20$, $n_2 = 20$, and $k = 1, 2$. Again, the data are ordered from low to high.

A comparison of these estimated cumulative probability distributions is shown in Figure 2.14. The center of an estimated cumulative distribution indicates the location of the sampled data and the rate of increase, displayed by the step-function, relates to the variability of the observations. Therefore, differences in locations and slopes of the estimated cumulative distribution functions reflect differences in means and the variances of the sampled distributions.

Table 2.4. Two empirical cumulative probability distributions——$\hat{F}_1(x)$ and $\hat{F}_2(x)$

	z_1	$\hat{F}_1(x_i)$	z_2	$\hat{F}_2(x_i)$
1	−2.293	0.05	−1.958	0.05
2	−1.349	0.10	−1.073	0.10
3	−1.005	0.15	−0.949	0.15
4	−0.683	0.20	−0.760	0.20
5	−0.434	0.25	−0.709	0.25
6	−0.235	0.30	−0.676	0.30
7	−0.204	0.35	−0.546	0.35
8	−0.193	0.40	−0.508	0.40
9	−0.117	0.45	−0.192	0.45
10	−0.102	0.50	−0.104	0.50
11	−0.010	0.55	−0.061	0.55
12	0.013	0.60	0.005	0.60
13	0.128	0.65	0.046	0.65
14	0.235	0.70	0.077	0.70
15	0.250	0.75	0.138	0.75
16	0.254	0.80	1.114	0.80
17	0.771	0.85	1.125	0.85
18	0.832	0.90	1.635	0.90
19	1.932	0.95	1.669	0.95
20	2.209	1.00	1.725	1.00

Cumulative distributions

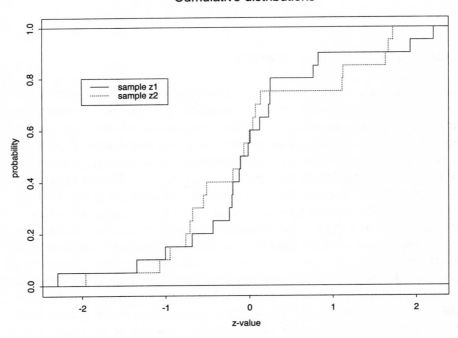

Figure 2.14

As before, an effective comparison is easily achieved by plotting the values from one cumulative distribution against the other. Such a comparison is produced by the S-function *qqplot(data1, data2)* where *data*1 and *data*2 represent input S-vectors each containing the data to be compared transformed to have means = 0 and variances = 1. Continuing the example (Table 2.4), the command

```
> qqplot(z1,z2,type="l",main = "S-qqplot -- z1 versus z2")
```

produces the plot in Figure 2.15 where $z1$ and $z2$ represent input data vectors (Table 2.4). The deviations from a straight 45°-line show the areas of dissimilarity in the "shape" of the two compared data sets.

For the case where the numbers of values observed in both samples are equal ($n_1 = n_2 = n$), plotting the ordered values in one sample against the ordered values in the other produces a qqplot, or

```
> # simple qqplot for equal sample sizes
> xx<- sort(x)
> yy<- sort(y)
> plot(xx,yy,type="l")
> abline(0,1)
```

S-qqplot -- z1 versus z2

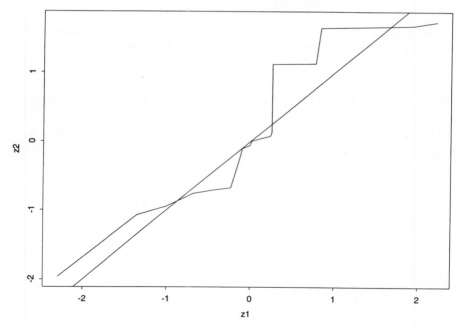

Figure 2.15

When the sample sizes are not equal, the plot is the same in principle but involves interpolating because of unequal sample sizes. The command $abline(0, 1)$ plots a comparison 45°-line (intercept = 0 and slope = 1). In general, the S-function $abline(a, b)$ plots a straight line over the range of the current plot with intercept = a and slope = b. Two special cases are: $abline(v = x0)$ plots a vertical line across the plotting range through the point x_0 and $abline(h = y0)$ plots a horizontal line across the plotting range through the point y_0.

The S-function $qqnorm(\ )$ is a special case of the S-function $qqplot(\ )$. The command $qqnorm(z, type = ``l'')$ is equivalent to

```
> cdf<- ((1:n)-1/3)/(n+1/3)
> qqplot(qnorm(cdf),z,type="l")
```

where z is an S-vector of data to be compared to a standard normal distribution. The S-functions that allow the calculation of specific cumulative probabilities (Table 1.4) make it possible to compare data-generated and theoretically generated cumulative probabilities for a variety of statistical distributions. For example, to address the question of whether the data contained in the S-vector x are consistent with a normal distribution with parameters m and s, then

```
> qqplot(qnorm(cdf,m,s),x,type="l")
```

To address the question of whether the data contained in the S-vector *sdata* are consistent with an exponential distribution with parameter *lam*, then

```
> qqplot(qexp(cdf,lam),sdata,type="l")
```

Comparisons of observed data to other specific distributions follow the same pattern.

To compare the white and black birth weight distributions the following S-functions produce three relevant plots; Figure 2.16 (density plots), Figure 2.17 (smoothed density plots), and Figure 2.18 (qqplot):

```
> # density plot
> plot(density(bwtw),type="l",ylab="density - bwt",
    xlab="birth weight",
    main="Birth weight distributions -- whites versus blacks")
> par(new=T)
> plot(density(bwtb),xlab="",ylab="",axes=F,type="l",lty=2)

> # density plot -- smoothed
> plot(density(bwtw,width=1000),type="l",ylab="density - bwt",
    xlab="birth weight",
    main="Birth weight distributions -- whites versus blacks")
> par(new=T)
> plot(density(bwtb,width=1000),xlab="",ylab="",axes=F,
    type="l",lty=2)
```

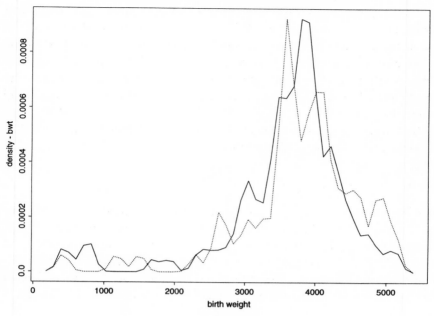

Figure 2.16

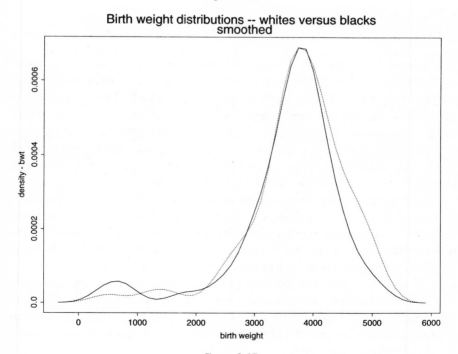

Figure 2.17

qqplot -- white versus black

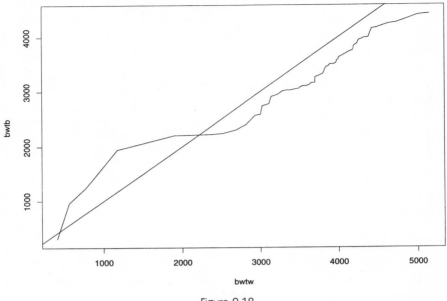

Figure 2.18

```
> # qqplot plot
> qqplot(bwtw,bwtb,type="l",main="qqplot -- white versus black")
> abline(0,1)
```

The first set of commands creates two density estimates (outlines of histograms) from the two birth weight samples (solid line = white infant birth weights and dotted line = black infant birth weights). The second set of commands displays the same density estimates but smoothed to represent more conceptually the underlying birth weight distributions. The third set of commands generates a qqplot again reflecting the differences between white and black birth weight distributions (white infants are heavier and slightly more variable when compared to black infants).

A few things are important to note about the three S-plots. The command *par(new = T)* ("par" for parameters) allows a second plot to be printed on the same set of axes as the current plot. The S-function *par( )* is an extensive S-tool designed to add specific parameters to plotting routines. For example, *par( )* invokes control over such graphic features as text and symbols (e.g., *cex*, *xlab*, or *ylab*), plotting area and axes (e.g., *xlim*, *ylim*, or *yaxt*), margins, page areas, and, in general, allows a large variety of ways to specifically tailor graphic output. A list and description of over 50 possible parameters used to control different features of a plot using *par( )* is produced with the "online" S-help command (see *?par*).

The plot options in Figures 2.16 and 2.17, *xlab*="", *ylab*="", and *axes* = *F*, suppress the *x*-label, the *y*-label, and the axes of the second plot so they do not overprint the values from the first plot. The different line styles result from the option *lty* = *k* ("lty" for line type) where *k* = 1, 2, 3, $\cdots$, 8 determines various line types (e.g., *lty* = 2 produces a dotted line). The second density plot uses the option *width* = 1000 to set the bandwidth parameter to produce smooth representations of the birth weight distributions. The third set of commands yields a qqplot contrasting white/black birth weight data. The three plots provide different perspectives on the same question—how do the birth weight distributions differ between white and black infants?

xy-PLOT

A natural extension of plotting a single variable is the simultaneous plotting of two variables. A two-dimensional plot (also called an *xy*-plot or a scattergram or scatter plot) is certainly among the most useful graphic techniques. The elements of a one-dimensional plot (e.g., histogram) are present in an *xy*-plot since the distribution of each variable is readily seen. Additionally, the relationship between two variables is displayed as a two-dimensional scatter of points. To illustrate, the expected length of life (described completely in Chapter 8) for white females and males is calculated for each of the 50 United States and the District of Columbia using 1980 mortality data from the National Center for Health Statistics and the 1980 United States Census Bureau population counts (Table 2.5). Also recoded is the percent of urban areas within each state (defined by the United States Census Bureau).

The following commands produce the plot in Figure 2.19 using the S-vectors *exwm* containing the expected length of life for white males, *exwf* containing the expected length of life for white females, and *urban* containing the percentage urban areas:

```
> postscript("temp.ps")
> plot(exwf[urban<75],exwm[urban<75],pch="+",
    ylim=range(exwm),xlim=range(exwf),
    ylab="expectation of life (wm)",
    xlab="expectation of life (wf)",
    main="Expectation of life -- males versus females")
> points(exwf[urban>=75],exwm[urban>=75],pch="o")
> abline(lsfit(exwf,exwm)$coef)
> points(mean(exwf[urban<75]),mean(exwm[urban<75]),
    pch="x",cex=1.5)
> points(mean(exwf[urban>=75]),mean(exwm[urban>=75]),
    pch="*",cex=1.5)
> legend(74.7,66,c("%urban<75","%urban>=75",
    "non-urban centroid","urban centroid"),pch="+ox*")
```

Table 2.5. Expectation of life for white males (exwm), females (exwf), and percent urban (urban) for the 50 United States plus District of Columbia

	exwm	exwf	urban		exwm	exwf	urban		exwm	exwf	urban		exwm	exwf	urban
AL	66.17	74.35	58.4	IN	67.25	73.81	64.9	NV	65.69	72.83	80.9	TN	66.68	74.31	58.8
AK	66.86	74.31	48.8	IA	68.40	74.98	57.2	NH	67.06	73.84	56.5	TX	67.24	74.36	79.8
AZ	66.97	74.19	79.5	KS	68.53	75.24	66.1	NJ	68.16	73.98	88.9	UT	68.96	75.18	80.6
AR	66.98	74.74	50.0	KY	66.24	73.60	52.4	NM	66.70	73.73	70.0	VT	67.32	74.27	32.2
CA	67.97	74.27	90.9	LA	66.16	73.93	66.1	NY	67.60	73.70	85.6	VA	67.27	74.38	63.1
CO	67.95	74.53	78.7	ME	66.75	73.42	50.9	NC	66.35	74.33	45.0	WA	67.93	74.56	72.6
CT	68.93	74.88	77.3	MD	67.48	74.16	76.6	ND	69.07	75.59	44.3	WV	65.35	72.82	39.0
DE	67.35	74.04	72.1	MA	67.80	74.20	84.6	OH	67.42	73.82	75.3	WI	68.71	74.75	65.9
DC	65.16	72.77	100.0	MI	67.57	73.94	73.9	OK	67.38	74.59	68.0	WY	66.19	74.08	60.4
FL	67.49	74.85	80.5	MN	68.87	75.26	66.4	OR	68.03	74.75	67.1				
GA	65.88	74.08	60.3	MS	65.74	74.06	44.5	PA	67.24	73.47	71.5				
HI	70.39	75.68	83.0	MO	67.32	74.17	70.1	RI	68.02	74.16	87.0				
ID	67.72	74.82	54.3	MT	66.74	74.08	53.6	SC	65.70	73.67	47.6				
IL	67.20	73.70	83.0	NE	68.53	75.23	61.6	SD	68.71	75.27	44.6				

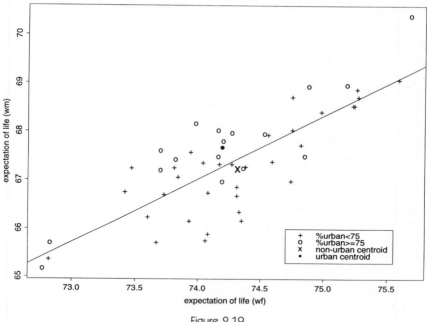

Figure 2.19

The command *postscript("exterior.file")* causes SPLUS to create a printable PostScript file containing all graphic output that follows the command. Execution of the *postscript( )* command cancels any open graphics window and directs the graphic output to an exterior file. When the S-session ends (i.e., type *q( )* to quit) the graphic results are found in the exterior PostScript file defined by the name between the quotes (e.g., *temp.ps,* in the example). The standard UNIX command *lpr* prints this file. If the user wishes the graphic output displayed at the terminal, a graphic output window is created by the UNIX S-commands *X*11( ), *motif( )* or Windows command *win.graph,* as noted. These graphic windows also have the option of directing current graphic output to a printer.

The command *plot(x,y)* causes points to be plotted at the coordinate values contained in the two argument vectors. For example, *plot(exwf,exwm)* plots the 51 pairs of expected lengths of life (values in Table 2.5). The plot character is set by *pch* ("pch" for plot character) where a symbol is defined by enclosing it in quotations marks (e.g., *pch* = "+" causes the symbol + to be plotted for each *xy*-pair). The option *pch* = *k* also produces up to 18 different symbols for $k = 1, 2, \cdots, 18$.

For the United States data, the command *points(exwf[urban $\geq$ 75], exwm[urban $\geq$ 75], pch* = "o") places points on the current plot (plot character is changed to "o") for states whose percent of urban areas equal or exceed 75%. The command *abline(lsfit(exwf, exwm)$coef)* is yet another application of the *abline( )* command and places a least squares estimated line on the current plot, where values of the independent variable are contained in the S-vector *exwf* (first argument) and values of the dependent variable are contained in *exwm* (second argument).

The last two *points( )* commands put two additional points on the plot. The centroids (bivariate mean—the pair of mean values $\bar{x}$ and $\bar{y}$) for states with less than 75% urban areas and for states with greater than or equal to 75% urban areas are plotted. The option $cex = f$ increases or decreases the plot character size by a factor of f ($f = 1.5$, in the example). The *cex* option can be applied to a specific graphics command, as illustrated, or the size of the plot characters can be defined by $par(cex = f)$ which then applies to all subsequent graphic commands until changed.

The last command creates a legend and places it on the plot. The S-function

$$legend(x_0, y_0, c(\text{'label 1''}, \text{''label 2''}, \cdots), pch = \text{''<symbols>''})$$

places a legend on the current plot where the first two arguments x_0, y_0 identify the location of the upper left corner of the legend box. The third argument is a vector of labels associated with the plot symbols defined by the fourth argument *pch* =<"symbols"> where the corresponding characters are placed between the quotes (one symbol for each label). To place the legend box in a completely determined position, the first argument is the two x-coordinates of the opposite corners (upper left and lower right) of the rectangular legend area and the second argument contains the two corresponding y-coordinates.

THREE-DIMENSIONAL PLOTS—PERSPECTIVE PLOTS

A natural extension of a two-dimensional plot is a three-dimensional plot. Occasionally it is important to display the interrelationships among three variables. The S-language allows a three-dimensional plot to be created from three variables with the S-function *persp( )*. Input is two sets of coordinate points ("floor") and an array of corresponding heights of the three-dimensional surface to be plotted. For example, birth weight (z—grams) is related to maternal height (x—centimeters) and weight (y— kilograms) by the following equation:

$$z_{ij} = 7627.0 - 72.0x_i + 25.0y_j + 0.25x_i^2 - 0.13y_j^2.$$

The coordinate points (x_i, y_j) and the corresponding heights z_{ij} serve as input to a three-dimensional plot produced by $persp(x, y, z)$. Example S-code that plots the birth weight surface is

```
> # coordinates (x=ht,y=wt)
> ht<- seq(130,200,1)
> wt<- seq(40,110,1)
> # height of the surface (z=bwt)
> bwt<- outer(ht,wt,function(ht,wt)
      {7627-72.0*ht+25.0*wt+0.25*ht^2-0.13*wt^2})
> persp(ht,wt,bwt/1000,xlab="height",ylab="weight",
      zlab="birth weight")
> title("Birth weight -- maternal height by weight")
```

where the S-array *bwt* contains the infant "birth weights" predicted from maternal height and weight. Figure 2.20 displays the three-dimensional surface. The S-function *outer*( ) is a primary tool for preparing the z-array from the x and y input vectors for a three-dimensional plot. The command *title*( ), not surprisingly, places a title at the top of the plot.

An input option of the *persp*( ) command makes it possible to view the plot from any perspective. Using the option labeled *eye*, coordinates of the viewpoint are communicated to the plot routine in terms of a three-valued vector where *eye*=$c(x0, y0, z0)$. Four perspectives of the birth weight relationship to maternal height and weight are given by

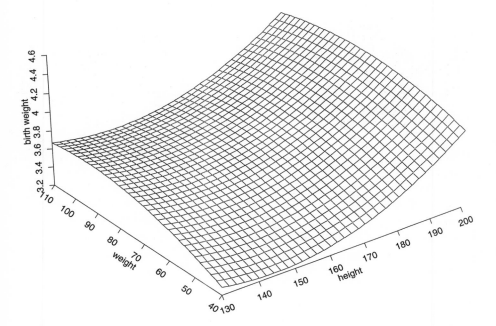

Birth weight -- maternal height by weight

Figure 2.20

Birth weight -- maternal height by weight

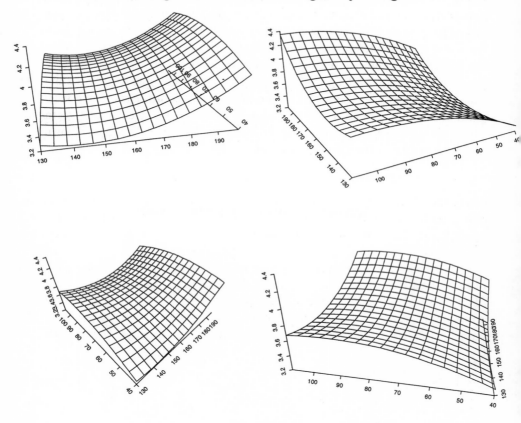

Figure 2.21

```
> par(mfrow=c(2,2))
> par(cex=0.4)
> persp(ht,wt,bwt/1000,xlab="ht",ylab="wt",zlab="bwt",
    eye=c(90,-210,4),box=F)
> persp(ht,wt,bwt/1000,xlab="ht",ylab="wt",zlab="bwt",
    eye=c(-90,210,4),box=F)
> persp(ht,wt,bwt/1000,xlab="ht",ylab="wt",zlab="bwt",
    eye=c(100,0,4),box=F)
> persp(ht,wt,bwt/1000,xlab="ht",ylab="wt",zlab="bwt",
    eye=c(-100,0,4),box=F)
```

and are displayed in Figure 2.21. If no perspective is specified, the plot is viewed from $c(-6, -8, 6)$ multiplied by the ranges of the x, y, and z values, respectively.

THREE-DIMENSIONAL PLOTS—CONTOUR PLOTS

The *persp*( ) command is one way of displaying the relationships among three variables. Another is the S-function *contour*( ). The general form of this S-function is

$$contour(x, y, z, nint = < number\ of\ contours >, \cdots)$$

where the input values x, y, and z are identical to those used in *persp*( ). The plot produces contour lines indicating equal values of the z-variable. The option *nint* = k ("nint" for number of intervals) dictates the number of contour lines plotted.

For example, concern was expressed about exposure levels of electromagnetic radiation from a microwave tower located in the city of San Francisco. Measurements were made where x and y represent the geographic locations around the tower and the amount of radiation at each point was measured (variable z; recoded in milligauss) for a large number of points (x, y). Plotted contours (Figure 2.22) are created using the S-function *contour*( ) and

```
> # contour plot: based on vectors x, y and array z
> par(pty="s")
> contour(x,y,z,xlim=c(1700,3100),ylim=c(1400,2700))
> title("Contours of emf exposure from Sutro
    tower -- milligauss")
```

The option *pty* = "*s*" ("pty" for plot type) makes the plot square.

A plot of the contours associated with the bivariate normal distribution illustrates another application of the S-function *contour*( ). The height at a point (x, y) of the bivariate normal distribution (i.e., the probability density) is given by the expression

$$f(x, y) = \frac{1}{\sqrt{2\pi\sigma_x^2\sigma_y^2(1 - \rho_{xy}^2)}} \times e^{-\frac{1}{2}q}$$

Contours of emf exposure from Sutro tower -- milligauss

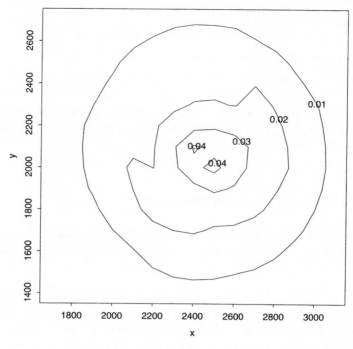

Figure 2.22

where

$$q = \left[\left(\frac{x-\mu_x}{\sigma_x}\right)^2 - 2\rho_{xy}\left(\frac{x-\mu_x}{\sigma_x}\right)\left(\frac{y-\mu_y}{\sigma_y}\right) + \left(\frac{y-\mu_y}{\sigma_y}\right)^2\right]/(1-\rho_{xy}^2)$$

and μ_x and σ_x^2 represent the mean and variance of the x-variable, μ_y and σ_y^2 represent the mean and variance of the y-variable, and ρ_{xy} represents the correlation between x and y. An S-function to compute these heights is

```
zht<- function(x,y){exp(-0.5*(((x-mx)^2/vx-2*r*(x-mx)*(y-my)
 /sqrt(vx*vy)+(y-my)^2/vy)/(1-r^2)))/sqrt(2*pi*vx*vy*(1-r^2))}
```

To plot bivariate normal contours,

```
> # contours of a bivariate normal distribution
> mx<- 0
> vx<- 1
> dx<- 0.1
> x<- seq(mx-3*sqrt(vx),mx+3*sqrt(vx),dx)
> my<- 0
> vy<- 1
> dy<- 0.1
> y<- seq(my-3*sqrt(vy),my+3*sqrt(vy),dy)
```

```
> r<- 0.5
> z<- outer(x,y,zht)
> contour(x,y,z,nint=10,pty="s")
> title("Contours for a bivariate normal distribution
    m={0,0} and v={1,1} with r = 0.5")
```

produces Figure 2.23.

A third example comes from the birth weight data depicted by the previous three-dimensional plot (Figure 2.20). The three-dimensional data relating estimated birth weight to maternal height and weight produces a contour plot when the same data input arguments used in the command *persp*( ) are employed in the command *contour*( ). Specifically, the S-function

```
> contour(ht,wt,bwt/1000,nint=16,labex=T,
    xlab="height (centimeters)",
    ylab="weight (kilograms)")
> title("bwt -- maternal height by weight")
```

plots 16 contour lines with labeling (*labex = F* suppresses S-labeling). Figure 2.24 consists of the contours (lines of equal estimated birth weights) for the birth weight relationship (previous expression).

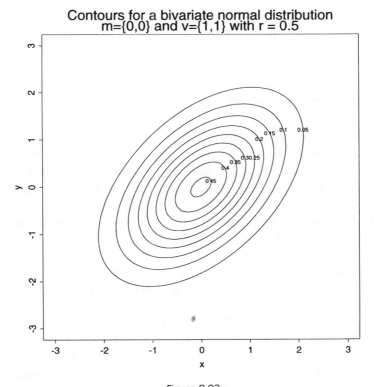

Figure 2.23

bwt -- maternal height by weight

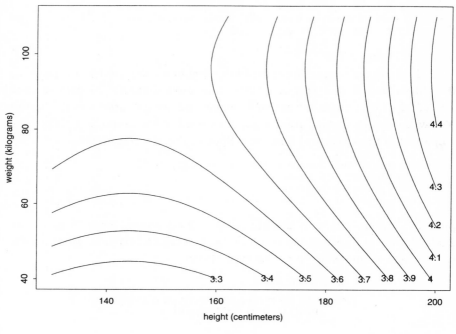

Figure 2.24

THREE-DIMENSIONAL PLOTS—ROTATION

A two-dimensional plot by definition requires two axes. When three variables x, y, and z are considered, three choices exist for displaying these variables on two axes (x and y or x and z or y and z). Two-dimensional plots are occasionally different ways to view multi-dimensional data. For example, if the three-dimensional data are viewed along the z-axis, the plot is in terms of x and y. In this context, a two-dimensional plot is a projection of the three-dimensional data on the plane perpendicular to the third axis (ignoring the third variable).

Plotting all possible pairwise combinations of variables is accomplished with the S-function *pairs( )*. The input argument is an $n \times k$ array where n = number of observations and k = number of variables per observation, which is a pattern used consistently by SPLUS. The S-function *pairs( )* plots all pairs of variables (columns) ignoring the existence of the other $k - 2$ variables.

Consider the data in Table 2.6 where the length of gestation (weeks), pattern of maternal weight gain (an index), and maternal weight gain (kilograms) are given for 79 extremely small infants with birth weights less than

Table 2.6. Length of gestation (weeks), pattern of maternal weight gain (index), and total maternal weight gain (kilograms) recorded for 79 infants weighing less than 1800 grams

gest	pattern	gain	gest	pattern	gain	gest	pattern	gain	gest	pattern	gain
29	−464.3	4.1	22	−44.7	6.0	27	377.3	10.4	25	−701.5	5.6
27	238.1	15.7	27	−784.3	0.6	26	−42.2	7.6	27	557.1	13.3
24	−693.7	3.3	23	−1598.1	−1.3	21	−1150.2	−1.6	31	−648.0	5.1
29	−645.4	9.2	27	−336.7	7.6	27	−285.7	8.4	27	302.2	14.7
29	421.5	13.5	25	−187.2	8.0	32	−305.6	5.5	28	154.7	7.9
24	749.7	14.1	33	−564.2	10.5	24	52.5	10.7	25	1455.0	18.9
24	−74.1	8.6	23	−101.8	6.4	27	125.5	11.8	25	−125.3	8.8
30	679.7	13.0	36	−726.2	8.0	31	−683.7	6.7	23	408.4	12.1
26	−330.7	6.9	26	239.7	13.2	29	357.9	15.7	26	−42.6	10.1
34	−1395.7	0.1	25	196.8	11.5	25	134.6	11.9	28	470.5	13.4
40	179.6	15.9	28	−49.4	14.0	32	472.1	17.1	27	46.4	12.9
26	−338.1	5.0	34	440.2	17.0	25	−307.6	3.9	26	−137.1	9.4
22	−463.7	4.4	25	82.7	12.6	30	769.8	15.6	29	1348.0	20.6
24	93.5	10.0	28	−257.7	7.7	30	−576.9	6.9	26	−582.5	6.9
29	27.4	14.1	30	1527.6	26.3	26	−52.1	11.5	25	6.7	9.6
24	−7.9	10.2	25	404.6	12.8	28	−303.9	8.1	31	−273.0	11.1
27	121.3	11.2	21	−180.2	5.8	26	−1639.6	0.3	31	−379.9	7.0
28	−338.7	9.0	34	−544.6	16.4	42	−733.8	9.7	28	−37.2	7.8
25	916.5	14.8	28	−138.4	9.1	24	−1202.5	1.6	24	161.9	12.0
40	−72.6	15.5	32	−107.5	12.4	29	−249.0	10.2			

1800 grams. The pattern of maternal weight gain is measured with an index reflecting the rate of gain, differentiating those mothers who slowed down in the last months of pregnancy (large negative values), who speed up in the last months (large positive values), or who followed a typical pattern (values near zero).

Figure 2.25 results from applying the command *pairs( )* to these data where

```
> # x = gestation
> x0<- (x-mean(x))/sqrt(var(x))
> # y = pattern index
> y0<- (y-mean(y))/sqrt(var(y))
> # z = total maternal weight gain
> z0<- (z-mean(z))/sqrt(var(z))
> pairs(cbind(x0,y0,z0),pch="*",cex=0.75)
```

The *pairs( )* command applies to an input array of any size, producing $k(k-1)$ plots for k variables (k column input array). Mechanically, the *pairs( )* command simply creates all possible plots of one variable plotted against the other.

The S-language contains an interactive function called *spin( )*. The input argument is again an array with rows $= n =$ number of observations and columns $= k =$ number of variables. The S-function *spin( )* displays a three-dimensional plot based on selecting three variables (e.g., columns of the input array). The user can view this display from any desired perspective. That is,

Growth, pattern, and gain for small infants

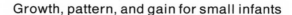

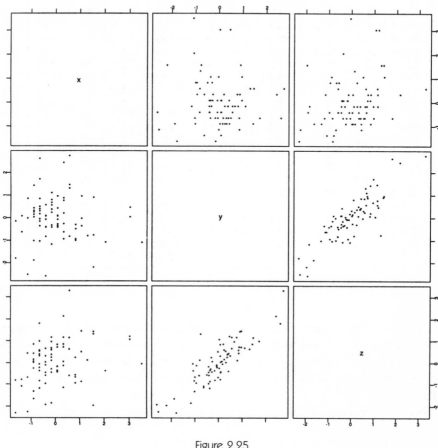

Figure 2.25

any set of axes can be chosen for plotting the data. The choice of the "view" axes is made by clicking the mouse cursor on the boxes marked "right," "left," "up," or "down." The end result is a cluster of points that appears to rotate in space. Rapidly "spinning" the plot of the (x, y, z)-points displays an apparent three-dimensional description of a "cloud" of three dimensional data.

"Spinning" results from an elementary mathematical transformation of the data points. To rotate three variables where the x-values are displayed on the vertical axis and the y and z values form the "floor" of the plot, the transformation

$$z' = z$$
$$x' = -x\sin(\theta) + y\cos(\theta)$$
$$y' = x\cos(\theta) + y\sin(\theta)$$

is used. The value (x, y, z) locates a point under the conventional coordinate system and (x', y', z') is the new location for the point when the coordinate axes have been rotated θ degrees to the left around the vertical axis. Figure 2.26 shows nine views of the data in Table 2.6 for selected values of θ (i.e., 0, 45, 90, 135, $\cdots$, 360 degrees). A simplified "spin" S-code illustrates:

```
> # x0 contains the standardized x-coordinates
> # y0 contains the standardized y-coordinates
> # z0 contains the standardized z-coordinates
> # means = 0, variances = 1
> tx<- seq(0,360,45)
> # parameters for 9 (3 by 3) square plots
> par(pty="s")
> par(mfrow=c(3,3))
> for(i in 1:length(tx)) {
  t0<- pi*tx[i]/180
# transformation
 znew<- z0
 ynew<- x0*cos(t0)+y0*sin(t0)
 xnew<- -x0*sin(t0)+y0*cos(t0)
# plotting the results
 temp<- paste("rotation in degrees =",tx[i])
 plot(ynew,znew,pch=".",xlab="",ylab="",
    xlim=c(-4,4),ylim=c(-4,4),main=temp)
# produces the "axes" and labels
lines(c(0,0),c(0,2))
lines(c(0,2*cos(t0)),c(0,0))
lines(c(0,2*cos(t0+pi/2)),c(0,0))
text(0,2,"Z")
text(2*cos(t0),-0.3,"Y")
text(2*cos(t0+pi/2),0.3,"X")
}
```

By modifying the S-code or changing the roles of the variables, data can be displayed rotated in any other chosen direction.

The S-functions *text*( ) and *lines*( ) place labeled representative axes on the plot. The *text*( ) command adds to a current plot the values or symbols given by the third argument of the function at the locations specified by the *xy*-coordinates given by the first two arguments. For example, *text*(0, 2, "Y") locates the symbol Y at the point (0, 2) on the current plot. The S-function *lines*( ) adds a line to a current plot described by the *x*-coordinates in the first argument and *y*-coordinates in the second argument. For example, the S-function *lines*($c(0, 0), c(0, 2)$) adds a solid line connecting the *xy*-point (0, 0) to (0, 2) on the current plot. In general, the S-function *lines*(*xpoints, ypoints, lty* = *k*) adds a line to a current plot of type *k* connecting the *xy*-points defined by the S-vectors *xpoints* and *ypoints*. To cause multiple plots to appear on the same page, the command *par*(*mfrow* = *c*(*r*, *c*)) is used

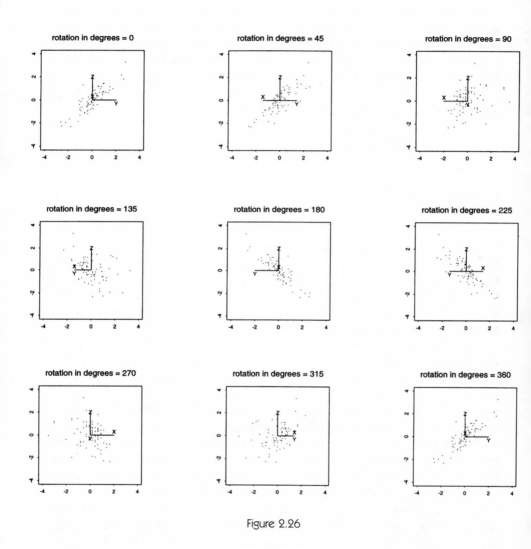

Figure 2.26

where r is the number of rows and c is a number of the columns in the layout format of a multiple plot screen or page. The nine views of the birth weight data (Figure 2.26) were formatted with the command $par(mfrow = c(3, 3))$. The command $paste(\ )$ combines character data and S-generated numeric values into a single variable. As the name implies, $paste(\ )$ pastes together any number of non-numeric characters (surrounded by quotes) and S-calcualted numeric values (seperated by commas), in any order, providing a convenient output variable. Like all S-functions, details of possible options and further examples of these graphics commands are found using the $help(\ )$ command. Note, as mentioned, that the trigonometry functions in SPLUS take radian arguments (radians $= \pi$ degrees/180).

SMOOTHING

A sequence of numeric values can be viewed as consisting of two components—a systematic component and a non-systematic component. The non-systematic component can be made up of a combination of such things as bias, random variation, outliers, and heterogeneity within the data. Regardless of the nature of the non-systematic component, it tends to obscure any systematic patterns. Smoothing techniques reduce this tendency to better reveal patterns within sampled observations.

Most smoothing techniques operate in the same fashion. Each observation is replaced by a more "typical" value. "Typical" is defined differently depending on the specific smoothing process. Nevertheless, all approaches combine adjacent observations producing a new, more "typical" observation whose value is influenced to some extent by its neighboring values. One such smoothing technique is called a median smooth. For the sequence of n observations $\{y_1, y_2, \cdots, y_n\}$ the ith smoothed value becomes the median of the three-value sequence $\{y_{i-1}, y_i, y_{i+1}\}$. To illustrate, $n = 18$ age-specific leukemia incidence rates are given in Table 2.7 and plotted in Figure 2.27 (broken line).

The median smoothed values are also shown in Table 2.7 (column 3—median smoothed). For example, the first three rates are 19.3, 1.4, and 4.0 making the second smoothed rate the median of these values; namely, the value 1.4 is replaced by new-$y_2 = 4.0$. The same process is sequentially applied to each of the 16 observations (the first and last values are not smoothed). Median smoothing effectively removes extreme values and outliers but tends to leave level spots in the sequence. Also, median smoothing has no effect on a sequence of increasing values. For example, the sequence of numbers $\{10, 50, 100, 1000, 2000\}$ is unaffected by the median smoothing process.

Table 2.7. Female age-specific leukemia incidence rates per 100,000, San Francisco, California, 1987

age	rate	median smoothed	mean smoothed
0–4	19.3	19.3	9.64
5–9	1.4	4.0	7.83
10–14	4.0	4.0	6.01
15–19	8.2	8.2	7.65
20–24	12.0	8.2	6.71
25–29	2.0	2.8	3.78
30–34	2.8	2.8	3.64
35–39	15.1	5.2	4.81
40–44	5.2	5.2	7.58
45–49	15.1	15.1	13.22
50–54	21.4	15.1	14.63
55–59	9.4	15.1	15.48
60–64	17.4	17.1	16.70
65–69	17.1	17.1	18.77
70–74	24.2	24.2	34.39
75–79	87.0	70.4	61.40
80–84	70.4	70.4	61.77
≥ 85	44.9	44.9	62.15

Female leukemia incidence rates per 100,000, San Francisco, 1987

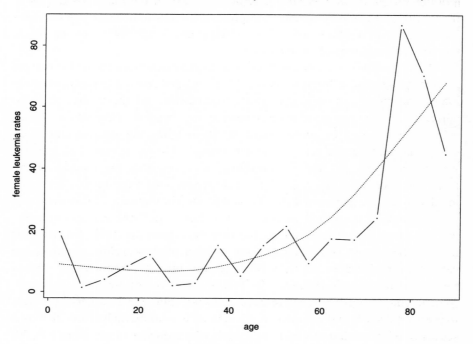

Figure 2.27

To improve the median smoothed values as a representation of the sequence of observed values, a moving average is applied. Already smoothed "data" are again smoothed. One version of a moving average involves calculating a new y_i-value (again from sets of three) where new-y_i = $(y_{i-1} + 2y_i + y_{i+1})/4$. For example, new-$y_2$ = (19.3 + 2(4.0) + 4.0)/4 = 7.83 replaces the already median smoothed value 4.0. These values are shown in Table 2.7 (column 4—mean smoothed). The first and last values are also not part of this moving average smoothing. Of course, using more than three values or different weightings produces a different moving average that can also be an effective description of a sequence of observations.

The first value y_1 can be smoothed by projecting the already smoothed points y_2 and y_3 to produce a smoothed value to replace y_1 where new-y_1 = $2y_2 - y_3$. For the leukemia data, new-y_1 = 2(7.83) − 6.01 = 9.64. Similarly, the last value can be smoothed, again based on projecting the already smoothed points, by new-y_n = $2y_{n-1} - y_{n-2}$ = 2(61.77) − 61.40 = 62.15.

Median/average smoothing can be repeated on the previously smoothed values until only small changes take place in the smoothed values (Figure 2.28 – dotted line). The results from one smoothing are input into the next sequence of median/average smoothing. Using an analogous scheme, the S-command *smooth()* produces a smoothed sequence of values. The leukemia data (Table 2.7) and the commands

```
> plot(age,rate,type="b",ylim=range(rate),ylab="female
      leukemia rates", main="Female leukemia incidence
      rates per 100,000, California, 1987")
> lines(age,smooth(rate),type="l"),lty=2)
```

produce the curves in Figure 2.27 where *age* and *rate* label the input S-vectors from the 18 leukemia observations (*age* = ages—column 1 and *rate* = age-specific leukemia rates—column 2 of Table 2.7).

Data from a cancer prevention study in Oakland, California (1985) provide a second example of smoothing. The question of interest is: what changes occurred in the frequency of regional and local colon cancer over the years 1974 to 1985 among black women surveyed as part of a study of cancer incidence?

Table 2.8. Frequencies of local and regional stages of colon cancer cases among black women, Oakland, California, 1974–1985

year	1974	1975	1976	1977	1978	1979	1980	1981	1982	1983	1984	1985
cases local	5	8	10	7	10	15	13	9	7	7	8	13
cases regional	4	3	2	1	3	3	1	1	4	5	3	2
percentage local	4.5	7.1	8.9	6.2	8.9	13.4	11.6	8.0	6.2	6.2	7.1	11.6
percentage regional	12.5	9.4	6.2	3.1	9.4	9.4	3.1	3.1	12.5	15.6	9.4	6.2

The observed proportions of local and regional cases (Table 2.8) are shown in the top plot of Figure 2.28 (local = solid line and regional = dotted line). The smoothed versions of the yearly proportions are given in the bottom plot.

A number of alternatives exist to smooth a sample of values using S-functions. The S-functions *less.smooth*( ), *smooth.spline*( ), and *supsu*( ) are three examples. These functions are a few of the many different ways to smooth a sequence of values. A discussion of the advantages and disadvantages of different smoothing techniques is found elsewhere [2]. Figure 2.29 contrasts four S-functions applied to smoothing 100 random pairs of values between 0 and 10 (correlation = 0.7) where

```
> n<- 100
> x0<- runif(n,0,10)
> y0<- x0+runif(n,0,10)
> xtemp<- order(x0)
> y<- y0[xtemp]
> x<- x0[xtemp]
> plot(x,y,pch=".",main="Four S-smoothing options")
> lines(x,smooth(y),lty=1)
> lines(supsmu(x,y),lty=2)
```

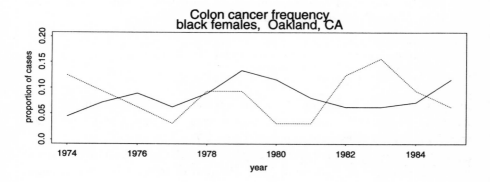

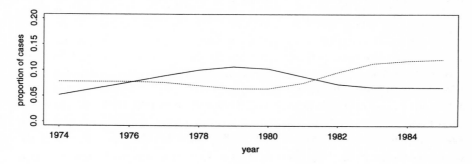

Figure 2.28

Four S-smoothing options

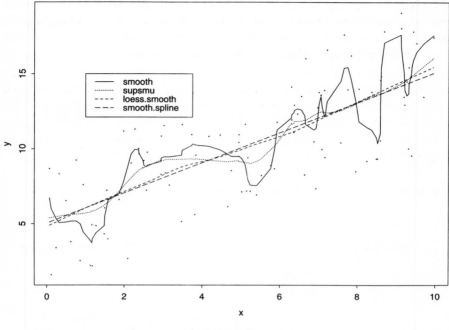

Figure 2.29

```
> lines(loess.smooth(x,y),lty=3)
> lines(smooth.spline(x,y),lty=4)
> legend(1,15,c("smooth","supsmu","loess.smooth",
      "smooth.spline"),lty=1:4)
```

TWO-DIMENSIONAL SMOOTHING OF SPATIAL DATA

Spatial data can be the location of specific types of plants or the location of cases of breast cancer or the location of any number of phenomena occurring over a defined geographic area. Much like the previous smoothing of a sequence of values, two-dimensional spatial data can be smoothed and displayed. In many situations, issues arise concerning the description of the distribution of spatial data and the location of any clustering. The same techniques used to estimate a one-variable density function can be extended to estimate a two-variable density function to address these issues. As before, each observation is summarized by a kernel function with a mean value at the location of the point being summarized. In the two-variable case, a two-dimensional kernel function is chosen. In the following illustration, the two-dimensional bivariate normal distribution is employed as the kernel function but other functions could be used. The bandwidth is a function of the standard deviations associated with the kernel bivariate normal distribution. The selected bandwidth determines again the degree of smoothness of the estimated density function. Hypothetical $n = 40$ points are:

```
> x0
[1]   3.5 5.6 4.8 4.4 2.5 4.4 0.8 4.0 3.5 1.2 2.1 2.4 5.5
[14]  3.2 4.2 6.0 6.6 7.0 5.6 5.8 7.2 6.9 7.7 4.0 5.6 2.5
[27]  4.0 2.0 8.6 4.2 5.7 3.3 8.7 7.8 7.6 7.7 9.1 3.6 6.5 6.4
> y0
[1]   9.2 7.4 1.7 4.8 9.1 9.2 2.6 4.8 3.7 6.2 6.8 2.6 3.9
[14]  8.0 8.2 3.7 2.6 3.7 3.2 3.0 2.7 3.2 3.8 3.4 1.4 4.2
[27]  8.9 2.5 8.5 1.8 9.3 3.6 4.1 5.0 3.0 4.3 1.3 8.2 1.2 8.7.
```

The points are plotted in Figure 2.30 (upper left).

Hypothetical data

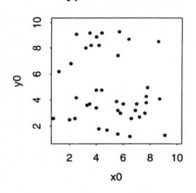

Perspective plot

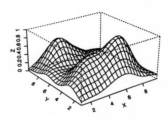

Contour plot

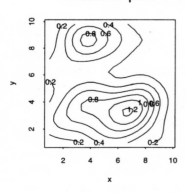

Areas of high incidence

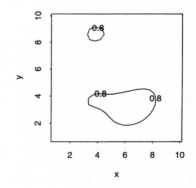

Figure 2.30

To estimate the bivariate density function that generated these 40 points, sums of the heights of the $n = 40$ kernel functions are calculated at a series of pairs of points (x and y) forming a smooth two-dimensional density estimate. The resulting sums (z) can be plotted with the S-function $persp(x, y, z)$. The plot displays the "hills" and "valleys" of the two-dimensional estimated density (Figure 2.30—h = bandwidth = $\sigma = 1.0$). The same estimated distribution can be displayed as a contour plot. The S-function $contour(x, y, z)$ provides another visual description of the two-dimensional estimated density. The S-function $contour(x, y, z)$ can also be used to select specific contours to identify areas of high or low frequency (option = *levels*). Three plots of the estimated density function based on the hypothetical data are generated with the example S-code:

```
> k<- length(x0)
> x<- seq(1,10,0.4)
> y<- seq(1,10,0.4)
> n<- length(x)
> # initialize the array z
> z<- array(0,c(n,n,k))
> #h = bandwidth = standard deviation
> h<- 1.0
> # bivariate normal distribution kernel function
> zfcn<- function(x,y){(exp(-0.5*(((x-m1)/h)^2
    +((y-m2)/h)^2)))/(2*pi)}
> # create the sums of the n kernel functions
> for(i in 1:k){
  m1<- x0[i]
  m2<- y0[i]
  z[,,i]<- outer(x,y,zfcn)
  }
> zsum<- apply(z,c(1,2),sum)
> # plot the results
> par(pty="s")
> par(mfrow=c(2,2))
> plot(x0,y0,pch="*",xlim=c(1,10),ylim=c(1,10))
> title("Hypothetical data")
> persp(x,y,zsum/max(zsum),cex=0.5)
> title("Perspective plot")
> contour(x,y,zsum,cex=0.7,nint=6)
> title("Contour plot")
> contour(x,y,zsum,cex=0.7,levels=0.8)
> title("Areas of high incidence")
```

A perspective plot and two contour plots are displayed in Figure 2.30. The process identifies two areas of high incidence ("clustering") where the contour heights exceed 0.8. Applying density estimation techniques and the two graphic S-functions $persp(\,)$ and $contour(\,)$ produces a three-dimensional descriptive of spatial data employing essentially the same commands and principles used in the two-dimensional case.

CLUSTERS AS A DESCRIPTION OF DATA

A fundamental description of collected data is often achieved by dividing the observations into homogeneous groups based on common characteristics. The process of grouping data frequently reveals differences and similarities within a data set leading to identifying what is important and not important among the measured variables. As might be expected, there are a number of approaches to this classification process. A popular technique based on hierarchical groupings classifies data into categories according to a measure of similarity. The process starts with as many "groups" as observations (one observation per "group") and ends up with one group containing all the observations. At each step of the process observations are added to existing groups or become the beginnings of new groupings, depending on their similarity. A classification "tree" is created to describe graphically the classification process. The "tree" is formally called a dendrogram and displays the number and types of groups formed at each level of similarity, potentially yielding insights into the structure underlying a data set.

A key element of grouping observations is the criterion used to decide when two values are similar. A simple method defines "closeness" in terms of the nearest neighbor distance. A nearest neighbor distance is pretty much what the name suggests. For a specific value, the distances to all other values are calculated. The nearest neighbor is then the observation with the minimum of these distances. Consider the hypothetical values $x_1 = 10$, $x_2 = 4$, $x_3 = 13$, $x_4 = 11$, $x_5 = 10$, $x_6 = 3$, and $x_7 = 19$. The array containing all possible distances between these seven values is

	x_1	x_2	x_3	x_4	x_5	x_6	x_7
x_1	0	6	3	1	0	7	9
x_2	6	0	9	7	6	1	15
x_3	3	9	0	2	3	10	6
x_4	1	7	2	0	1	8	8
x_5	0	6	3	1	0	7	9
x_6	7	1	10	8	7	0	16
x_7	9	15	6	8	9	16	0

Using this array, groups are formed based on the 21 distances. The smallest nearest neighbor distance is between x_1 and x_5 (distance = 0), identifying the first group. The next smallest nearest neighbor distance is between x_1 and x_4 (distance = 1) indicating that x_4 joins x_1 and x_5 as a group since x_4 is "closest" to the x_1/x_5-group among all other nearest neighbor distances. Also at distance = 1, values x_2 and x_6 form another group. Then, x_3 is the nearest neighbor to x_4 making it a member of the first group (distance = 2). Finally, x_2 is distance 6 from x_5 and x_7 is distance 6 from x_3 so both the second group (x_2 and x_6) and x_7 are added to the first group. This process is neatly summarized by the dendrogram in Figure 2.31.

A more realistic example is given by exposure measurements made on six individuals who perform differing tasks in the production and sale of gasoline (attendant, transportation worker type 1, transportation worker type 2, works outside, works inside, maintenance worker). Each individual was measured for exposure to six different potentially toxic compounds (n-butene, isopentane, n-pentane, isobutane, n-hexane, and 2-methyl-2-butene). The data are presented in Table 2.9.

Table 2.9. Exposure levels to six specific compounds (ppm) for six types of workers

	n-butene	isopentane	n-pentane	isobutane	n-hexane	methylbutene
attendant	0.97	0.10	0.94	0.77	3.00	0.65
transportation 1	0.97	0.35	0.14	0.85	0.88	0.76
transportation 2	1.96	2.36	2.11	0.83	3.04	3.61
outside	1.15	2.43	2.45	0.93	4.00	4.46
inside	1.35	2.73	2.68	1.06	4.19	2.81
maintenance	1.81	1.67	1.83	1.73	2.03	2.29

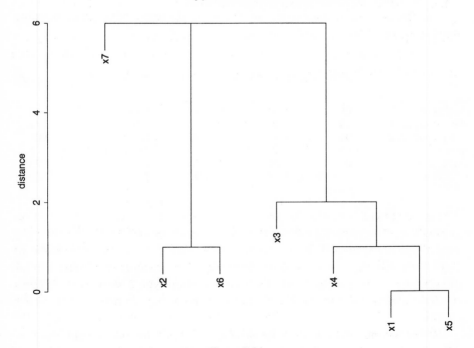

Figure 2.31

For the gasoline workers the meaning of distance between individuals is not perfectly clear. Distance between two multivariate observations can be measured in several ways [3]. Perhaps the simplest of these methods consists of calculating the geometric distance using an xy-coordinate system. Distance between two observations (x_1, y_1) and (x_2, y_2) is

$$d_{12} = \sqrt{(x_1 - x_2)^2 + (y_1 - y_2)^2}.$$

If three values are considered $(x, y,$ and $z)$, then the distance between two observations (x_1, y_1, z_1) and (x_2, y_2, z_2) is

$$d_{12} = \sqrt{(x_1 - x_2)^2 + (y_1 - y_2)^2 + (z_1 - z_2)^2}.$$

A general definition of distance between two multivariate observations made up of k measurements (i.e., i^{th} observation $= \{x_{i1}, x_{i2}, \cdots, x_{ik}\}$ and j^{th} observation $= \{x_{j1}, x_{j2}, \cdots, x_{jk}\}$) follows the same pattern where the distance between the ith and j^{th} observation is

$$d_{ij} = \sqrt{\sum (x_{il} - x_{jl})^2} \qquad l = 1, 2, 3, \cdots, k$$

called Euclidean distance. Euclidean distance can be calculated with the S-function $dist(\ )$.

For the gasoline worker data, the Euclidean distances between all possible pairs of workers are:

	attendant	transportation 1	transportation 2	outside	inside	maintenance
attendant	0.00	2.28	3.97	4.83	4.03	2.92
transportation 1	2.28	0.00	4.61	5.76	5.24	3.12
transportation 2	3.97	4.61	0.00	1.57	1.71	2.01
outside	4.83	5.76	1.57	0.00	1.72	3.26
inside	4.03	5.24	1.71	1.72	0.00	2.73
maintenance	2.92	3.12	2.01	3.26	2.73	0.00

The nearest neighbor criterion used in the one-measurement per observation example equally applies to these Euclidean distances and again the grouping process is summarized by a classification "tree." All possible pairs of Euclidean distances forms a similarity array. For example, the most similar observations are the outside and the transportation type 2 workers (1.57) and the least similar are the outside worker and the transportation worker type 1 (5.76).

Three S-functions calculate the similarity and plot the pattern of clustering ($dist(\ )$, $hclust(\ )$, and $pclust(\ )$ functions). First, the Euclidean distances are computed with *dist*(*input.array*) where the data are contained in an $n \times k$ input array. The S-function *dist*( ) calculates all possible pairs of multivariate distances between the column variables. In general,

$$dist(input.array, metric = <type>, \cdots)$$

calculates multivariate distance where *input.array* is an array of data (e.g., rows = n = workers and columns = k = measurements). The option *metric* provides a choice of ways to measure distance ("euclidean," "maximum," "manhattan," and "binary"—see ?*dist*). Then, the analytic values necessary to classify the data into groups are computed by the S-function *hclust*( ) ("h" stands for hierarchical) followed by *plclust*( ) ("pl" stands for plot) which plots the dendrogram. An option *method* is available in *hclust*( ) that provides different ways to measure similarity ("connected," "average," and "compact"—see ?*hclust*). Figure 2.32 was created with the four commands,

Exposure to gasoline components

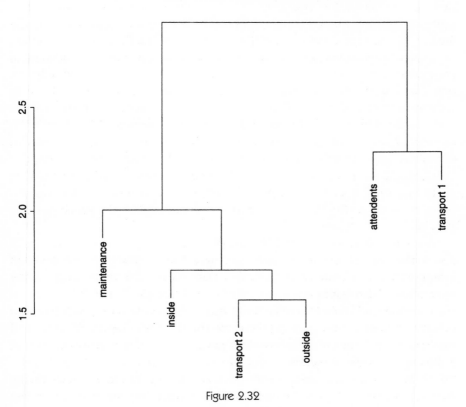

Figure 2.32

```
> dd<- dist(x,metric="euclidean")
> htemp<- hclust(dd,method="connected")
> # create labels for the plot
> ltemp<- c("attendants","transport 1","transport 2",
     "outside","inside","maintenance")
> plclust(htemp,labels=ltemp,
     main="Exposure to gasoline components")
```

where x is the 6×6 input array of data (Table 2.9) and "connected" is another term for the nearest neighbor criterion. The transportation type 2 and outside workers are the most similar observations (distance = 1.57) producing the first grouping. This group is joined next by the inside worker and then the maintenance worker. Lastly, the attendant and the transportation type 1 worker form a second group at a fairly large nearest neighbor distance (2.28; not very similar), implying that the attendant and transportation type 1 worker likely have different exposure experiences than the other four workers.

Euclidean distance tends to be most influenced by those variables with the greatest variability. To classify data eliminating influences from unequal variances, measurements can be normalized by dividing each measurement by its estimated standard deviation. The transformed variables then have the same variance as well as the same measurement units (unitless) and classification proceeds as before. In the case of the gasoline workers data, standardizing the data to equalize the variability for all measurements has little influence on the subsequent cluster analysis. These data are measured in the same units, parts per million (ppm). However, when the k measurements are made in different units, it is probably advantageous but not necessary to define multivariate distance in terms of standardized data. Distances between observations measured in different ways influences the pattern of clustering. Also, there are a number of choices of ways to measure similarity of the calculated distances, which also influences the pattern of groupings of the observations. Descriptive statistical methods usually involve subjective decisions such as these. One advantage of a descriptive approach such as hierarchical cluster analysis stems from the ability to use subjective criteria to explore the properties of a data set.

A more extensive example of using hierarchical cluster analysis as a descriptive tool comes from classifying breakfast cereals by the nutritional information on the side of the package. Data on $n = 30$ cereals each with $k = 11$ measurements per cereal are given in Table 2.10.

The analysis is based on adjusting 10 measurements so that each brand of cereal is compared for an equivalent weight (i.e., 30 grams). The price is calculated for "regular" size box (450 grams). The relative size (volume) of a 30 gram serving is included as a variable, labeled *size*. The classification "tree" reveals the clustering pattern among the 30 different cereals in the data set (Figure 2.33). Using an S-array labeled *cdata* containing the data

Table 2.10. Data on 30 breakfast cereal nutritional contents

	company	name	size	calories	%fat	fat	Na*	K*	carbo	fiber	sugar	protein	cost
1	post	honey bunches	0.78	134.48	31.03	3.10	186.21	67.24	24.83	1.03	6.21	3.10	4.13
2	g mills	kix	1.33	120.00	10.00	1.00	270.00	50.00	26.00	1.00	3.00	2.00	2.97
3	kelloggs	raisin squares	0.41	98.18	2.73	0.55	0.00	114.55	14.73	2.73	6.55	2.18	2.32
4	safeway	corn flakes	1.11	111.11	0.00	0.00	311.11	27.78	25.56	1.11	2.22	2.22	2.21
5	safeway	bran flakes	0.75	100.00	5.00	0.50	200.00	170.00	24.00	5.00	5.00	3.00	3.45
6	g mills	basic	0.55	114.55	16.36	2.73	169.09	87.27	22.91	1.64	6.55	2.18	2.37
7	kelloggs	nutrigrain	0.68	109.09	13.64	0.00	180.00	98.18	24.00	2.18	6.55	2.18	2.36
8	post	bran flakes	1.06	95.24	0.00	0.00	222.22	201.06	24.34	5.29	5.29	4.23	3.33
9	kelloggs	all-bran	0.50	120.00	7.50	0.75	180.00	405.00	34.50	12.00	10.50	6.00	5.38
10	kelloggs	corn flakes	1.00	110.00	0.00	0.00	330.00	35.00	26.00	1.00	2.00	2.00	2.09
11	kashi	puffed rice	1.20	84.00	6.00	1.20	0.00	0.00	22.80	2.40	0.00	3.60	2.34
12	kelloggs	corn pops	1.00	110.00	0.00	0.00	95.00	20.00	27.00	1.00	13.00	1.00	4.29
13	g mills	cheerios	1.00	110.00	15.00	2.00	280.00	90.00	22.00	3.00	1.00	3.00	4.29
14	kelloggs	rice krispies	1.00	110.00	0.00	0.00	360.00	35.00	26.00	1.00	3.00	2.00	4.15
15	g mills	whole grain	0.75	110.00	10.00	1.00	200.00	100.00	24.00	3.00	5.00	2.00	5.09
16	nabisco	shredded wheat	0.61	104.08	3.06	0.31	0.00	122.45	25.10	3.06	0.00	3.06	2.97
17	kelloggs	healthy choice	0.68	103.64	5.45	0.55	3.27	103.64	24.55	3.27	4.36	2.73	2.34
18	g mills	wheaties	1.00	110.00	10.00	1.00	220.00	110.00	24.00	3.00	4.00	3.00	2.99
19	kelloggs	specialk	1.00	110.00	0.00	1.00	250.00	55.00	21.00	1.00	3.00	6.00	5.19
20	post	coca pebbles	0.79	116.40	10.58	1.06	148.15	47.62	26.46	5.29	11.64	1.06	4.10
21	kelloggs	bran flakes	0.75	100.00	5.00	0.50	230.00	180.00	25.00	5.00	6.00	3.00	3.45
22	quaker	natural(honey)	0.29	129.41	35.29	4.12	5.88	123.53	21.18	2.35	8.24	2.94	2.94
23	quaker	natural(crispy)	0.30	114.00	15.00	1.80	2.40	132.00	24.00	1.80	9.60	2.40	2.99
24	quaker	oat squares	0.54	117.86	13.39	1.34	139.29	123.21	23.04	2.14	4.82	3.75	2.83
25	kelloggs	golden wheat	0.75	100.00	5.00	0.50	240.00	140.00	24.00	4.00	6.00	3.00	3.23
26	g mills	honey nut cheerios	1.00	120.00	15.00	1.50	270.00	95.00	24.00	2.00	11.00	3.00	4.95
27	g mills	nut+honey	0.66	120.00	15.00	2.00	200.00	40.00	25.00	0.00	10.00	2.00	4.79
28	post	frosted wheat	0.58	109.62	5.77	0.58	5.77	103.85	25.96	2.88	6.35	2.31	2.36
29	g mills	apple/cinn cheerios	0.75	120.00	25.00	2.50	190.00	70.00	24.00	1.00	12.00	2.00	3.95
30	g mills	frosted mini wheats	1.33	120.00	10.00	1.00	270.00	45.00	26.00	1.00	3.00	2.00	4.39

*Na = sodium, K = potassium and carbo = carbohydrates

Multivariate cereal data

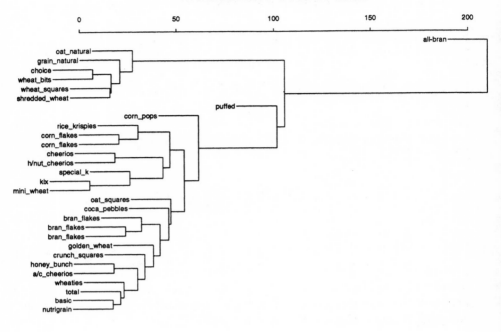

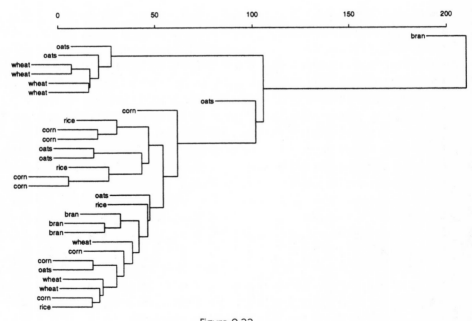

Figure 2.33

(rows = n = 30 = cereal brands and columns = k = 11 = variables = cereal measurements), the key commands for plotting the classification tree are

```
> dd<- dist(cdata,metric="euclidean")
> htemp<- hclust(dd,method="connected")
> par(mfrow=c(1,2))
> plclust(htemp,cex=0.5,labels=cnames,
      main="cereal classification")
> plclust(htemp,cex=0.5,labels=grains,
      main="cereal classification")
```

and produce Figure 2.33.

The vector *cnames* contains the names of the cereals; that is,

```
> cnames
 [1] "honey_bunch"  "kix"           "wheat_squares" "corn_flakes"
 [5] "bran_flakes"  "basic"         "nutrigrain"    "bran_flakes"
 [9] "all-bran"     "corn_flakes"   "puffed_rice"   "corn_pops"
[13] "cheerios"     "rice_krispies" "total"         "shred_wheat"
[17] "choice"       "wheaties"      "special_k"     "coca_pebbles"
[21] "bran_flakes"  "oat_natural"   "grain_natural" "oat_squares"
[25] "golden_wheat" "nut_cheerios"  "crunch_squares" "wheat_bits"
[29] "a/c_cheerios" "mini_wheat"
```

The underscore is a trick to connect several words into a single computer "word" to simplify the character data (one "word" per label). The vector *cnames* is read into the S-program with the command *scan*( ) using an option designed to read character data. For the example,

```
> cnames<- scan("cereal.names",what="")
```

where the cereal names are contained in an exterior file labeled "cereal.-names." The grain types are similarly read, creating the character S-vector *grains* to label the second plot in Figure 2.33. The S-vectors *cnames* and *grains* containing character data identifying the n = 30 cereals are incorporated into the cluster analysis employing the option *labels* in the *pclust*( ) command.

Types of cereal (left side of Figure 2.33) appear to cluster regardless of the manufacturer or price. The right-hand plot is the same plot but labeled by the type of grain which begins to indicate reasons for some of the observed clustering. Three bran cereals form a group and two brands of corn flakes form another "close" group. Four cereals made of wheat form another cluster. Three cereals are last to be grouped. Puffed Rice and Corn Pops due to their low densities and All-bran due to its high density make these cereals rather different from the other 27 brands regardless of the grain type. In general, groups appear to be roughly based on the type of grain (e.g., oats, wheat, bran, rice, and corn).

Another multivariate classification scheme is achieved with the S-function *faces*( ), which is based on a technique originated by H. Chernoff [4] where the characteristics of a cartoon face graphically identify similarities and differences among k measurements on n multivariate observations (one face per observa-

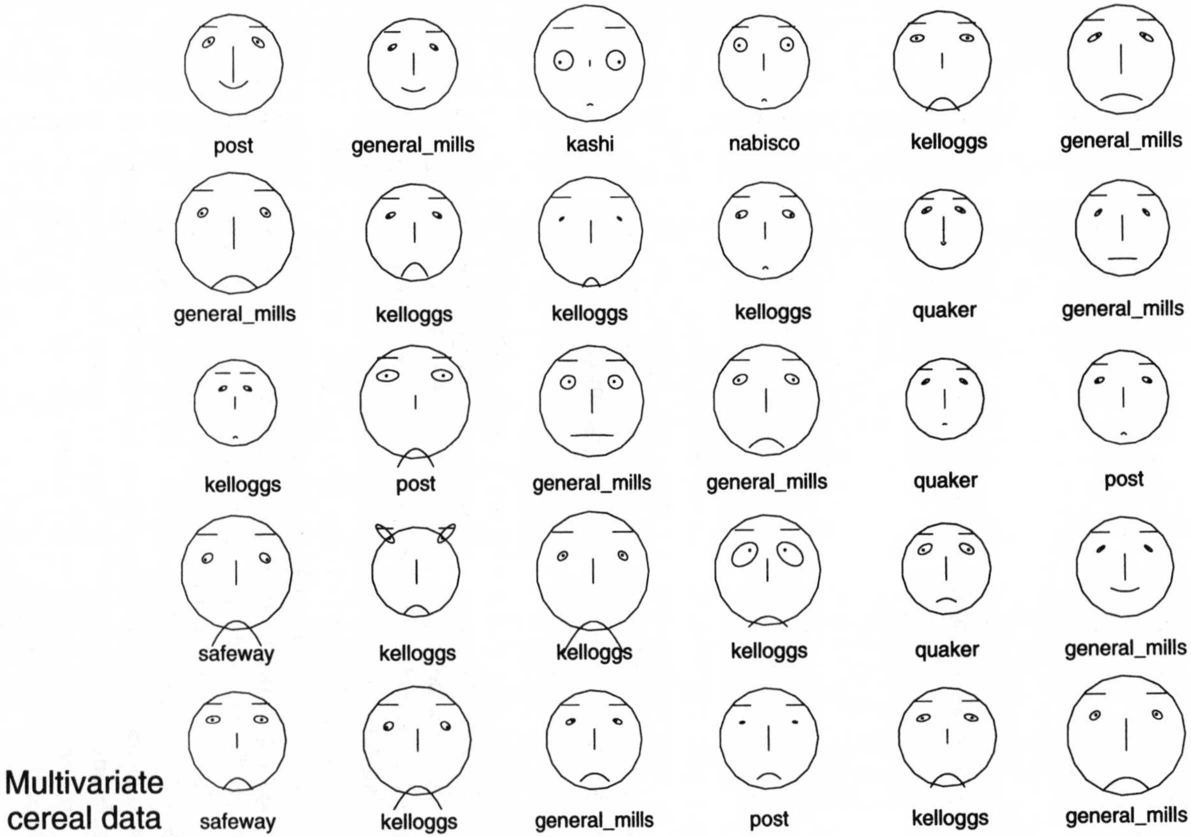

Figure 2.34

Multivariate
cereal data

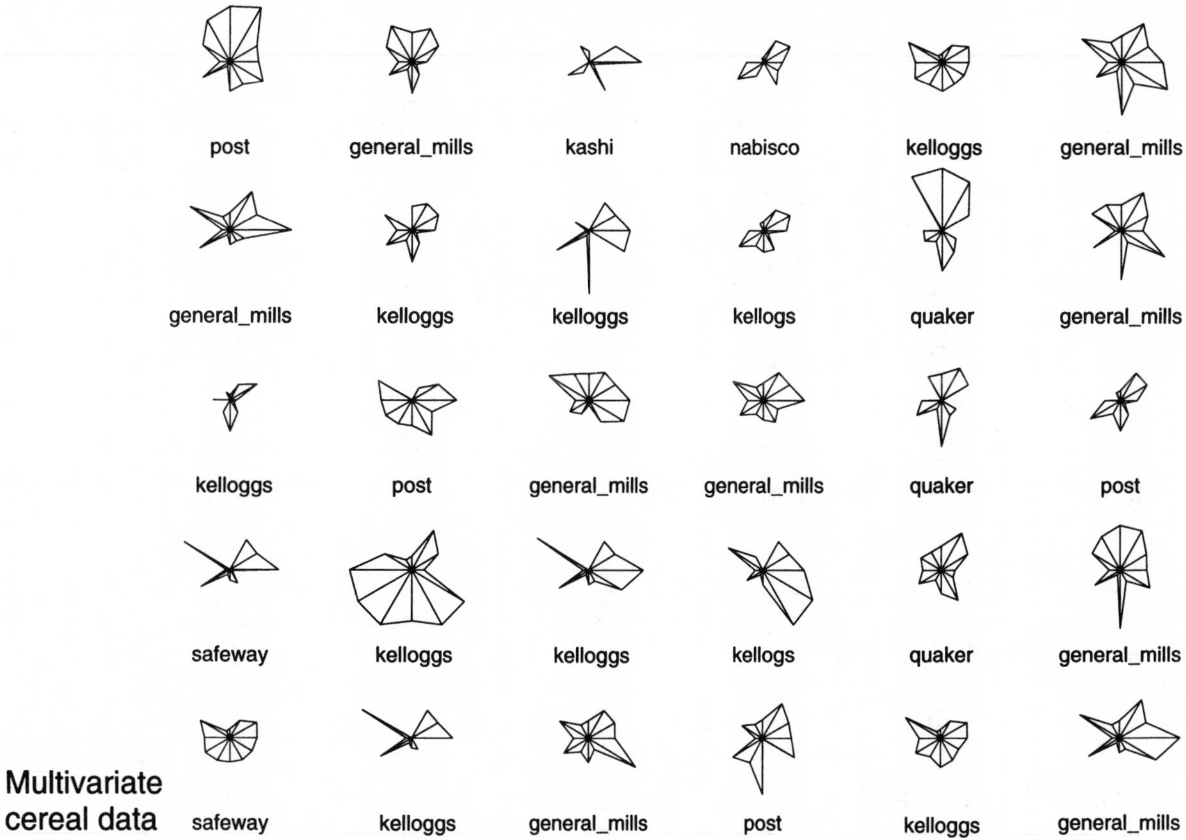

Multivariate
cereal data

Figure 2.35

tion). Features of a face such as eyes, nose, mouth, and head shape represent different aspects of a k-variable measurement with the hope that the multidimensional observation is captured by a one-dimensional multi-faceted picture. For example, each cereal has $k = 11$ characteristics and the $n = 30$ faces (one of each cereal) are displayed in Figure 2.34. The command that created the plot is *faces(cdata, labels = cnames)* where again *cdata* is the array of cereal data and *cnames* is a character vector containing the cereal names. Yet another but similar display is created by *stars(cdata, names = cnames)*. Figure 2.35 displays again the cereal data where each multivariate observation is depicted with lines forming a star (11 lines = number of variables for each cereal brand).

As mentioned, a number of schemes exist to classify multivariate data [5]. For example, the S-function *tree( )* uses regression and classification techniques to classify the observations and also produces a "tree" diagram (see *?tree*). However, there is no generally accepted "best" method. The goal is a subjective but useful description of the multivariate data and not a rigorous inference (i.e., a statistical test leading to a significance probability). Experience plus trial and error are often the best guides to selecting an effective description.

ADDITIVITY—"SWEEPING" AN ARRAY

Tables are themselves summaries of sampled values but tables typically need further analysis to understand fully the relationships among the variables used to generate the tabular data (independent variables). One approach contrasts the observed values in a table to values generated that conform perfectly to an additive relationship. Additive relationships within a two-dimensional table require the cell values to be the sum of three components, represented by a, r, and c. In symbols,

$$f_{ij} = a + r_i + c_j + e_{ij}$$

where f_{ij} represents a measured characteristic found in the ith and j^{th} cell. The term r_i represents a level of influence of the ith row variable, c_j represents a level of influence of the jth column variable, and the symbol a represents an overall "background" level. The term e_{ij} represents the influence of statistical variation (an "error" term). Illustrative numbers that perfectly conform to an additive structure ($e_{ij} = 0$) are:

	column 1	column 2	column 3	column 4	column 5	mean values
row 1	1	3	7	13	21	9
row 2	5	7	11	17	25	13
row 3	15	17	21	27	35	23
mean values	7	9	13	19	27	15

For these artificial values, model parameter a is 15, the parameters for the rows are $r_1 = -6$, $r_2 = -2$, and $r_3 = 8$ and the column parameters are $c_1 = -8$, $c_2 = -6$, $c_3 = -2$, $c_4 = 4$, and $c_5 = 12$. For example, $f_{33} = a + r_3 + c_3 = 15 + 8 - 2 = 21$. Note that: a = overall mean, r_i = (i^{th} row mean) $- a$, c_j = (j^{th} column mean) $- a$, and $f_{ij} = a + r_i + c_j$ exactly, for these "observations."

Additivity means that the variables used to classify observations have separate influences on the measured quantities within each cell of the table. As a consequence, differences among rows are unaffected by the column variable and, similarly, differences among columns are unaffected by the row variable. The perfectly additive "data" illustrate. The difference between row 2 and row 3, for example, is 10 for each column and the difference between column 1 and column 5 is 20 for each row. When either the row values or column values are plotted, they form parallel lines. A direct consequence of additivity is that the row and column mean values from a two-way table reflect the relationships within the table except for random variation. For the perfectly additive data (no random variation), the difference in the mean values between columns 2 and 4, for example, is 10, which perfectly duplicates the same differences in all the rows.

Contrasting observed values to theoretical values derived to have perfect additive relationships produces two possibilities: a close fit where only small inconsequential values remain after accounting for the additive effects or a lack of fit of some or all the observed values identifying non-additive relationships between row and column variables, called an interaction. A close fit indicates evidence of "independent" influences from the row and column variables on the measured outcome f_{ij}. The influences of the row variable are then entirely separate from the influences of the columns variable and vice versa. Areas of lack of fit indicate where and how two variables depend on each other. It is fundamental in describing relationships between two variables to know whether the variables have separate independent influences on the observed outcome (additivity) or whether the influences of one variable depend on levels of the other (interaction).

Like most statistical descriptions of data, a number of ways exist to compare the observed values to the values expected from an additive relationship. The S-function *sweep*( ) is useful in this context. The command *sweep*( ) has the general form

$$sweep\,(input.\,array,\ indicator,\ sweep.out,\ ``operator").$$

The input data are contained in either a two- or three-dimensional array. The named operator is applied to the rows (indicator = 1), the columns (indicator = 2), or the levels (indicator for the three-dimensional case). The sweep-operator (fourth argument) uses the values in *sweep.out* (third argument) and applies these values to the input array (first argument) according to the indicator (second argument). Some examples are:

```
> # test array
> a<- matrix(1:35,5,7)
> a
     [,1] [,2] [,3] [,4] [,5] [,6] [,7]
[1,]    1    6   11   16   21   26   31
[2,]    2    7   12   17   22   27   32
[3,]    3    8   13   18   23   28   33
[4,]    4    9   14   19   24   29   34
[5,]    5   10   15   20   25   30   35
> # divide each column by 10
> sweep(a,2,10,"/")
     [,1] [,2] [,3] [,4] [,5] [,6] [,7]
[1,]  0.1  0.6  1.1  1.6  2.1  2.6  3.1
[2,]  0.2  0.7  1.2  1.7  2.2  2.7  3.2
[3,]  0.3  0.8  1.3  1.8  2.3  2.8  3.3
[4,]  0.4  0.9  1.4  1.9  2.4  2.9  3.4
[5,]  0.5  1.0  1.5  2.0  2.5  3.0  3.5
> #divide each column by the values 1, 2, 3, 4, 5, 6 and 7
> sweep(a,2,c(1,2,3,4,5,6,7),"/")
     [,1] [,2]     [,3] [,4] [,5]     [,6]     [,7]
[1,]    1  3.0 3.666667 4.00  4.2 4.333333 4.428571
[2,]    2  3.5 4.000000 4.25  4.4 4.500000 4.571429
[3,]    3  4.0 4.333333 4.50  4.6 4.666667 4.714286
[4,]    4  4.5 4.666667 4.75  4.8 4.833333 4.857143
[5,]    5  5.0 5.000000 5.00  5.0 5.000000 5.000000
> #subtract the row means from each column
> mtemp<- apply(a,1,mean)
> mtemp
[1] 16 17 18 19 20
> # sweep(a,1,mtemp,"-") = sweep(a,1,mtemp)
> sweep(a,1,mtemp,"-")
     [,1] [,2] [,3 [,4] [,5] [,6] [,7]
[1,]  -15  -10   -5    0    5   10   15
[2,]  -15  -10   -5    0    5   10   15
[3,]  -15  -10   -5    0    5   10   15
[4,]  -15  -10   -5    0    5   10   15
[5,]  -15  -10   -5    0    5   10   15.
```

Along the same lines, the S-function *sweep*( ) can be used to calculate the row percentages or the column percentages for a table of counts. For a table denoted as *tab.data*, the row percentages are computed with

```
> 100*sweep(tab.data,1,apply(tab.data,1,sum),"/")
```

and the column percentages with

```
> 100*sweep(tab.data,2,apply(tab.data,2,sum),"/")
```

Applying the command *sweep*( ) to an array *x* to remove the values expected from an additive structure leaves a set of residual values measuring lack of fit and is accomplished with two consecutive commands:

```
> xx<- sweep(x,2,apply(x,2,mean))
> xx<- sweep(xx,1,apply(xx,1,mean))
```

For example, if x is

	column 1	column 2	column 3	column 4
row 1	6	3	12	9
row 2	13	16	19	22
row 3	11	14	11	22

then the values that remain after an additive relationship is "removed" from the observed values are

```
> x
      [,1] [,2] [,3] [,4]
[1,]    6    3   12    9
[2,]   13   16   19   22
[3,]   11   14   11   22
> xx<- x
> # residuals -- lack of fit
> xx<- sweep(xx,1,apply(xx,1,mean))
> xx<- sweep(xx,2,apply(xx,2,mean))
> round(xx,4)
         [,1]     [,2]     [,3] [,4]
[1,]   1.6667  -2.3333   3.6667   -3
[2,]  -1.3333   0.6667   0.6667    0
[3,]  -0.3333   1.6667  -4.3333   3.
```

Perfectly additive "data" are calculated by subtracting the values that remain after the estimated additive values have been "removed" from the original data. For the example,

```
> # perfect additive values
> round(x-xx,4)
          [,1]      [,2]     [,3] [,4]
[1,]    4.3333    5.3333   8.333  312
[2,]   14.3333   15.3333  18.333  322
[3,]   11.3333   12.3333  15.333  319.
```

For these model generated "data" values, the row and column influences are perfectly additive. The "sweep" process divides each observation (x) into a residual component (xx) and an additive component ($x - xx$). For example, $f_{11} = 6 = 1.667$(residual) + 4.333(additive).

The values in the residual array (after "sweeping") are the same as the residual values that emerge from an analysis of variance applied to a two-way table (Chapter 7). Using *sweep*( ) to produce residual values and exactly additive "data" is strictly a descriptive approach with no assumptions about the population from which the sample is selected. An inspection of the residuals (without any statistical tests) is all that is suggested. If the observations f_{ij} are normally distributed or, at least, approximately normally distributed, analysis of variance techniques (Chapter 7) allow an extensive analysis of the roles of the row and column variables, along with rigorous statistical tests.

An alternative approach based on the median is achieved by replacing the mean function with the median function in the *sweep()* command. The resulting process is called a "median polish" [6] and usually gives much the same results as applying the mean. However, the median polish requires a number of iterations of the *sweep()* function to produce stable residual values (usually four or five iterations). For example, again using the 3×4 array *x*,

```
> # residual -- lack of fit
> xx<- x
> for(i in 1:5) {
  xx<- sweep(xx,1,apply(xx,1,median))
  xx<- sweep(xx,2,apply(xx,2,median))
  }
> # residual values
> round(xx,4)
      [,1]     [,2]     [,3]     [,4]
x1  3.0000 -2.8125  3.1875 -2.8125
x2 -0.1875  0.0000  0.0000  0.0000
x3  0.0000  0.1875 -5.8125  2.1875
> # additive values
> round(x-xx,4)
    [,1]      [,2]      [,3]      [,4]
x1  3.0000  5.8125  8.8125 11.8125
x2 13.1875 16.0000 19.0000 22.0000
x3 11.0000 13.8125 16.8125 19.8125
> twoway(x,iter=5)$resid
      [,1]     [,2]     [,3]     [,4]
x1  3.0000 -2.8125  3.1875 -2.8125
x2 -0.1875  0.0000  0.0000  0.0000
x3  0.0000  0.1875 -5.8125  2.1875.
```

The S-function *twoway()* is a more extensive application of the "median polish" technique (see *?twoway*).

The choice between using a mean or a median to estimate the row and column influences becomes, as usual, primarily one of deciding on the weight to be given to extreme values. The median effectively minimizes any disproportionate influences of extreme or outlier observations where employing the mean incorporates the influence of each observation proportional to its magnitude.

To describe the influence of smoking and behavior type on the risk of coronary heart disease, data on 3154 men aged 40–50 (Table 2.11) were collected. These data yield the array of rates in Table 2.12. Applying *sweep()* to establish the residual and additive components for these coronary heart disease rates gives

```
> # data contained in x
> x
        [,1]       [,2]       [,3]       [,4]
[1,] 89.28571 113.06533 155.25114 154.25532
[2,] 32.25806  61.42506  86.02151  96.15385
> xx<- sweep(x,1,apply(x,1,mean))
> xx<- sweep(xx,2,apply(xx,2,mean))
```

Table 2.11. Coronary heart disease (CHD) frequency classified by smoking and behavior type (A/B)

cigs/day	0	1 to 20	21 to 30	>30	total
			TYPE-A		
CHD	70	45	34	29	178
no CHD	714	353	185	159	1411
total	784	398	219	188	1589
			TYPE-B		
CHD	28	25	16	10	79
no CHD	840	382	170	94	1486
total	868	407	186	104	1565

```
> # residual values -- lack of fit
> round(xx,3)
        [,1]   [,2]    [,3]    [,4]
[1,] -0.986 -3.68   5.115 -0.449
[2,]  0.986  3.68  -5.115  0.449
> # additive expected values
> round(x-xx,3)
        [,1]     [,2]     [,3]     [,4]
[1,]  90.272 116.745 150.136 154.705
[2,]  31.272  57.745  91.136  95.705
```

where x contains the 2×4 array of input data (rates of CHD over an eight-year period) from Table 2.12.

In some situations a multiplicative structure is used to describe the impact of a series of variables on a specific outcome. In epidemiology, biology, and medicine, risk factors of disease are frequently thought to act in a multiplicative fashion. For example, the influence of smoking and behavior type could increase the risk of coronary heart disease multiplicatively. If smoking increases the risk of heart disease by factors of 1.5 and behavior type doubles the risk, then both factors could increase the total risk by a factor of $1.5 \times 2 = 3$ times and the logarithm of the total risk is increased (additive) by log(3) = 1.099. When factors act multiplicatively, the corresponding logarithms produce an additive relationship (e.g., log(1.5) + log(2) = log(3) when 1.5×2.0 = 3). Under multiplicative conditions, the influences of one independent variable on the measured outcome is not affected by the other independent

Table 2.12. Coronary heart disease (CHD) rates per 1000 individuals classified by smoking and behavior type (A/B)

	non-smokers	1–20 cigs/day	21–30 cigs/day	>30 cigs/day
type-A	89.29	113.07	155.25	154.26
type-B	32.26	61.43	86.02	96.12

variables in the model (no interaction). Each independent variable multiplies the outcome value by a specific amount regardless of the other values of the other independent variables.

To evaluate multiplicative relationships in tabular data, the logarithm of the cell frequency is used and these transformed values are contrasted to an additive structure. For the coronary heart disease data, a multiplicative structure is analyzed by

```
> xx<- log(x)
> xx<- sweep(xx,1,apply(xx,1,mean))
> xx<- sweep(xx,2,apply(xx,2,mean))
> # residual values -- lack of fit
> round(exp(xx),3)
      [,1]  [,2]  [,3]  [,4]
[1,] 1.188 0.969 0.960 0.905
[2,] 0.841 1.032 1.042 1.105
> # multiplicative expected values
> round(exp(log(x)-xx),3)
        [,1]    [,2]   [,3]    [,4]
[1,] 75.130 116.665 161.78 170.493
[2,] 38.336  59.530  82.55  86.996.
```

The basic technical difference from the additive approach is that the input array contains not the CHD rates but logarithms of the CHD rates and the resulting output "data" array will have constant row and column ratios.

Both analyses show that additive or multiplicative structures accurately describe the influences of behavior type and smoking on CHD rates (small residual values). For example, the multiplicative structure implies that type-A behavior increases the rate of disease by a factor of 1.96 relative to type-B behavior regardless of the level of smoking (constant ratios within rows—all row ratios are the same for the multiplicative "data"). Smoking increases CHD risk by a factor of 1.5, 2.15, and 2.27 for each smoking category relative to the non-smokers regardless of behavior type. As mentioned, both additive and multiplicative structures imply that the row and column variables act separately. The dotted lines (Figure 2.36) represent the perfectly additive "data" and are, therefore, perfectly parallel. The relatively small residuals (absence of interactions) in the description of the coronary heart disease rates (Figure 2.36) indicate that considering smoking exposure and behavior type as having separate influences on the risk of CHD (i.e., either additive or multiplicatively) is consistent with the observed data.

The choice between using an additive or a multiplicative structure to model the relationships between the independent variables (rows and columns) and the dependent variable (cell observations) is basically non-statistical. The decision is influenced by such considerations as knowledge of the biologic/physical mechanism underlying the data, goodness-of-fit of more

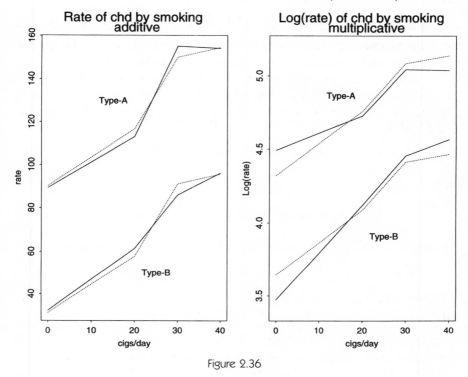

Figure 2.36

complex models [7], and, sometimes, simply the patterns established by previous analyses.

EXAMPLE—GEOGRAPHIC CALCULATIONS USING S-FUNCTIONS

A strength of the S-language is the ability to coordinate graphic display with computations. To further illustrate this property, an S-program is created that calculates and plots several important features of a geographic area. The area and the perimeter of an arbitrary polygon described in terms of xy-coordinates are calculated from the following:

$$area = \frac{1}{4}\sum w_i \qquad i = 1, 2, 3, \cdots, m = \text{ number of polygon segments}$$

where $w_i = S_{yi}D_{xi} - S_{xi}D_{yi}$ when the sum S and the difference D are defined by

$$S_{xi} = x_{i+1} + x_i \quad \text{and} \quad D_{xi} = x_{i+1} - x_i$$

for the x-coordinates. Similarly, the corresponding sum and difference are

$$S_{yi} = y_{i+1} + y_i \quad \text{and} \quad D_{yi} = y_{i+1} - y_i$$

for the y-coordinates. There are m segments to the polygon and, by convention, $x_{m+1} = x_1$ and $y_{m+1} = y_1$. The length of the perimeter is

$$perimeter = \sum \sqrt{D_{xi}^2 + D_{yi}^2} \qquad i = 1, 2, 3, \cdots, m.$$

The geographic centroid (the center of a polygon) is given by

$$x\text{-coordinate of the centroid} = \frac{1}{12A} \sum w_i S_{xi}$$

and

$$y\text{-coordinate of the centroid} = \frac{1}{12A} \sum w_i S_{yi}.$$

An outline of a California county is defined by the relative coordinates:

$x = \{3, 3, 1, 6, 11, 13, 23, 23, 8\}$ and $y = \{8, 13, 18, 18, 10, 8, 8, 1, 1\}$.

The following S-program plots the county boundaries, calculates the area, the perimeter, and the centroid coordinates (placed on the plot):

```
> # area, perimeter and centroid of a polygon
> x<- c(3,3,1,6,11,13,23,23,8)
> y<- c(8,13,18,18,10,8,8,1,1)
> # plots the polygon using the S-function polygon()
> par(pty="s")
> plot(x,y,type="n",main="A California county")
> polygon(x,y,density=10)
> # computation of the area
> sx<- (c(x,x[1])+c(1,x))[-1]
> sy<- (c(y,y[1])+c(1,y))[-1]
> dx<- (c(x,x[1])-c(1,x))[-1]
> dy<- (c(y,y[1])-c(1,y))[-1]
> w<- sy*dx-sx*dy
> area<- sum(w)/4
> # computation of the perimeter
> p<- sum(sqrt(dx^2+dy^2))
> text(3.5,2,paste("area =",round(area,3)))
> text(3.5,3,paste("perimeter =",round(p,3)))
> # computation of the centroid
> ex<- sum(w*sx)/(12*area)
> ey<- sum(w*sy)/(12*area)
> points(ex,ey,pch="*",cex=1.5)
> # label the centroid
> text(ex+2,ey+2,"centroid")
> lines(c(ex,ex+1.7),c(ey,ey+1.7))
```

The results are shown in Figure 2.37. The plot option $type="n"$ allows the creation of the plotting region but suppress the plotting of any points or lines. The S-function $polygon(x, y, density = k, \cdots)$ adds a polygon to a current plot where the argument vectors x and y are the coordinate points of the m vertices of the polygon listed in sequential order. The shading of the polygon is deter-

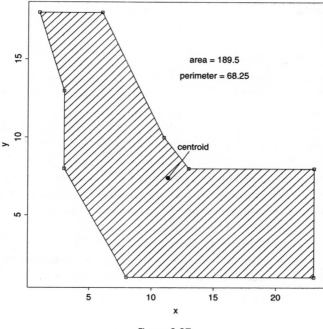

A California county

area = 189.5

perimeter = 68.25

centroid

Figure 2.37

mined by the option *density* = *k* where *k* determines the number of lines per inch of the fill (*density* = 0 produces no shading). A related but more general S-function is *segments*( ) (see ?*segments*) which also can be used to plot a polygon but does not require the segments to be in any specific order.

ESTIMATION OF THE CENTER OF A TWO-DIMENSIONAL DISTRIBUTION

A convex hull is roughly defined as the smallest polygon (smallest perimeter) that encloses all the points in a two-dimensional plot [8]. The S-function *chull*(*xpoints, ypoints, · · ·*) ("chull" for convex hull) identifies the points of the convex hull for data described by points whose *xy*-coordinates are contained in the S-vectors *xpoints* and *ypoints*. For *n* = 100 pairs of random normal points (circular bivariate normal distribution; pairs of uncorrelated, normally distributed values with means = 0 and variances = 1), example S-code that calculates a convex hull and provides an additional illustration of the S-function *polygon*( ) is

```
> n<- 100
> x<- rnorm(n)
> y<- rnorm(n)
> plot(x,y,pch="*")
> # hpoints contains the positions of the convex hull
> hpoints<- chull(x,y)
> polygon(x[hpoints],y[hpoints],density=0)
```

The S-vector *hpoints* contains the positions of the convex hull points extracted from the 100 pairs of x and y coordinates. Based on these points, the S-function *polygon*( ) plots the convex hull.

It has been suggested that the "center" of a two-dimensional distribution of points can be estimated by calculating a sequence of convex hulls. This two-dimensional "median" is estimated without any assumptions about the structure of the sampled data. The process starts by finding the convex hull for the entire data set. Then these points are removed from consideration and a next convex hull is computed based on the remaining points and the associated points removed. The process is repeated and each time a convex hull is calculated the associated points are removed. The result is a sequence of polygons, each smaller in size than the previous one, that converges to the "center" of the observed distribution. Such a sequence is created by

```
> # x = x-coordinates of the data points
> # y = y-coordinates of the data points
> for(i in 1:100){
    x0<- x
    y0<- y
    hpoints<- chull(x,y)
    x<- x[-hpoints]
    y<- y[-hpoints]
    if(length(x)<=3) break
    }
> polygon(x0[hpoints],y0[hpoints],density=0)
```

Figure 2.38 contains four plots displaying the application of *chull*( ) and *polygon*( ) to estimate a bivariate centroid. The first plot is 100 random points sampled from a circular bivariate normal distribution (upper left). The second plot (upper right) shows the convex hull based on these 100 points. The third plot (lower left) shows the sequence of nested convex hulls. The last plot (lower right) is the smallest convex hull providing an estimate of the location of the "center" of the two-dimensional distribution of points.

ADDENDUM: S-GEOMETRY

The plotting routines in System-S are sufficiently flexible to produce not only plots associated with statistical analyses but a variety of geometric figures. Six examples are

Convex hull estimation

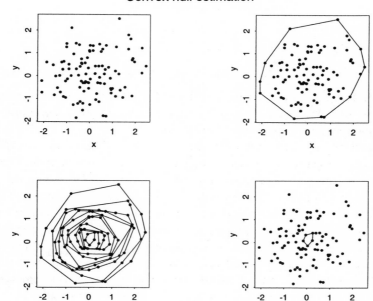

Figure 2.38

```
par(mfrow=c(3,2))

#sin*cos
x<- seq(-2*pi,2*pi,0.25)
y<- x
z<- outer(x,y,function(x,y){sin(x)*cos(y)})
persp(x,y,z,box=F,axes=F)
title("sin*cos")

#sin(1/x)
x1<- seq(-0.1,0.001,0.001)
x2<- seq(0.001,0.1,0.001)
x<- c(x1,x2)
y<- x*sin(1/x)
plot(x,y,type="l",main="x*sin(1/x)")
abline(h=0)
abline(v=0)

#limacon
x<- seq(-2*pi,2*pi,0.01)
y<- 2*(1-4*sin(x))
plot(y*cos(x),y*sin(x),type="l",main="limacon")

#hyperbolic paraboloid
x<- seq(-1,1,0.1)
y<- x
z<- outer(x,y,function(x,y){x^2/4-y^2/4})
persp(x,y,z)
title("hyperbolic paraboloid")
```

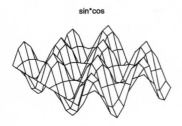

sin*cos

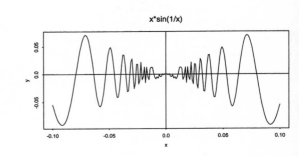

x*sin(1/x)

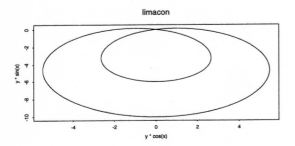

limacon

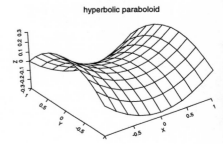

hyperbolic paraboloid

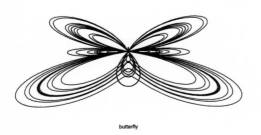

butterfly

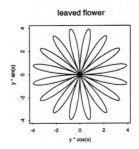

leaved flower

Figure 2.39

138

```
#butterfly[9]
tt<- seq(0,24*pi,len=2000)
rr<- exp(cos(tt))-2*cos(4*tt)+sin(tt/12)^5
plot(rr*sin(tt),-rr*cos(tt),type="l",axes=F,
     xlab="butterfly",ylab="")

#flower
x<- seq(-2*pi,2*pi,0.01)
y<- 4*sin(8*x)
par(pty="s")
plot(y*cos(x),y*sin(x),type="l",main="leaved flower")
```

producing Figure 2.39.

Problem set II

1. Plot the function $f(x) = xlog(x)$ for $0 < x < 1$. Use the *arrows*( ) S-command to point out the minimum of $f(x)$ and the value of x at which the minimum occurs (see *?arrows*).

2. Plot four distributions using the *density*( ) function on the same set of axes based on $n = 200$ observations sampled at random from each of four normal distributions with the same variance ($\sigma = 2$) but with mean values = $\mu_i = \{2, 4, 6, 8\}$.

   Also plot four distributions using the *density*( ) function on the same set of axes based on $n = 200$ observations sampled at random from each of four normal distributions with the same mean ($\mu = 2$) but with standard deviations = $\sigma_i = \{2, 2.5, 3, 3.5\}$.

   Repeat the two plots with n increased to $n = 2000$.

3. Suppose a needle with length l is tossed on a grid with horizontal lines spaced d units apart. Plot the 11 horizontal lines between 0 and 1, $d = 0.1$ units apart. Then, "drop" $n = 50$ random needles on the grid with $l = 0.05$.

   This plot is a display of Buffon's classic problem where he calculated the probability that a needle tossed on such a grid intersects a horizontal line (probability of an intersection = $l/[\pi d]$).

4. Plot the bivariate normal density with *persp*( ) and *contour*( ) where $\mu_x = 0$, $\sigma_x = 1$, $\mu_y = 2$, $\sigma_y = 3$ for $\rho_{xy} = \{0.1, 0.5, 0.9\}$ (see chapter for the mathematical expression of the density function).

5. The S-commands $x <- runif(n)$ and $y <- runif(n)$ generate a set of n random points on the unit square. Divide the x-axis into 10 intervals and calculate the median for values x and y in each interval. Generate three plots with $n = 100, 1000$, and 10,000 random points. Connect the median values to form a median trace (showing, if any, trends in the generated data). Plot the points and the smoothed median traces.

6. Generate a random sample from a normal distribution of $n = 10,000$ values. Test the boxplot definition, of an "outlier" which should produce about 0.7% or 70 generated values as "outliers."

7. The first smoothed observation is a combination of the next two smoothed observations. Justify* that $new - y_1 = 2y_2 - y_3$.

8. Plot the function

$$f(x,y) = \frac{sin(x)}{\sqrt{1 + cos^2(y)}}$$

over the ranges $-2\pi < x < 2\pi$ and $-2\pi < y < 2\pi$ using *persp*( ) and *contour*( ).

9. Consider the data describing prostatic cancer by age and year of death (rates/100,000):

age	1930	1935	1940	1945	1950	1955
45–49	3.5	4.9	6.6	7.2	4.7	4.7
50–54	5.4	11.4	16.0	15.7	23.3	16.3
55–59	18.8	22.4	32.1	41.4	39.0	44.4
60–64	24.0	45.9	50.2	60.4	77.7	84.2
65–69	35.1	60.2	72.3	74.1	74.1	141.1
70–74	60.7	66.5	90.1	126.0	148.0	168.5
75–79	47.5	90.6	151.4	130.0	219.2	234.4
80+	56.7	124.5	152.1	155.6	299.1	328.6

Separate each rate into an additive and a residual component using *sweep*( ).

Assume the effects on the disease rate from year and age are additive. Calculate and inspect the residual pattern (e.g., plot the residuals).

Plot the additive "data" (each year = a line) and the observed rates on the same set of axes.

Repeat the same analysis, assuming the year and age influences have multiplicative influences on the rate of prostatic cancer.

*Solve theoretically and not with a computer program.

REFERENCES

1. Hoaglin, D. C., Mosteller, F., and Tukey, J. W. (eds), *Understanding Robust and Exploratory Data Analysis*. John Wiley & Sons, New York, NY, 1985.
2. Tukey, J. W., *Exploratory Data Analysis*. Addison-Wesley Publishing Company, Reading, MA, 1977.
3. Manly, B. F. J., *Multivariate Statistical Methods—A Primer*. Chapman and Hall, New York, NY, 1986.
4. Chernoff, H., (1973) The use of Faces to Represent Points in k-Dimensional Space Graphically. Journal of the American Statistical Association, 68:361–368.
5. Anderson, T. W., *An Introduction to Multivariate Statistical Analysis*. John Wiley & Sons, New York, NY, 1958.
6. McNeil, D. R., *Interactive Data Analysis*. John Wiley & Sons, New York, NY, 1977.
7. Breslow, N. E. and Day N. E., *Statistical Methods in Cancer Research*. vol 2. Oxford University Press, New York, NY, 1980.
8. Barnett, V., (1976) The ordering of multivariate data. Journal of the Royal Statistical Society, Series A 139:318–354.
9. Venables, W. N. and Ripley, B. D., *Modern Applied Statistics with S-Plus*. Springer-Verlag, New York, NY, 1994.

3

Simulation: Random Values

Parallel to the development of modern computing technology is the growth of interest in using this technology to simulate biological, physical, and statistical phenomena. Simulation on a computer is frequently achieved with a few lines of code producing simple quantities. On the other hand, there are huge program systems to model such things as weather patterns and air pollution. Simple or complex simulation programs, at best, only approximate the real-world process. Even a rough approximation, however, produces benefits in terms of organizing theory, improving understanding, checking analyses, assessing modifications of existing theory, and, perhaps, producing useful predictions. These benefits are achieved at relatively little cost and without risk or expensive experimentation.

The key to simulation techniques is a sequence of random numbers. Randomness is not an easy concept to define. It is usually defined by what it is not. A random sequence is taken to be a sequence of numbers with no detectable pattern. Historically random values have come from a wide range of sources—cosmic radiation, military draft numbers, and color beads are some early tools used to develop "random" numbers. Forty years ago the Rand Corporation published a book containing one million random digits. These digits are actually pseudo-random numbers because all sequences starting at the same point produce the same sequence of values. Even the concept of pseudo-random numbers is not perfectly clear. The term "pseudo" is not explicit in the following since it is understood that a computer employs a deterministic process to produce "random" values. The process is systematic and reproducible; two properties definitely not part of the concept of randomness. Once numbers with no detectable pattern are available, it is possible to use these values to generate other random values with specific statistical properties. These variables are then applied to such tasks as selecting samples of data, testing differences among groups, making estimates of parameters and, more and more, are becoming a vital part of data analysis in general. Generation of apparently random statistical values is the topic of this chapter.

RANDOM UNIFORM VALUES

The high speed and large integer capability of modern computers allow extremely long sequences of numbers to be produced before values repeat. A sequence of integers that does not repeat until several billion values are generated frequently provides smaller sequences that appear as "random" and serve as pseudo-random numbers.

An early method proposed to generate a sequence of random integers is based on extracting the middle portion of the squared value of a large integer. For example,

$$(3712)^2 = 13[7789]44 \text{ yielding } 7789,$$
$$(7789)^2 = 60[6685]21 \text{ yielding } 6685,$$
$$(6685)^2 = 44[6892]25 \text{ yielding } 6892,$$

and so forth. This mid-square process, although simple, is flawed. Sequences with only a few non-repeating values tend to occur rather frequently [1]. Continuing the process,

$$(6892)^2 = 47[4996]64 \text{ yielding } 4996,$$
$$(4996)^2 = 24[9600]16 \text{ yielding } 9600,$$
$$(9600)^2 = 92[1600]16 \text{ yielding } 1600,$$

yields the clearly "non-random" repeating sequence 1600, 5600, 3600, 9600, 1600, $\cdots$.

Modulo arithmetic produces integers that, under certain conditions, do not repeat until all integers in the sequence have been exhausted. The form of such a sequence of integers is

$$x_{i+1} = (ax_i + c)[\text{mod}(m)]$$

where a and c are constants determined to make the sequence of the integers, modulo m, $x_0, x_1, x_2 \cdots$ as long as possible before repeating. The phrase "modulo m" means (repeating from Chapter 1) the integer value that remains after removing multiples of m. The set of generated integers is called a linear congruential sequence and is referred to as mixed-congruential since the expression that yields x_{i+1} involves both multiplication (a) and addition (c).

A small example illustrates where $a = 13$, $c = 7$, and $m = 3$, then

$$x_{i+1} = (13x_i + 7)[\text{mod}(3)].$$

Starting at $x_0 = 3$, the next value is $x_1 = (13(3) + 7)[\text{mod}(3)] = 1$ and the sequence continues

2 0 1 2 0 1 2 0 1 2 0 1 2 0 1 2 0 1 2 0 1 2 0 1 2 0 1 2 0 1 2 0 $\cdots$

and has a period of 3 (repeats after three values). The sequence modulo 10 ($x_0 = 3$ and $m = 10$)

$$x_{i+1} = (13x_i + 7)[\mod(10)]$$

is

6 5 2 3 6 5 2 3 6 5 2 3 6 5 2 3 6 5 2 3 6 5 2 3 $\cdots$

and has a period of 4. A sequence that has full period is

$$x_{i+1} = (13x_i + 7)[\mod(9)]$$

and starting at $x_0 = 3$ yields

1 2 6 4 5 0 7 8 3 1 2 6 4 5 0 7 8 3 1 2 6 4 5 0 7 8 3 1 2 6 $\cdots$

with a period of 9 (repeats after 9 values) and appears "random." Full period means that the number of non-repeating sequential integers equals m before repeating. Clearly, the choice of a and c is important; if $a = 1$, $c = 1$ (modulo 8), then if $x_0 = 2$,

3 4 5 6 7 0 1 2 3 4 5 6 7 0 1 2 3 4 5 6 7 $\cdots$

which is full period but certainly not acceptably "random."

Selection of constants a and c for a specific m dictates the length of the non-repeating sequence (period). The value for m is usually set at the limit of the integer representation of the computer (frequently about 2^{32} for a machine with 32-bit integer representation—over 4 billion). Choosing m in the neighborhood of 2^{32} allows non-repeating sequences to be generated with extremely long cycles (also in the neighborhood of 2^{32}). Furthermore, for certain values of a and c, sequences appear to have no detectable pattern among the integers generated and become ideal sources of "random" values.

Two choices of a and c illustrate: $a = 2^{10} + 3$ or $a = 2^{10} + 1$ with $c = 0$ and $m = 2^{20}$. Theoretical considerations make possible optimum choices of a and c for a specified value of m [1]. Practically every computer system has at least one optimum random number generator. Nevertheless, it is instructive to compare the two illustrative choices with the SPLUS random number generator *runif*( ).

The following S-code generates $n = 1000$ "random" values using the constants $a = 2^{10} + 3$, $c = 0$, and $m = 2^{20}$:

```
> n<- 1000
> k<- 29983
> a0<- 2^10
> m<- 2^20
> ran0<- NULL
> for (i in 1:n) {
  k<- (a0+3)*k
  k<- k%%m
```

```
ran0[i]<- k/(m-1)
}
```

The S-vector labeled *ran0* contains 1000 potentially random integers trans-formed to values between 0 and 1 by dividing by the maximum possible value that can be generated. The S-variable k (29983, for the example) is called the seed and is the starting point of the random sequence. The seed value is simply a positive integer. A useful property of the seed is that the same seed produces the same sequence. This property is handy when checking for errors. As long as the same seed value is used, computer generated values do not change, making the process of checking the computer code for errors less confusing. The S-function *runif*() employs a rather complicated seed value. However, this seed value is saved in the user's working S-directory each time random values are generated and can be recalled. When it is necessary to repeat exactly a calculation that includes random values, the seed can be restored (see *Random.seed*). Also, if the need arises, a seed value can be spe-cified with the S-function *set.seed*(). For example,

```
> set.seed(111)
> round(runif(9),3)
[1] 0.833 0.575 0.994 0.434 0.191 0.858 0.107 0.117 0.156
> # same seed
> set.seed(111)
> round(runif(9),3)
[1] 0.833 0.575 0.994 0.434 0.191 0.858 0.107 0.117 0.156
> # seed not set
> round(runif(9),3)
[1] 0.330 0.806 0.351 0.996 0.805 0.866 0.609 0.820 0.821.
```

Contrasting three sets of 1000 possibly random values ($a = 2^{10} + 3$ produces the S-vector *ran0*, $a = 2^{10} + 1$ produces the S-vector *ran1* with $c = 0$, and the S-function *runif*() produces the S-vector *ran2*) gives

```
> describe(ran0)
         n    xbar     md      s2      s      se
[1,] 1000  0.5043  0.5016  0.0818  0.2860  0.0090
     xmin    xmax     rng
   0.0013  0.9978  0.9965

> describe(ran1)
         n    xbar     md      s2      s      se
      1000  0.4994  0.4988  0.0833  0.2887  0.0091
     xmin    xmax     rng
   0.0002  0.9992  0.9990

> describe(ran2)
         n    xbar      md      s2      s      se
[1,] 1000  0.4939   0.4755  0.0861  0.2935  0.0093
     xmin    xmax     rng
   0.0000  0.9999  0.9994
```

where *describe*() is the specially created S-function from Chapter 2. The expected mean and median value of a continuous uniform random value bounded between 0 and 1 is 0.5 and the variance is $1/12 = 0.0833$.

There are a variety of methods to test a sequence of values for evidence of non-randomness. A good place to start is a table or histogram. For example, using the $n = 1000$ observations stored in *ran0*, then

```
> tab<- table(cut(ran0,seq(0,1,0.1)))
> tab
 0.0+ thru 0.1 0.1+ thru 0.2 0.2+ thru 0.3
            92            106            91
 0.3+ thru 0.4 0.4+ thru 0.5 0.5+ thru 0.6
           104            106           105
 0.6+ thru 0.7 0.7+ thru 0.8 0.8+ thru 0.9
            92            110            88
 0.9+ thru 1.0
           106.
```

The tabled values are consistent with a uniform distribution of values between 0 and 1. The expected number of values in any one cell of the table is $n/10 = 1000/10 = 100$. To add a bit more rigor to assessing this table, a chi-square statistic produces the likelihood that the observed variation in cell frequency arose by chance (significance probability), or

```
> x2<- sum(((tab-n/10)^2/(n/10)))
> probability<- 1-pchisq(x2,9)
> cbind(x2,probability)
        x2    probability
[1,] 6.02      0.7379149.
```

This chi-square statistic has nine degrees of freedom, one less than the number of cells in the table.

A clever method to assess randomness is based on counting the numbers of runs-up and runs-down. Each value in a sequence is compared to the previous value in the sequence; if it is larger, the run continues up and if it is smaller, the run continues down. A count of increasing (runs-up) and decreasing (runs-down) sequences is made. For the sequence $x = \{1, 4, 5, 3, 6, 7, 9, 8, 3, 1,$ and $2\}$, there are three runs-up and two runs-down giving a total of five. A large number or a small number of runs should not appear in a random sequence. Large or small is judged relative to the expected number of runs calculated for a random sequence. The expected number of runs in a sequence of n values is

$$\textit{expected number of runs} = r_0 = \frac{2n - 3}{3}$$

with associated variance of the observed total number of runs (represented by r) given by

$$\textit{variance}(r) = \frac{16n - 29}{90}$$

when the sequence is random [2]. Example S-code producing a run test using $n = 10,000$ values from the S-function *runif*( ) is

```
> n<- 10000
> x<- runif(n)
> test<- diff(sign(diff(x)))
> r<- sum(ifelse(test!=0,1,0))+1
> r0<- (2*n-3)/3
> v<- (16*n-29)/90
> z<- (r-r0)/sqrt(v)
> cat("r =",r,"r0 =",round(r0,3),"z =",round(z,3),"\n")
  r = 6679 r0 = 6665.667 z = 0.316
> cat("p-value = ", round(pnorm(z),3),"\n")
  p-value = 0.624
```

and gives an observed number of runs of $r = 6679$ with an expected number of $r_0 = 6665.667$ yielding $z = 0.316$. The test-statistic z has an approximate standard normal distribution when the sequence is uniformly random; therefore, implying that a smaller number of runs than the one observed occurs with probability 0.624 by chance alone. The deviation of the observed number of runs from the value expected when the sequence is random is likely, leading to the inference that no reason exists to suspect that the sequence is not random. Tests of randomness frequently produce a "not guilty" verdict. One can never absolutely determine whether the sequence is random or whether the test does not yield sufficient evidence of non-randomness.

The same analytic process used to compare a sample of data to a normal distribution (qqnorm—Chapter 2) can be used to compare a sample of data to a uniform distribution. The question is: are the sampled values random? The answer lies again in comparing a theoretically derived cumulative probability distribution $F(x)$ to an empirically derived cumulative probability distribution $\hat{F}(x)$.

For a uniformly distributed random variable X ($0 \leq x \leq 1$), the cumulative probability function is $F(x) = P(X \leq x) = x$. A plot of the cumulative distribution function consists of a straight line from $(0, 0)$ to $(1, 1)$ ($45°$ slope). This cumulative probability distribution is shown in Figure 3.1 (dotted line). A small illustrative data set is

$$x = \{0.15, 0.16, 0.18, 0.22, 0.23, 0.29, 0.34, 0.65, 0.77, 0.92\}$$

where the values have been ordered from low to high. The "+" symbols marked on the plot (Figure 3.1) represent the theoretical cumulative probabilities at each observation x_i under the hypothesis that the data are sampled from a uniform distribution. For example, $F(x_7) = P(X \leq x_7) = P(X \leq 0.34) = 0.34$.

The empirical cumulative probabilities are estimated by the proportion of values less than or equal to a specific observed value divided by the total number of values observed (Chapter 2). Specifically, the empirical cumulative probability function is again $\hat{F}(x_i) = \hat{P}(X \leq x_i) = i/n$ for the ordered sample of observations $x_1 \leq x_2 \leq x_3 \leq \cdots \leq x_n$. For example, $\hat{F}(x_7) = \hat{P}(X \leq x_7) = 7/10$

Kolmogorov-test -- plot

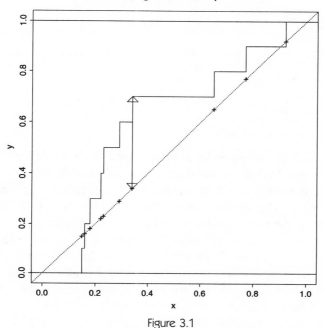

Figure 3.1

= 0.7. The empirical cumulative probability distribution is also plotted in Figure 3.1 (solid line). The empirical distribution is again a step function, rising an amount $1/n$ at each observed value of x in the ordered sample. The points defining a step-function are calculated with the S-function *stepfun*$(x, y, ...)$ where x and y are S-vectors containing the coordinates of the points to be plotted. For the example data,

```
> stepfun(x,y)
$x:
 [1] 0.15 0.16 0.16 0.18 0.18 0.22 0.22 0.23 0.23 0.29
     0.29 0.34 0.34 0.65 0.65 0.77 0.77 0.92 0.92

$y:
 [1] 0.1 0.1 0.2 0.2 0.3 0.3 0.4 0.4 0.5 0.5 0.6 0.6 0.7
     0.7 0.8 0.8 0.9 0.9 1.0
```

where x is the vector of data values and $y = \{0.1, 0.2, 0.3, 0.4, 0.5, 0.6, 0.7, 0.8, 0.9, 1.0\}$ is a vector of estimated cumulative probabilities (i.e., $y_i = i/n$, $i = 1, 2, 3, \cdots, n$). Figure 3.1 contrasts these two cumulative distribution functions and is created by

```
> x<- c(0.15,0.16,0.18,0.22,0.23,0.29,0.34,0.65,0.77,0.92)
> n<- length(x)
> x<- sort(x)
> y<- x
```

```
> plot(x,y,pch="+",xlim=c(0,1),ylim=c(0,1),
    main="Kolmogorov-test -- plot ")
> abline(0,1,lty=2)
> par(new=T)
> y0<- (1:n)/n
> plot(stepfun(c(0,x),c(0,y0)),type="l",xlim=c(0,1),ylim=c(0,1),
    xlab="",ylab="",axes=F)
> abline(h=0)
> abline(h=1)
> dif<- abs(y-y0)
> m<- order(dif)[n]
> arrows(x[m],y[m],x[m],y0[m])
> arrows(x[m],y0[m],x[m],y[m])
```

A measure of lack of correspondence between the two cumulative probability functions $F(x)$ and $\hat{F}(x)$ is the maximum observed distance between the "+"-values and the steps. Each "+" (theoretical) and step (empirical) corresponds to an observation. The double arrow (Figure 3.1) indicates the maximum distance between the two cumulative probability distributions.

The maximum distance (denoted $\hat{K}$) serves as a test statistic. For the example data, $\hat{K} = |0.34 - 0.70| = 0.36$. If the maximum estimated distance is small, then the sampled data are consistent with a uniform distribution and if it is large, the hypothesis of randomness becomes suspect. The theoretical distribution of the maximum distance $\hat{K}$ was derived by the Russian statistician Kolmogorov. Probabilities that the maximum distance $\hat{K}$ results only from random variation are found in tables [3] for small samples of data. Approximations exist for the quantiles of the distribution of $\hat{K}$, accurate for moderately large sample sizes ($n > 40$). Some examples are (two-sided probability):

$$P(K \geq 1.07/\sqrt{n}) = 0.2, P(K \geq 1.22/\sqrt{n}) = 0.1$$

$$P(K \geq 1.36/\sqrt{n}) = 0.05, \text{ and } P(K \geq 1.63/\sqrt{n}) = 0.01$$

when the data are sampled from a uniform distribution. For the example data,

```
> K<- max(abs(y-(1:n)/n))
> cat("maximum distance = ",round(K,3),"\n")
 maximum distance = 0.36.
```

From a table of the distribution of the Kolmogorov statistic [3], p-value = 0.12 = $P(\hat{K} \geq 0.36)$ for $n = 10$.

The approximate quantiles make it a simple matter to test large samples of data for evidence of non-randomness. For example, $n = 2000$ values from the S-function *runif*( ) are analyzed by

```
> n<- 2000
> y<- sort(runif(n))
> K<- max(abs(y-(1:n)/n))
> K20<- 1.07/sqrt(n)
> K10<- 1.22/sqrt(n)
> K5<- 1.36/sqrt(n)
```

```
> K1<- 1.63/sqrt(n)
> round(cbind(K,K20,K10,K5,K1),3)
         K    K20    K10     K5     K1
[1,] 0.024  0.024  0.027  0.030  0.036.
```

The probability that a maximum deviation $\hat{K} = 0.024$ or greater arising by chance alone from data sampled from a uniform distribution is p-value = 0.2, approximately. Similarly, the $n = 1000$ values from $ran0$ can be tested for randomness and

```
> y<- sort(ran0)
> n<- length(y)
> K<- max(abs(y-(1:n)/n))
> K20<- 1.07/sqrt(n)
> K10<- 1.22/sqrt(n)
> K5<- 1.36/sqrt(n)
> K1<- 1.63/sqrt(n)
> round(cbind(K,K20,K10,K5,K1),3)
       K    K20    K10     K5     K1
   0.017  0.034  0.039  0.043  0.052
```

also shows no evidence of non-randomness (p-value > 0.2).

Another assessment of randomness comes from simply plotting the generated values. Figure 3.2 displays the odd values of the sequence $ran0$ plotted

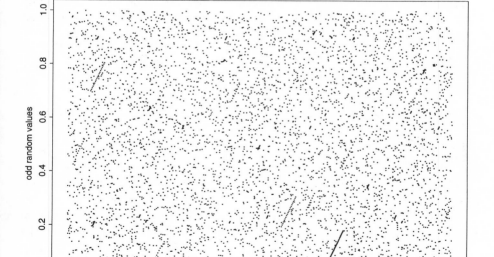

Random values from ran0

Figure 3.2

against the even values. The plot shows areas of non-randomness (small sets of values falling on diagonal lines) that would be difficult to detect with a statistical test. Figure 3.3 shows that the values contained in *ran*1 are far from acceptably "random" since the generated values fall on one of two straight lines emphasizing the importance of choosing the *a*, *c*, and *m* components of the congruential random number generator. As expected, *runif*( ) shows no evidence of non-randomness (Figure 3.4).

The type of "nonrandom" pattern displayed in Figure 3.3 associated with *ran*1 can be identified with a serial correlation coefficient. A measure of randomness within a sequence of numbers comes from estimating the correlation between a series of values at different distances apart. This measure of randomness is called a serial correlation coefficient or an autocorrelation coefficient. Values from a random sequence regardless of the distance apart will very likely have a serial correlation coefficient in the neighborhood of zero. Large deviations from zero indicate a pattern associated with a specific distance.

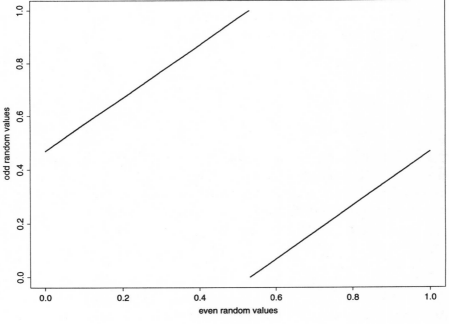

Figure 3.3

Random values from ran2

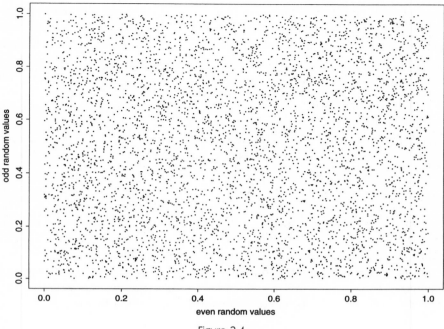

Figure 3.4

An approximate autocovariance for a sequence $\{x_1, x_2, x_3, \cdots, x_n\}$ of n values ($n > 100$ or so) is defined as

$$c_k = \frac{1}{n}\sum(x_i - \bar{x})(x_{i+k} - \bar{x}) \qquad i = 1, 2, 3, \cdots, n - k$$

with

$$c_0 = \frac{1}{n}\sum(x_i - \bar{x})^2 \qquad \text{where } \bar{x} = \frac{1}{n}\sum x_i \qquad i = 1, 2, 3, \cdots, n.$$

The estimated serial correlation coefficient is $r_k = c_k/c_0$. The quantity r_k is the estimated serial correlation coefficient at lag k ($-1 \le r_k \le 1$). The term lag identifies the distance between the values correlated. An S-function to compute a serial correlation coefficient is

```
rserial<- function(x,k) {
  n<- length(x)
  ck<- sum((x[1:(n-k)]-mean(x))*(x[(1+k):n]-mean(x)))
  c0<- sum((x-mean(x))^2)
  ck/c0
}
```

Applying a "serial correlation test" to the three sets of $n = 1000$ values ($ran0$, $ran1$, and $ran2$) at four different lag values yields

```
> # lag = 2
> round(c(rserial(ran0,2),rserial(ran1,2),rserial(ran2,2)),3)
[1]  -0.012 -0.478 -0.017
> # lag = 3
> round(c(rserial(ran0,3),rserial(ran1,3),rserial(ran2,3)),3)
[1] -0.026 0.197 -0.028
> # lag = 4
> round(c(rserial(ran0,4),rserial(ran1,4),rserial(ran2,4)),3)
[1]   0.007 0.361 0.005
> # lag = 5
> round(c(rserial(ran0,5),rserial(ran1,5),rserial(ran2,5)),3)
[1] -0.002 -0.441 0.038.
```

The S-function $acf()$ ("acf" for autocovariance function) is a general time series command that also can be used to compute autocovariances and serial correlation coefficients for any given lag period.

The lack of "randomness" in $ran1$ is obvious from the large (nonzero) values of the serial correlation coefficients at different lag values. A serial correlation coefficient can be tested against the expectation zero [4]. However, for computer random values where very large samples are easily generated, statistical tests for randomness are often unnecessary.

Many other tests for randomness exist ([1] or [4]) but most computer languages come with a reliable, fast and useful random number generator. The S-function $runif()$ is one of these and is used in the following.

AN EXAMPLE

Before discussing computer simulated random values with specific distributions, an example of using simulation to answer a question arising from collected data illustrates a general approach. Figure 3.5 shows hypothetical data surrounding a point (dot in Figure 3.5—pch = "*"). The point could be a source of electromagnetic radiation or a toxic waste site and the "+"-symbol could represent locations of cases of disease or deaths (pch = "+"). The question: is the configuration of observed points likely to have occurred by chance or is there evidence of spatial clustering associated with the point?

The xy-coordinates of the $n = 18$ data values (x_i, y_i) and the specific point (x_0, y_0) in Figure 3.5 are

```
> x
 [1]  0.25 0.84 0.39 0.59 0.76 0.40 0.26 0.41 0.47
      0.75 0.40 0.34 0.72 0.61 0.31 0.90 0.90 0.82
> y
 [1]  0.47 0.83 0.38 0.80 0.67 0.68 0.57 0.63 0.38
      0.12 0.21 0.28 0.36 0.87 0.28 0.24 0.88 0.14
> x0
 [1]   0.60
> y0
 [1]   0.65.
```

Distance data

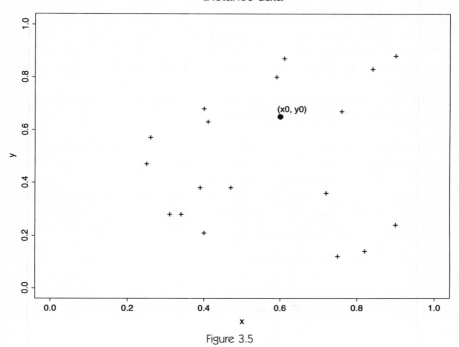

Figure 3.5

The observed mean distance from the point (x_0, y_0) based on the 18 observations is

```
> d0<- sqrt((x-x0)^2+(y-y0)^2)
>  mean(d0)
  [1] 0.3511924.
```

To judge whether this distance is particularly small (evidence of clustering) or a value likely to have occurred by chance, it is necessary to know the distribution of distances from the point of interest ($x_0 = 0.60$, $y_0 = 0.65$) when no spatial pattern exists. Such a distribution is estimated by generating samples of $n = 18$ independent random points. A random point consists of a value x and a value y between 0 and 1 selected independently from a uniform distribution. Each sample of $n = 18$ random points produces a mean distance and 5000 random mean distances are generated by

```
> xx<- matrix(runif(5000*18),18,5000)
> yy<- matrix(runif(5000*18),18,5000)
> d<- sqrt((xx-x0)^2+(yy-y0)^2)
> dbar<- apply(d,2,mean)
```

Figure 3.6 is a histogram of the 5000 random mean distances contained in the vector labeled *dbar*. To repeat, these mean distances have no association with the point (x_0, y_0). Differences among these mean values reflect only random variability. Without a computer simulation approach, it requires sophisticated statistical theory to define even an approximate distribution of these sample mean values.

The mean distance $(\bar{d})$ and its associated variance estimated from this "null distribution" of 5000 random mean distances are

```
> mean(dbar)
[1] 0.4109727
> var(dbar)
[1] 0.00164894.
```

The likelihood (p-value) of observing a distance smaller than the observed mean ($\bar{d}_0 = 0.351$) when no spatial pattern exists is estimated by counting the number of "null" mean values that are smaller than $\bar{d}_0$ or

```
> sum(ifelse(dbar<mean(d0),1,0))
[1] 365.
```

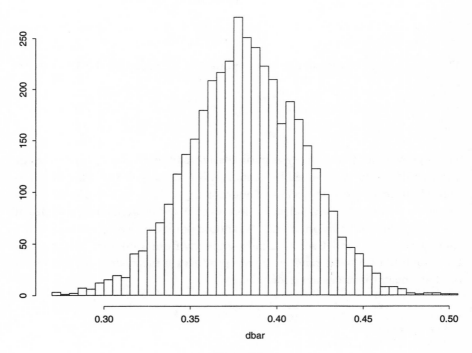

Histogram of simulated mean values (n = 18)

Figure 3.6

Without assumptions about the distribution of the population sampled or complicated mathematics, the probability of a mean value less than $\bar{d}_0 = 0.351$ occurring by chance is estimated as $365/5000 = 0.073$ when no spatial pattern exists.

The shape of the histogram (Figure 3.6) indicates an approximate normal distribution of mean distances, which is expected since mean values typically have approximate normal distributions. Based on a normally distributed estimated mean, then

```
> z<- (mean(d0)-mean(dbar))/sqrt(var(dbar))
> pvalue<- pnorm(z)
> cbind(z,pvalue)
            z     pvalue
[1,] -1.472161    0.07048875.
```

The two approaches (one nonparametric and the other parametric) yield almost the same results. This example is simple but contains many of the elements of more complicated simulation approaches used to answer specific questions about observed data.

SAMPLING WITHOUT AND WITH REPLACEMENT

A sample of n elements selected from a population of N elements is achieved with the S-function *sample*( ). When it is required that a sample be selected so that no population element appears more than once in the sample, the sampling scheme is called sampling without replacement. A common example of sampling without replacement is a lottery. For the California lottery, there are 51 possible numbers and each lottery drawing consists of sampling six random numbers (n) from the 51 (N) without replacement. The S-statement

$$s0 \; <- \; sample(x, n, replace = F)$$

samples without replacement n values from the N values contained in the vector x and places them in the S-vector $s0$. This sample is also achieved by $s0 <- x[rank(runif(N))][1 : n]$. To simulate a lottery pick, $sample(1 : 51, 6, replace = F)$ or $(1 : 51)[rank(runif(51))][1 : 6]$ could be used.

A random permutation of the elements of a vector is related to sampling without replacement. The S-function *sample*(n) produces a random permutation of the integers 1 to n. A command that produces a random permutation of a vector x containing N elements is then $x <- x[sample(N)]$ or equivalently $x <- x[rank(runif(N))]$. A random permutation of the N values contained in the vector x is also achieved by $sample(x, N, replace = F)$ and the "default" version of the same command is $sample(x)$.

Sampling with replacement does not change the sampled population. Duplicate sampled values are possible and, in some cases, probable among the n elements selected with replacement from a population of N elements. The S-command

$$s1 \; <- \; sample(x, n, replace = T)$$

produces n elements sampled from x (length $= N$) with replacement. A fragment of S-code that achieves the same thing is $s1<-x[ceiling(N * runif(n))]$. For example, rolling a pair of dice is sampling with replacement from six (N) values where the sample size is two (n). Computer "dice" are simulated by $sample(1:6, 2, replace = T)$ or $ceiling(6 * runif(2))$. To generate a sequence of 2000 rolls of two "dice" and compute the sum of the two outcomes:

```
> # rolls[1,] first n tosses of two dice
> # rolls[2,] second n tosses of two dice
> n<- 2000
> rolls<- matrix(ceiling(6*runif(2*n)),2,n)
> # or rolls<- matrix(sample(1:6,2*n,replace=T),2,n)
> tosses<- apply(rolls,2,sum)
> # frequency of observed outcomes
> o<- table(tosses)/n
> # expected frequency of outcomes
> e<- c(1,2,3,4,5,6,5,4,3,2,1)/36
> round(cbind(o,e),4)
            o        e
   2   0.0255   0.0278
   3   0.0650   0.0556
   4   0.0805   0.0833
   5   0.1175   0.1111
   6   0.1430   0.1389
   7   0.1635   0.1667
   8   0.1350   0.1389
   9   0.1080   0.1111
  10   0.0745   0.0833
  11   0.0550   0.0556
  12   0.0325   0.0278.
```

As expected, the proportions of observed and expected outcomes associated with the 11 possible sums of two dice hardly differ.

RANDOM SAMPLE FROM A DISCRETE PROBABILITY DISTRIBUTION— ACCEPTANCE/REJECTION SAMPLING

A discrete random variable X is described by the probability distribution $P(X = x) = p_x$ where $x = 1, 2, 3, \cdots, k$ or

$$P(X = 1) = p_1$$
$$P(X = 2) = p_2$$
$$P(X = 3) = p_3$$

$$\cdot$$
$$\cdot$$
$$\cdot$$

$$P(X = k) = p_k.$$

It is important to keep clear the distinction between the mean and variance of a probability distribution and the mean and variance estimated from data. The mean of a probability distribution gets a special name, expectation. The expectation is the measure of location of a probability distribution analogous to the mean from a sample of data but depends only on the probabilities defining the probability distribution (i.e., the p_x-values). For a discrete probability distribution, the expectation of a random variable X is defined as

$$\text{expectation of } X = \sum x p_x$$

summed over all possible values of x. The variance associated with a discrete probability distribution is defined as

$$\text{variance}(x) = \sum (x - \text{expectation})^2 p_x$$

again summed over all possible values of x.

To use acceptance/rejection sampling to produce a random value from a specific discrete probability distribution two uniformly distributed random variables are generated. The first variable u_1 takes on the discrete values to be generated $x = 1, 2, 3, \cdots, k$ with equal probability, $1/k$. The second value u_2 is a continuous and uniformly distributed variable over the interval 0 to 1. If $u_1 = x$ and $u_2 < p_x$, then the value x is a random observation from the defined discrete probability distribution; otherwise a new pair of values (u_1, u_2) is selected and tested. The process is repeated until a value x is accepted. The accepted value x is then a random selection from the distribution defined by the probability distribution $p_1, p_2, p_3, \cdots, p_k$.

Consider a simple example. Say a value X has the following discrete probability distribution:

$$X = 1 \text{ with probability } P(X = 1) = p_1 = 0.4,$$
$$X = 2 \text{ with probability } P(X = 2) = p_2 = 0.3,$$
$$X = 3 \text{ with probability } P(X = 3) = p_3 = 0.2,$$
$$X = 4 \text{ with probability } P(X = 4) = p_4 = 0.1.$$

The expected value for this probability distribution is 2 and the associated variance is 1. Then, the following acceptance/rejection procedure produces a random variable X with the defined distribution:

Let the symbols u_1 and u_2 represent two independent uniform random variables where u_1 takes on each of the values of the variable to be generated (1, 2, 3, and 4) with equal probability (0.25) and the value u_2 is continuous and uniformly distributed between 0 and 1. Generate a pair of random values (u_1, u_2) and

if $u_1 = 1$ and $u_2 < p_1 = 0.4$, then assign $x = u_1$; otherwise select another (u_1, u_2) pair,

if $u_1 = 2$ and $u_2 < p_2 = 0.3$, then assign $x = u_1$; otherwise select another (u_1, u_2) pair,

if $u_1 = 3$ and $u_2 < p_3 = 0.2$, then assign $x = u_1$; otherwise select another (u_1, u_2) pair,

if $u_1 = 4$ and $u_2 < p_4 = 0.1$, then assign $x = u_1$; otherwise select another (u_1, u_2) pair,

Then,

$$P(X = 1) = P(\mu_2 < 0.4 | \mu_1 = 1)P(\mu_1 = 1) = 0.4(0.25)/P$$
$$P(X = 2) = P(\mu_2 < 0.3 | \mu_1 = 2)P(\mu_1 = 2) = 0.3(0.25)/P$$
$$P(X = 3) = P(\mu_2 < 0.2 | \mu_1 = 3)P(\mu_1 = 3) = 0.2(0.25)/P$$
$$P(X = 4) = P(\mu_2 < 0.1 | \mu_1 = 4)P(\mu_1 = 4) = 0.1(0.25)/P$$

and $P = 0.4(0.25) + 0.3(0.25) + 0.2(0.25) + 0.1(0.25) = 0.25$ is the probability of accepting a value $u_1 = x$. Therefore, $P(X = 1) = 0.4$, $P(X = 2) = 0.3$, $P(X = 3) = 0.2$, and $P(X = 4) = 0.1$.

The probability of acceptance P is increased by dividing each probability p_x by the maximum probability from the distribution sampled. That is, accept $u_1 = x$ when $u_2 < p_x/p_{max}$; reject $u_1 = x$ otherwise. Continuing the example, $p_{max} = p_1 = P(X = 1) = 0.4$ is the maximum and

$$P(X = 1) = (0.4/0.4)(0.25)/P = 0.0250/0.625 = 0.4$$
$$P(X = 2) = (0.3/0.4)(0.25)/P = 0.1875/0.625 = 0.3$$
$$P(X = 3) = (0.2/0.4)(0.25)/P = 0.1250/0.625 = 0.2$$
$$P(X = 4) = (0.1/0.4)(0.25)/P = 0.0625/0.625 = 0.1.$$

Now, the value $P = (0.4/0.4)(0.25) + (0.3/0.4)(0.25) + (0.2/0.4)(0.25) + (0.1/0.4)(0.25) = 0.625$ is the probability of accepting a value $u_1 = x$. Dividing by the maximum probability increases the efficiency of the process by increasing the likelihood of accepting a generated value (0.25 versus 0.625, in the example) and does not change the probabilities associated with the selected value.

Figure 3.7 shows the geometry of acceptance/rejection sampling for the example probability distribution. A value 1, 2, 3, or 4 is selected with probability 0.25 determining a rectangle representing one of the four outcomes.

Simple probability distribution

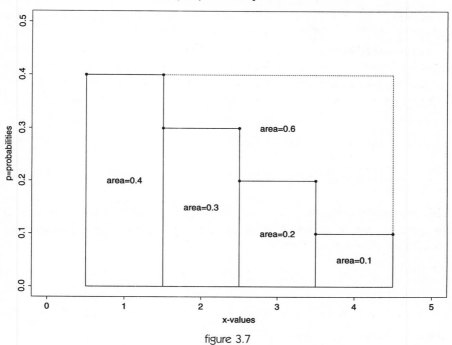

figure 3.7

Once a rectangle is selected, the second uniform variable is either in the acceptance or in the rejection region (i.e., $\mu_2 < p_x/p_{max}$, then accept or $\mu_2 \geq p_x/p_{max}$, then reject). Given a specific rectangle, the probability is $p_x/p_{max} = p_x/$ 0.4 that the value is accepted or 1.0, 0.75, 0.50, or 0.25, respectively. The overall probability of being in one of the four acceptance regions is $1.0/1.6 =$ 0.625 (ratio of acceptance area to total area—Figure 3.7). The acceptance/rejection method appears more complex than necessary for this small example but the approach applies to any discrete probability distribution and, as will be seen, also applies to variables sampled from a continuous distribution.

The following example S-code generates a sample of 5000 random values from the illustrative probability distribution, tabulates these values, and computes the estimated mean and variance as well as a z-statistic to assess the deviation of the sample mean from the expected value of 2:

```
> n<- 10000
> # probability distribution
> p<- c(4,3,2,1)/10
> p
[1] 0.4 0.3 0.2 0.1
> u<- ceiling(4*runif(n))
> ran1<- ifelse(runif(n)<p[u]/max(p),u,999)
```

```
> # proportion accepted
> sum(ifelse(ran1==999,0,1))/n
[1] 0.632
> # ran1=vector of random values (1,2,3 and 4)
> ran1<- ran1[ran1!=999]
> ran1<- ran1[1:5000]
> table(ran1)/5000
      1      2      3      4
 0.3972 0.3006 0.2038 0.0984
> mean(ran1)
[1] 1.992089
> var(ran1)
[1] 1.015132
> ztest<- (mean(ran1)-2)*sqrt(n)
> ztest
[1] -0.5594199
> 2*(1-pnorm(abs(ztest)))
[1] 0.5758752.
```

This example S-code illustrates the general acceptance/rejection approach. If the goal is only to generate 5000 random values from the given discrete probability distribution, then

```
> x0<- rep(1:4,4:1)
> ran2<- sample(x0,5000,replace=T)
> table(ran2)/5000
      1      2      3      4
 0.4058 0.2998 0.1912 0.1032
```

simply provides such a sample.

RANDOM SAMPLE FROM A DISCRETE PROBABILITY DISTRIBUTION— INVERSE TRANSFORM METHOD

Despite the complicated sounding name, using an inverse transformation to generate a discrete random variable with a specific probability distribution is straightforward. The first step is to divide the interval between 0 and 1 into a series of segments. The length of each segment is equal to a probability from the specified discrete probability distribution. The first segment has length equal to p_1, the second segment has length equal to p_2, and so forth until the last segment has length equal to p_k. Since the sum of probabilities p_i from a probability distribution is equal to one ($\sum p_i = 1$), the lengths perfectly divide the unit interval into the required k segments. That is,

segment 1 has length p_1 and covers from 0 to p_1
segment 2 has length p_2 and covers from p_1 to $p_1 + p_2$
segment 3 has length p_3 and covers from $p_1 + p_2$ to $p_1 + p_2 + p_3$
segment 4 has length p_4 and covers from $p_1 + p_2 + p_3$ to $p_1 + p_2 + p_3 + p_4$
and so forth.

The interval cut-points are the cumulative probabilities for the given discrete probability distribution or $F(x) = P(X \leq x) = p_1 + p_2 + p_3 + \cdots + p_x$. The second step is to generate a continuous, uniformly distributed random variable u between 0 to 1. The location of this variable determines the value selected for the random variable X. If u is found in the first segment, then $X = 1$; if u is found in the second segment, then $X = 2$; if u is found in the third segment, then $X = 3$, and so on. The value X is then a random selection from the discrete probability distribution used to construct the line segments.

Continuing the example where X takes on the values 1, 2, 3, or 4. The cumulative probabilities are $P(X \leq 1) = 0.4$, $P(X \leq 2) = 0.7$, $P(X \leq 3) = 0.9$, and $P(X \leq 4) = 1.0$ (cumulative probability distribution $F(x)$—Figure 3.8). Example S-code that produces 5000 random values of X with the example probability distribution is

```
> n<- 5000
> # probability distribution
> p<- c(4,3,2,1)/10
> p
> # cumulative probability distribution
[1] 0.4 0.3 0.2 0.1
> f<- c(0,cumsum(p))
```

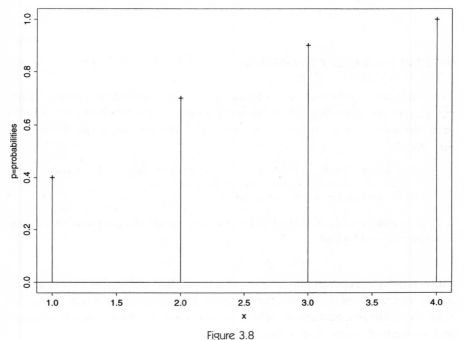

Cumulative probabilities for x = 1, 2, 3, and 4

Figure 3.8

```
> f
[1] 0.0 0.4 0.7 0.9 1.0
> ran2<- cut(runif(n),f,labels=c(1,2,3,4))
> table(ran2)/n
       1       2       3       4
  0.4084 0.2916 0.1988 0.1012
> mean(ran2)
[1] 1.9886
> var(ran2)
[1] 0.984667
> ztest<- (mean(ran2)-2)*sqrt(n)
> ztest
[1] -0.8061017
> 2*(1-pnorm(abs(ztest)))
[1] 0.4201842.
```

The following describes the inverse transformation method geometrically: a random discrete value is found by extending a line horizontally from a randomly selected point between 0 and 1 on the vertical axis until it intersects the cumulative probability function. The point on the x-axis directly below the intersection is then a randomly selected value from the distribution used to construct the cumulative probability function. Again, the pattern of generating a random variable in this simple case generalizes to more complicated discrete cases and, furthermore, the inverse transformation approach can be used to generate random continuous variables with given probability distributions (to be discussed).

BINOMIAL PROBABILITY DISTRIBUTION

The binomial distribution is a centrally important discrete probability distribution and the following defines some of its properties. A binomially distributed variable is a summary of a series of variables with two outcomes. Specifically,

1. a binary variable X_i is either 1 or 0 with probabilities p or $1 - p$, respectively,
2. each X_i variable is statistically independent, and
3. the probability p is the same for all values X_i.

The binomial variable X is the sum of n binary values of X_i (sometimes called a Bernoulli variable) or

$$X = X_1 + X_2 + \cdots + X_n.$$

More simply, X represents the count of the number of times X_i equals 1. The binary character of X_i makes the variable X applicable to a wide range of situations with two outcomes—alive or dead, male or female, case or control, and, in general, event A or event not A.

The probability associated with a specific outcome $X = x$, denoted as p_x, is given by

$$p_x = P(X = x) = \binom{n}{x} p^x (1 - p)^{n-x} \quad \text{where } x = 0, 1, 2, \cdots, n.$$

The term $\binom{n}{x}$ is the number of different ways x values of 1 and $n - x$ values of 0 can occur among n values of X_i and is evaluated in the usual way, $n!/[(n - x)!x!]$ (Chapter 1—binomial coefficients). The quantity $p^x(1 - p)^{n-x}$ is the probability of a specific configuration of 1's and 0's. The product of these two quantities is the probability that x values of 1 and $n - x$ values of 0 occur in any order making $X = x$.

The $n + 1$ binomial probabilities can be calculated with the S-function *dbinom( )* (Table 1.4). To illustrate, for $n = 10$, $p = 0.4$, and $x = 0, 1, 2, 3, \cdots,$ 10, the binomial probabilities are given by

```
> # probability distribution
> n<- 10
> p<- 0.4
> x<- 0:n
> round(dbinom(x,n,p),3)
[1] 0.006 0.040 0.121 0.215 0.251 0.201 0.111
    0.042 0.011 0.002 0.000.
```

Example S-code that also produces binomial probabilities is

```
choose<- function(n,x){gamma(n+1)/(gamma(x+1)*gamma(n-x+1))}
round(choose(n,x)*p^x*(1-p)^(n-x),3)
[1] 0.006 0.040 0.121 0.215 0.251 0.201 0.111
    0.042 0.011 0.002 0.000.
```

The cumulative binomial probabilities are $P(X \leq x)$ and *pbinom(x, n, p)* produces these probabilities:

```
> # cumulative probability distribution
> round(pbinom(x,n,p),3)
[1] 0.006 0.046 0.167 0.382 0.633 0.834 0.945 0.988
    0.998 1.000 1.000.
```

or

```
> round(cumsum(dbinom(x,n,p)),3)
[1] 0.006 0.046 0.167 0.382 0.633 0.834 0.945 0.988
    0.998 1.000 1.000.
```

Formally, $p_x = P(X = x) = \binom{10}{x}(0.4)^x(1 - 0.4)^{10-x}$.

A direct result from these binomial probabilities is that the expected value of X for a series of n observations is

$$\text{expected value of } X = np$$

and the associated variance (derived in [5] or [6]) is

$$\text{variance}(X) = np(1 - p).$$

The expected value is $np = 10(0.4) = 4$ and the variance is $np(1 - p) = 10(0.4)(0.6) = 2.4$ when $n = 10$ and $p = 0.4$. Since the expected value is $ex = \sum xp_x$ and the variance is $\sum(x - ex)^2 p_x$ for any discrete probability distribution, then

```
> px<- dbinom(x,n,p)
> ex<- sum(x*px)
> v<- sum((x-ex)^2*px)
> cat("expectation =",round(ex,3)," variance =",
    round(v,3),"\n")
  expectation = 4 variance = 2.4.
```

Random binomial values are produced in the usual way with the S-function r + root.name or $rbinom(number, size, probability)$. For 20 random binomial values with $n = 10$ and $p = 0.4$, then

```
>  rbinom(20,n,p)
[1] 4 2 3 5 6 2 3 2 3 3 4 5 2 5 3 3 6 4 4 3.
```

A fragment of S-code that also generates $k = 20$ random binomial values is

```
> k<- 20
> rtemp<- matrix(ifelse(runif(n*k)<p,1,0),n,k)
> apply(rtemp,2,sum)
 [1] 1 5 3 2 4 3 3 5 3 5 5 1 4 2 5 2 4 3 3
```

where again $n = 10$ with $p = 0.4$. Acceptance/rejection or inverse transformation sampling can also be used to generate binomial random variables for specified values of n and p.

Analyses of observations with two outcomes are frequently based on the binomial distribution. The outcome is then required to occur or not occur with a constant probability and these occurrences must be independent. Data collected on the presence and absence of a specific genetic trait detected in blood called Esterase D illustrate (Table 3.1).

Assuming the measured individuals are independently sampled and individuals within the same racial group have the same probability of possessing the trait (EsD), then statistical tests and $(1 - \alpha)\%$ confidence intervals constructed from the estimated proportions of EsD-positive individuals can be constructed using the S-function $prop.test(\,)$ In other words, the properties of the estimated summary values are based on the conjecture or knowledge that the observations within racial categories have a binomial distribution.

Table 3.1. Frequency of Esterase D in four racial groups

	white	black	Hispanic	Asian
EsD positive	794	626	1077	56
EsD negative	231	144	401	867
total	1025	770	1478	923

For whites, the proportion of individuals with the *EsD* trait is $\hat{p}_{white} = 794/1025 = 0.775$ with a 95% confidence interval of

```
> prop.test(794,1025,conf.level=0.95)$)conf.int
[1] 0.7475518    0.7996267.
```

Two proportions can be compared with *prop.test*( ). For example, comparing the proportion of *EsD* among whites (0.775) with the same value observed in the Hispanic sample (0.729) is achieved by

```
> x<- c(794,1077)
> n<- c(1025,1478)
> prop.test(x,n,conf.level=0.99)

      2-sample test for equality of proportions
            with continuity correction

data: x out of n
X-squared = 6.5286, df = 1, p-value = 0.0106
alternative hypothesis: two.sided
99 percent confidence interval:
  0.0002035023    0.0916899595
sample estimates:
 prop'n in Group 1    prop'n in Group 2
          0.7746341              0.7286874.
```

Like many S-functions, specific values can be extracted from the *prop.test*( ) command. For example, a confidence interval based on the observed difference between these two proportions $\hat{p}_{white} - \hat{p}_{hispanic} = 794/1025 - 1077/1478 = 0.775 - 0.729 = 0.046$ is

```
> prop.test(x,n,conf.level=0.99)$conf.int
[1] 0.0002035023 0.0916899595
```

or, the *p*-value from the test of the difference $\hat{p}_{white} - \hat{p}_{hispanic}$ $(p_{white} = p_{hispanic}?)$ is

```
> prop.test(x,n)$p.value
[1] 0.01061548.
```

To repeat, these examples and other applications of *prop.test* require the data to have at least an approximate binomial distribution.

HYPERGEOMETRIC PROBABILITY DISTRIBUTION

A hypergeometric probability distribution, like the binomial distribution, describes a count from a sample of values with two outcomes. The fundamental difference between a hypergeometric and a binomial variable concerns the way the population is sampled. The sampling process associated with a binomial variable leaves the population unchanged (sampling with replacement—each binary event has the same probability). In the hypergeometric case, each sampled observation reduces the population size by one (sampling without replacement—each binary event has a different probability). It is sampling from a constantly changing population that produces the characteristics of a hypergeometric variable. Formally, a hypergeometric distributed variable is made up of a series of variables with two outcomes where

1. a binary variable X_i is either 1 or 0,
2. each X_i variable is statistically independent, and
3. the probability associated with X_i depends only on the composition of the population at the time each observation is selected (not constant).

The hypergeometric variable X is also the sum of n binary values of X_i or

$$X = X_1 + X_2 + \cdots + X_n$$

where the sample size is n. Like a binomial variable, the variable X represents the count of the number of times X_i equals 1.

Consider a population of size N where m members have a specific characteristic and $N - m$ do not. A sample of n individuals is selected from this population. The random variable X represents the number sampled with the characteristic where each sampled observation is selected independently, without replacement. The word "independently" in this context means that the probability that any individual is selected depends only on the composition of the population at the time of selection and does not depend in any way on whether the individual possesses or does not possess the characteristic. The minimum value of X is the larger of 0 or $n + m - N$ and the maximum value of X is the smaller of the values m or n. The discrete probability distribution describing X, called the hypergeometric distribution, is given by

$$p_x = P(X = x) = \frac{\binom{m}{x}\binom{N-m}{n-x}}{\binom{N}{n}} = \frac{\binom{n}{x}\binom{N-n}{m-x}}{\binom{N}{m}}.$$

For a population size N, m members with the characteristic and $(N - m)$ without the characteristic, a sample of size n produces a description of the population in terms of a 2×2 table (Table 3.2).

Table 3.2. The notation for a sample of size n from a population of size N sampled without replacement

	with the characteristic	without the characteristic	total
sampled	X	$n - X$	n
not sampled	$m - X$	$(N - m) - (n - X)$	$N - n$
total	m	$N - m$	N

A classic application of the hypergeometric probability distribution involves a capture/recapture strategy for estimating population size. To estimate the size of a "closed" population, a preliminary sample is collected and the "captured" observations are marked. These marked observations are returned to the population, which is then resampled. The number of marked observations ("recaptured") in the second sample relates to the size of the population. If a high proportion of the resampled observations are marked, then the population is likely to be relatively small; if a low proportion of the second sample are marked, then the population is likely to be large. The first sample produces m marked population members and $N - m$ unmarked population members. The second sample of n observations produces X marked members and the count X has a hypergeometric distribution (Table 3.2) when the population members are sampled independently. In fact, there are problems with applying this model to many populations, particularly the assumption that the "tagged" observations have the same probability of being selected on the second sampling as the "non-tagged" observations. That is, in applied situations it is not always possible to collect independent observations. Nevertheless, this capture/recapture approach frequently provides estimates of the size of free living animal populations such as whales, mountain lions, and wild dogs.

Hypergeometric probabilities ($N = 20$, $m = 10$, and $n = 6$) are calculated with the following S-functions:

```
> N<- 20
> m<- 10
> n<- 6
> x<- max(0,n+m-N):min(m,n)
> # probability distribution
> round(dhyper(x,m,N-m,n),3)
[1] 0.005 0.065 0.244 0.372 0.244 0.065 0.005

> # cumulative probability distribution
> round(phyper(x,m,N-m,n),3)
[1] 0.005 0.070 0.314 0.686 0.930 0.995 1.000
> round(cumsum(dhyper(x,m,N-m,n)),3)
[1] 0.005 0.070 0.314 0.686 0.930 0.995 1.000.
```

Using hypergeometric probabilities, the expected value of the hypergeometric distribution is (derived in [5] or [6])

$$expected\ value\ of\ X = n\left(\frac{m}{N}\right)$$

with associated variance

$$variance(x) = n\left(\frac{m}{N}\right)\left(1 - \frac{m}{N}\right)\left(\frac{N - n}{N - 1}\right).$$

The term $(N - n)/(N - 1)$ is called the finite population correction factor. This factor causes the variance of x to decrease as the proportion of the population sampled increases (as n/N becomes closer to 1.0). Ultimately, when the entire population is sampled ($n = N$), the variance is zero since x must always equal m for any sample ($variance(x) = 0$).

If N is much larger than n, the finite correction factor has negligible influence and the hypergeometric and the binomial probability distributions become approximately equal. Not surprisingly, the expectation and variance of the hypergeometric distribution are also essentially the same as the expectation and variance associated with a binomial distribution when $N >> n$ and $n/N = p$.

The expected value and the variance associated with the hypergeometric distribution are calculated by the usual expressions. For example when $N = 20$, $m = 10$, and $n = 6$, then

```
> px<- dhyper(x,m,N-m,n)
> ex<- sum(x*px)
> v<- sum((x-ex)^2*px)
> cat("expectation =",round(ex,3)," variance =",
    round(v,3),"\n")
  expectation = 3    variance = 1.105.
```

An S-function to select a random value from a hypergeometric distribution is

```
hprob<- function(N,m,n){
xtemp<- c(rep(0,N-m),rep(1,m))
id<- rank(runif(N))[1:n]
sum(xtemp[id])
}
```

and, as usual, the S-function $rhyper(nsample, m, N - m, n)$ also produces $nsample$ random values from a hypergeometric distribution (Table 4.1). For example, $nsample = 20$ random hypergeometric values are

```
>rhyper(nsample,m,N-m,n)
[1] 3 2 5 2 2 3 3 2 2 3 2 3 3 3 4 3 3 2 4 3
```

where again $N = 20$, $m = 10$, and $n = 6$.

POISSON PROBABILITY DISTRIBUTION

The Poisson distribution, like the binomial and hypergeometric distributions, is an important discrete statistical distribution and also describes a count from a series of binary outcomes. The maximum value for a binomial or hypergeometric variable is the total number of sampled observations where, in principle, a Poisson variable can take on any integer count. Formally, a Poisson distributed random variable is made up of a series of variables with two outcomes where

1. a binary variable X_i is either 1 or 0 occurring with probability p and $1 - p$,

2. each X_i variable is statistically independent, and
3. the probability p is constant while the number of binary variables X_i is large (n is large—in theory, $n = \infty$).

The Poisson variable X is also the sum of values of X_i or

$$X = X_1 + X_2 + X_3 + \cdots.$$

Like the binomial and hypergeometric variables, the count X represents the number of times X_i equals 1. The probabilities associated with a Poisson distributed variable X are given by

$$p_x = P(X = x) = \frac{\lambda^x e^{-\lambda}}{x!}$$

where $x = 0, 1, 2, 3, \cdots$. A single parameter (represented by λ) determines the Poisson probability distribution.

The expectation and variance are derived from the probabilities p_x. The expected value of a Poisson distributed variable X is

expected value of $X = \lambda$

with associated variance (derived in [5] or [6]) given by

variance$(X) = \lambda.$

For example, for $\lambda = 2$, the Poisson probabilities are

```
> # probability distribution
> x<- 0:10
> lam<- 2
> round(dpois(x,lam),3)
[1] 0.135 0.271 0.271 0.180 0.090 0.036 0.012
     0.003 0.001 0.000 0.000

> # cumulative probability distribution
> round(ppois(x,lam),3)
[1] 0.135 0.406 0.677 0.857 0.947 0.983 0.995
     0.999 1.000 1.000 1.000.
```

To verify that the expectation and variance of a Poisson distribution is the parameter λ, for $\lambda = 2$ the expectation and variance calculated by applying the general expressions for discrete probability distributions are

```
> x<- 0:30
> px<- dpois(x,lam)
> ex<- sum(x*px)
> v<- sum((x-ex)^2*px)
> cat("expectation =",round(ex,3)," variance =",
        round(v,3),"\n")
 expectation = 2 variance =2.
```

Decay of radioactive particles is a classic example of a phenomenon accurately described by a Poisson distribution. Each atom in a piece of radioactive material either decays or not (binary variable X_i). Clearly the number of possible observations n is huge (equal to the number of atoms). However, the probability p of any one atom decaying is small (detected by a counter). It is assumed that p is constant, which is equivalent to postulating that the atoms within the observed radioactive material decay randomly. The variable X is the count of decays per unit time and has been observed to be closely approximated by a Poisson distribution.

Early data collected by Rutherford and Geiger in 1910 [7] show the counts of decaying α-particles observed for intervals of an eighth of a minute. The values x_j represent the counts per unit time and have frequency denoted by f_j (Table 3.3). Table 3.3 is a shorthand summary of $n = 2608$ individual counts—0 occurs 57 times, 1 occurs 203 times, 2 occurs 383 times $\cdots$.

The estimate of the parameter λ is the mean of the 2608 observed counts. The count of nine or more within an interval (9^+) is coded as 9 for simplicity of estimation, incurring a slight downward bias. In symbols, $\hat{\lambda} = \bar{x} = \sum f_j x_j / n = 10070/2608 = 3.861$ (justified in Chapter 5) where $j = 1, 2, 3, \cdots, 10 =$ the number of categories.

```
> # Poisson data?
> f<- c(57,203,383,525,532,408,273,139,45,43)
> n<- length(f)
> x<- rep(0:(n-1),f)
> table(x)
   0   1   2   3   4   5   6   7  8  9
  57 203 383 525 532 408 273 139 45 43
> lam<- mean(x)
> lam
 [1] 3.861196
> p<- dpois(0:(n-2),lam)
> p[n]<- 1-sum(p)
> ex<- round(sum(f)*p,1)
> cbind(f,ex)
          f     ex
 [1,]    57   54.9
 [2,]   203  211.9
 [3,]   383  409.1
 [4,]   525  526.5
 [5,]   532  508.3
 [6,]   408  392.5
 [7,]   273  252.6
 [8,]   139  139.3
 [9,]    45   67.2
[10,]    43   45.7.
```

The comparison of the observed (f) to the expected (ex) counts based on the Poisson distribution shows a close correspondence ("fit"). Empirical evidence

Table 3.3. α-particles counts

x_j	0	1	2	3	4	5	6	7	8	9^+	total
f_j	57	203	383	525	532	408	273	139	45	43	2608

such as these data indicates that decay of radioactive material frequently appears to conform to the requirements of a Poisson distribution.

The binomial distribution becomes indistinguishable from the Poisson distribution when n (the number of X_i-values) is large and $P(X_i = 1) = p$ is small. The expectation and variance of a Poisson distribution are then essentially equal to the expectation and variance associated with a binomial distribution. Situations arise where the variable observed is binary, the number of observations n is large, and p is small and constant, implying that the Poisson distribution can essentially replace a binomial distribution as a description of a phenomenon with two outcomes. For the application of a Poisson distribution knowledge of p and n is unnecessary; only the parameter λ must be known or estimated to generate Poisson probabilities. A partial list of phenomena observed to fit a Poisson distributions is: cases of leukemia, deaths by horse kicks, numbers of radioactive decay particles, arrivals of patients at a doctor's waiting rooms, typographical errors, numbers of individuals over 100 years old, supreme court appointments, occurrences of suicide, telephone calls arriving at a switchboard, $\cdots$.

Random Poisson variables are generated efficiently with either the acceptance/rejection or the inverse transformation sampling. The example S-programs that follow illustrate both approaches for $\lambda = 2$:

Acceptance/rejection

```
> # acceptance/rejection sampling
> n<- 10000
> lam<- 2
> u<- ceiling(10*runif(n))
> # S-function generates Poisson probabilities
> p<- dpois(0:10,lam)
> round(p,3)
[1] 0.135 0.271 0.271 0.180 0.090 0.036 0.012
    0.003 0.001 0.000 0.000
> x<- ifelse(runif(n)<p[u]/max(p),u-1,999)
> x<- x[x!=999]
> x<- x[1:2000]
> # x-values have a Poisson distribution
> mean(x)
[1] 2.007853
> var(x)
[1] 2.191288
```

Inverse transformation method

```
> # inverse transformation sampling
> n<- 2000
> lam<- 2
> # S-function generates cumulative Poisson probabilities
> pp<- c(0,ppois(0:10,lam),1)
> round(pp,3)
[1] 0.000 0.135 0.406 0.677 0.857 0.947 0.983
    0.995 0.999 1.000 1.000 1.000
```

```
> x<- cut(runif(n),pp)
> x<- x-1
> #x-values have a Poisson distribution
> mean(x)
[1] 1.965
> var(x)
[1] 1.900725.
```

Both S-programs result in S-vectors x containing 2000 random values with Poisson distributions ($\lambda = 2$). Of course, the S-function *rpois*( ) achieves the same result.

SPLUS—rpois( )

```
# SPLUS function rpois
> n<- 2000
> lam<- 2
> x<- rpois(n,lam)
> mean(x)
[1] 1.945
> var(x)
[1] 2.059005.
```

GEOMETRIC PROBABILITY DISTRIBUTION

The geometric probability distribution is another discrete probability distribution and the following defines some of its properties. A geometric distributed random variable is again made up of a series of variables with two outcomes. Formally,

1. a binary variable X_i is either 1 or 0 with probabilities p or $1 - p$, respectively,
2. each X_i variable is statistically independent, and
3. the probability p is the same for all X_i.

But unlike the previous discrete distributions, X is the count of the number of times X_i equals 0 preceding the first time X_i equals 1. This probability distribution is an example of a waiting time distribution since it involves the probabilities of waiting until a specified event occurs. For example, say a mythical country exists where citizens are subject to the family planning rule that all couples must continue to have children until a male child is born and once a male is born these families are not allowed to have further children. The probability that a family contains a specific number of female children (all families have one male) is then described by a geometric probability distribution.

The probability associated with a specific outcome of X is given by the expression

$$p_x = P(X = x) = p(1 - p)^x \qquad x = 0, 1, 2, 3, \cdots.$$

In words, p_x is the probability that x events ($x_i = 0$) occur before the occurrence of a specific complementary event ($x_i = 1$). The probabilities p_x yield the expectation of X for a geometric distribution (parameter $= p$) from the previously given expression and

$$\text{expectation of } X = \frac{1-p}{p}$$

with associated variance

$$\text{variance}(X) = \frac{1-p}{p^2}.$$

The expectation shows, perhaps surprisingly, that the family planning rule in the mythical country produces an equal number of males and females. The expected number of female children born before a male is one when $p = P(\text{male}) = P(\text{female}) = 0.5$, yielding an expected family size of two.

Computationally using the S-root name *geom*, the geometric probabilities for $p = 0.5$ are

```
> probability distribution
> x<- 0:10
> p<- 0.5
> round(dgeom(x,p),3)
[1] 0.500 0.250 0.125 0.062 0.031 0.016 0.008
    0.004 0.002 0.001 0.000

> # cumulative probability distribution
> round(pgeom(x,p),3)
[1] 0.500 0.750 0.875 0.938 0.969 0.984 0.992
    0.996 0.998 0.999 1.000.
```

The S-calculated expected value and variance follow as

```
<- 0:30
> px<- dgeom(x,p)
> ex<- sum(x*px)
> v<- sum((x-ex)^2*px)
> cat("expectation =",round(ex,3)," variance =",
    round(v,3),"\n")
  expectation = 1   variance = 2.
```

A tricky way to generate random values from a geometric distribution is

```
> n<- 20
> p<- 0.5
> x<- trunc(log(runif(n))/log(1-p))
> x
[1] 0 0 4 0 0 0 0 0 0 1 1 1 0 1 0 1 0 1 2 2.
```

The S-vector x contains $n = 20$ geometrically distributed random variables where $p = 0.5$. The S-function *rgeom*(n, p) also produces n random values from a geometric distribution with parameter p and, for example,

```
> rgeom (n,p)
[1] 1 0 2 0 0 2 0 0 0 0 0 4 1 1 0 0 6 4 3.
```

RANDOM SAMPLES FROM A CONTINUOUS DISTRIBUTION

Unlike a discrete probability distribution, continuous variables cannot be characterized in terms of discrete probabilities, $P(X = x) = p_x$. In fact, the probability that a continuous variable equals any particular value is zero. However, a continuous probability function is effectively characterized by cumulative probabilities where $F(x) = P(X \leq x)$ provides a description of the probability distribution. As before, these cumulative probabilities are calculated with S-functions by placing a p before the root name of the probability distribution (Table 1.4).

Probabilities associated with a continuous variable are equally expressed in terms of a density function. A probability density function describes a continuous variable in much the same way a histogram describes a sample of data (Chapter 2). The area under a density function curve reflects the cumulative probabilities. The area to the left of a specific value corresponds to the probability of observing an equal or smaller random value. The entire area enclosed by a probability density function is exactly one, since the probability of being smaller than or equal to the largest possible value is necessarily one, $F(x_{largest}) = 1$. More rigorously, the area to the left of a specified point x is represented by $F(x)$ and

$$cumulative\ probability\ distribution = P(X \leq x) = F(x) = \int_a^x f(u)du$$

where $f(u)$ is the density function associated with a specific probability distribution and a represents the smallest possible value of the random variable X. It is, therefore, generally true that the probability density function is

$$density\ function = f(x) = \frac{d}{dx}F(x).$$

The quantity $f(x_0)$ is called the ordinate of the density function at the value x_0. Ordinate values are calculated by placing the symbol d in front of the S-function root name of the probability distribution. Figure 3.9 shows these two versions of a probability distribution ($f(x)$ and $F(x)$ distributions) for two cases—the positive triangular distribution and the normal distribution. For the normal distribution, the density function $f(x)$ is described by $dnorm(x)$ and the cumulative distribution function $F(x)$ is described by $pnorm(x)$.

The expectation of a continuous variable X has an expression analogous to the discrete probability distribution function and is defined by

$$expectation\ of\ X = \int_a^b uf(u)du$$

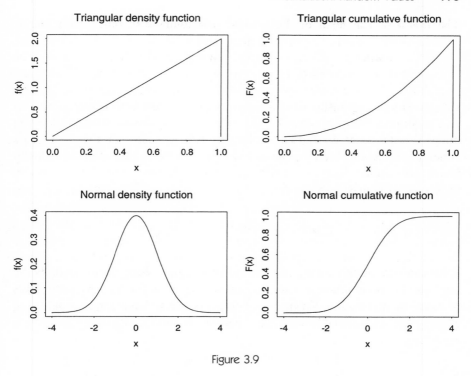

Figure 3.9

where the symbols a and b represent the smallest and largest possible values of the variable X. The variance of a continuous probability distribution is defined as

$$variance(x) = \int_{a}^{b} (u - expectation)^2 f(u) du.$$

A simple probability distribution is the positive triangular distribution (Figure 3.9—top). The cumulative probability function has a triangular shape describing the probabilities associated with a variable x between 0 and 1 where large values of x are more likely than small. The mathematical expression of the cumulative probability function $F(x)$ is found with plane geometry. The area of a right triangle is *half* × *base* × *height*. For the triangular distribution, $F(x) = P(X \leq x) = \frac{1}{2} \times x \times 2x = x^2$ is the area to the left of a value x (right triangle, base = x) for x between 0 and 1. Therefore, $dF(x)/dx = dx^2/dx = 2x = f(x)$ is the probability density for $0 \leq x \leq 1$ (Figure 3.9—top). For the positive triangular distribution: *total area* = 1.0, *expectation* = 2/3, and *variance* = 1/18.

Also shown in Figure 3.9 (bottom) are the density function $f(x)$ and the cumulative probability distribution $F(x)$ for the standard normal distribution.

The mathematical form of the normal probability distribution function is derived elsewhere [8]. The normal density function is

$$normal\ density\ function = f(x) = \frac{1}{\sigma\sqrt{2\pi}}e^{-\frac{1}{2}\left(\frac{x-\mu}{\sigma}\right)^2} \qquad -\infty < x < \infty.$$

The density function $f(x)$ describes a symmetric curve with center (mean) μ and maximum height $= 1/\sigma\sqrt{2\pi}$. The parameter σ (standard deviation) determines the spread of the normal probability function and is a measure of the variability associated with the variable X. The corresponding cumulative probability distribution function remains the area under the density function curve to the left of a given value and is

$$cumulative\ probability\ distribution = P(X \le x_0) = F(x_0) = \frac{1}{\sigma\sqrt{2\pi}} \int\limits_{-\infty}^{(x_0-\mu)/\sigma} e^{-\frac{1}{2}z^2}\,dz.$$

Numerical methods exist to evaluate an integral. Using these methods the cumulative probabilities, the mean, and the variance for a given continuous probability distribution can be calculated. For example, an expression called Bode's rule approximates an integral with a sum and is

$$A_i = \int\limits_{x_i}^{x_{i+4}} f(u)du \approx \frac{2h}{45}[7f(x_i) + 32f(x_{i+1}) + 12f(x_{i+2}) + 32f(x_{i+3}) + 7f(x_{i+4})]$$

where h is the difference between the five equally spaced x-values (i.e., $x_{i+1} - x_i = h$). The integral from x_0 to x_n is then

$$area = \sum A_i \approx \int\limits_{x_0}^{x_n} f(u)du \qquad i = 0, 4, 8, \cdots, 4k,$$

where k values of A_i are summed. The accuracy of Bode's rule increases as the number of intervals k used to approximate the integral increases. Bode's rule yields approximate values for the expectation $= \int uf(u)du$ and the variance $= \int(u - expectation)^2 f(u)du$ and can be computed with a specially designed S-function. For example,

```
moments<- function(x0,xn,k,f){
#integral of f(x) from x0 to xn divided into k intervals
b<- c(7,rep(c(32,12,32,14),k))
b[length(b)]<- 7
x<- seq(x0,xn,length=length(b))
h<- x[2]-x[1]
area<- sum((2*h/45)*b*f(x))
mean<- sum((2*h/45)*b*x*f(x))
variance<- sum((2*h/45)*b*(x-mean)^2*f(x))
round(cbind(area,mean,variance),3)
}
```

and

```
> # normal distribution mean = 1 and variance = 2
> f<- function(x){exp(-.5*(x-1)^2/2)/sqrt(2*pi*2)}
> moments(-10,10,10,f)
      area mean variance
[1,]     1    1    2.000
> # normal distribution mean = 3 and variance = 0.5
> f<- function(x){exp(-.5*(x-3)^2/0.5)/sqrt(2*pi*0.5)}
> moments(-10,10,30,f)
      area mean variance
[1,]     1    3      0.5
> # positive triangular distribution
> f<- function(x){2*x}
> moments(0,1,10,f)
      area   mean variance
[1,]     1  0.667    0.056
> # uniform distribution (0,1)
> f<- function(x){1}
> moments(0,1,10,f)
      area mean variance
[1,]     1  0.5    0.083
> # uniform distribution (0,5)
> f<- function(x){1/5}
> moments(0,5,5,f)
      area mean variance
[1,]     1  2.5     2.08
> #exponential distribution -- parameter lambda = 0.5
> f<- function(x){0.5*exp(-0.5*x)}
> moments(0,50,50,f)
      area mean variance
[1,]     1    2       4.
```

Numerical methods are frequently not necessary since the expectations and variances can be derived in closed-form expressions for many continuous probability functions. For example, the expectation of a uniform distribution on the interval a to b is $(a+b)/2$ and the associated variance is $(b-a)^2/12$ from direct integration.

INVERSE TRANSFORM METHOD

For a continuous probability distribution the inverse transformation method of generating a random variable is easy, fast and provides values for most common probability distributions. The approach does not differ in principle from the previous discrete case. Let X represent a continuous random variable with a cumulative probability distribution function $F(x)$. If U is a uniformly distributed random variable between 0 and 1, then

$$X = F^{-1}(U)$$

where X has the probability distribution function determined by F. The relationship shows that a uniform variable can be transformed into a variable with the cumulative distribution function $F(x)$ if the inverse function of F (denoted F^{-1}) is known or can be closely approximated. To indicate why, the following is straightforward: when $X = F^{-1}(U)$, then

$$P(X \leq x) = P(F^{-1}(U) \leq x) = P(U \leq F(x)) = F(x).$$

To illustrate, for the positive triangular distribution $F(x) = x^2$, therefore $F^{-1}(x) = \sqrt{x}$. To generate a random value, first a random value u between 0 and 1 with a uniform distribution is selected, then $x = F^{-1}(u) = \sqrt{u}$ has a positive triangular distribution. To generate a random value from a positive triangular distribution where the smallest possible observation is a and the largest b, then $x = a + (b - a)\sqrt{u}$.

A useful continuous distribution function defined by the probability density

$$f(x) = \lambda e^{-\lambda x} \qquad 0 \leq x \leq \infty$$

is called an exponential probability distribution. The exponential distribution is frequently applied in the analysis of survival or failure time data (Chapter 8). A single parameter λ defines the exponential density. This distribution provides another example of applying an inverse transformation to produce random variables with specific statistical properties. The cumulative distribution function is

$$F(x) = \int_0^x \lambda e^{-\lambda u} du = 1 - e^{-\lambda x},$$

making the inverse function

$$F^{-1}(x) = -\log(1 - x)/\lambda.$$

When

$$x = -\log(1 - u)/\lambda = -\log(u)/\lambda,$$

the value x is a random selection from an exponential distribution with parameter λ when, as before, u is a random uniform variable between 0 and 1. Selection of a variable or variables from an exponential distribution for a given value of the parameter λ is also accomplished with an S-function following the usual pattern, *rexp(number of values, parameter value)*.

Geometrically, the inverse transformation method is no more than reading the cumulative distribution function backwards. Instead of a value x leading to a probability of $F(x)$, a value of u is selected at random leading to a value $F^{-1}(u) = x$, which is a random value with the cumulative probability distribution $F(x)$. A set of $n = 10$ random uniform variables is

$$u = \{0.89, 0.67, 0.78, 0.51, 0.34, 0.40, 0.74, 0.61, 0.98, 0.84\}.$$

To produce 10 corresponding random values with an exponential distribution (parameter = λ = 0.5), then $x = -\log(1-u)/0.5$ and

$$x = \{4.41, 2.22, 3.03, 1.43, 0.83, 1.02, 2.69, 1.88, 7.82, 3.67\}.$$

Figure 3.10 displays geometrically the process of transforming the 10 random uniform values u to the 10 random exponential values x.

The S-language defines an inverse cumulative distribution function by placing a q before the root name of the distribution (Table 1.4). For example, the inverse of the cumulative standard normal distribution function is given by $q + norm(\ )$ and, therefore, the S-functions $qnorm(runif(n))$ produces n random variables with a standard normal distribution. The S-function $qnorm(runif(n), m, s)$ produces n random values from a normal distribution with mean = m and standard deviation = s. For a chi-square distribution, $qchisq(runif(n), df)$ similarly produces n random values selected from a chi-square distribution with df degrees of freedom or $qt(runif(n), df)$ yields n values from a t-distribution with df degrees of freedom. As noted earlier, the inverse transformation approach also applies to discrete distributions.

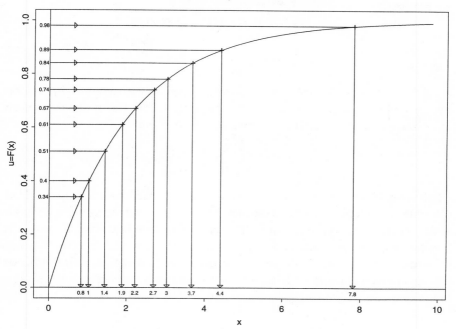

Figure 3.10

SIMULATING VALUES FROM THE NORMAL DISTRIBUTION

The normal distribution is fundamental to many statistical procedures. It plays a role as a model for the distribution of observed data but, more importantly, it plays a fundamental role as the distribution or approximate distribution of quantities calculated or estimated from observed data. Simulating values with a normal distribution is, not surprisingly, a significant part of statistical simulation in general.

The S-function that generates random normal values, as discussed, is

rnorm(number of observations, mean, standard deviation).

Since the variable $X = Z\sigma + \mu$ has a normal distribution with mean μ and standard deviation σ when Z has a standard normal distribution, two equivalent S-commands are

```
> x<- rnorm(100,4,2)
```
and
```
> x<- 2*rnorm(100)+4.
```

Both commands produce 100 random values from a normal distribution with mean = μ = 4 and standard deviation = σ = 2. A number of other ways to generate random normal values are worth exploring since they demonstrate specific approaches to this central problem.

The expression, derived by the mathematician Polya,

$$F(z) = \frac{1 + [1 - e^{-2z^2/\pi}]^{\frac{1}{2}}}{2} \qquad 0 \le z \le \infty$$

is a good but not excellent approximation to the cumulative normal probability distribution function. The inverse function allows the generation of an approximate random standard normal variate z where

$$z = F^{-1}(u) = s\sqrt{-\frac{\pi}{2}\log[1 - (2u - 1)^2]}$$

when $s = 1$ with probability 0.5 and $s = -1$ with probability 0.5. It is simple to generate a random uniform value between 0 and 1 and employ this approximate inverse function to generate an approximate standard normal value or a series of approximate standard normal values.

A better approximation to the inverse standard normal cumulative distribution function is achieved by employing a Hasting's approximation [9]. The approximation is

$$z = t - \frac{c_0 + c_1 t + c_2 t^2}{1 + b_1 t + b_2 t^2 + b_3 t^3} \qquad 0 \le z \le \infty$$

where $t = \sqrt{\log(1/u^2)}$ and

$$
\begin{aligned}
c_0 &= 2.515517 & b_1 &= 1.432788 \\
c_1 &= 0.802853 & b_2 &= 0.189269 \\
c_2 &= 0.010328 & b_3 &= 0.001308.
\end{aligned}
$$

A uniformly distributed value u is converted to t and z is then calculated. If $u < 0.5$, z is set to $-z$ giving z a standard normal distribution. The Hasting's approximation of $z = F^{-1}(p)$ has a maximum difference between the actual value and the approximate value of less than 0.0008 for all values of z.

An extremely efficient transformation that produces a pair of random standard normal variables, referred to as the Box-Muller [4] transformation, is

$$
z_1 = \sqrt{-2\log(u_1)}\cos(2\pi u_2)
$$

$$
z_2 = \sqrt{-2\log(u_1)}\sin(2\pi u_2)
$$

where u_1 and u_2 are two independent uniformly distributed random variables. The values z_1 and z_2 are then two independent random selections from a standard normal distribution.

The central limit theorem states that sums of independent variables have approximate normal distributions. The approximation is particularly accurate when the values summed come from a symmetric distribution. The sum of 12 independent uniform random variables has a mean value of 6, variance of 1 (each variate generated has expectation 0.5 and variance 1/12) and results from sampling a symmetric distribution. Therefore,

$$
z = \sum u_i - 6 \qquad i = 1, 2, 3, \cdots, 12
$$

has an approximate standard normal distribution where u_i represents the ith independent random uniform variable between 0 and 1.

Acceptance/rejection sampling also produces random values with a standard normal distribution. The density function of a standard normal distribution is given by

$$
f(z) = \frac{1}{\sqrt{2\pi}} e^{-\frac{1}{2}z^2}
$$

and the maximum value is $m = 1/\sqrt{2\pi}$ occurring at $z = 0$. To generate a random standard normal value, two independent uniform variables (u_1 and u_2) are used. The first variate (u_1) covers the range of the variable to be generated (e.g., between -3 and 3; approximate but reasonable range for the standard normal distribution). The second variate (u_2) is a uniform variable between 0 and 1. Then, if $u_2 < f(u_1)/m = e^{-0.5u_1^2}$ set $z = u_1$; if not, resample until a value z is accepted. The value z is then a random selection from a standard normal distribution. This process is essentially the same as the acceptance/rejection method described for a discrete probability distribution and applies to continuous distributions when the density function $f(x)$ is known.

Example S-code contrasting seven methods of generating n random standard normal values follows:

```
> n<- 1000

> # S-function
> z0<- rnorm(n)
> round(c(mean(z0),var(z0)),3)
[1] -0.007 1.041

> # inverse function
> z1<- qnorm(runif(n))
> round(c(mean(z1),var(z1)),3)
[1] -0.006 0.928

> # Polya's approximation
> ztemp<- sqrt((-pi/2)*log(1-(2*runif(n)-1)^2))
> z2<- ifelse(runif(n)<0.5,-ztemp,ztemp)
> round(c(mean(z2),var(z2)),3)
[1] -0.028 0.888

> # Hasting's approximation
> t<- sqrt(log(1/runif(n)^2))
> temp1<- 2.515517+0.802853*t+0.010328*t^2
> temp2<- 1+1.432788*t+0.189269*t^2+0.001308*t^3
> ztemp<- t-temp1/temp2
> z3<- ifelse(runif(n)<0.5,-ztemp,ztemp)
> round(c(mean(z3),var(z3)),3)
[1] 0.087 0.985

> # Box-Muller transformation
> u1<- runif(n)
> u2<- runif(n)
> z4<- sqrt(-2*log(u1))*cos(2*pi*u2)
> z5<- sqrt(-2*log(u1))*sin(2*pi*u2)
> round(c(mean(z4),var(z4)),3)
[1] 0.030 1.031
> round(c(mean(z5),var(z5)),3)
[1] 0.010 1.003

> # central limit theorem
> temp<- matrix(runif(12*n),12,n)
> z6<- apply(temp,2,sum)-6
> round(c(mean(z6),var(z6)),3)
[1] 0.048 0.986

> # acceptance/rejection
> u1<- runif(5*n,-3,3)
> u2<- runif(5*n)
> x<- ifelse(u2<exp(-0.5*u1^2),u1,999)
> z7<- x[x!=999][1:n]
> round(c(mean(z7),var(z7)),3)
[1] 0.059 0.942.
```

FOUR OTHER STATISTICAL DISTRIBUTIONS

The chi-square distribution, the t-distribution, the F-distribution, and the lognormal distribution are derived from different combinations of normally distributed variables. Capitalizing on these relationships makes it possible to generate random variables from these distributions using random normal values.

Chi-square distribution

A chi-square distribution is a sum of squared independent standard normal values. If $\{z_1, z_2, z_3, \cdots, z_k\}$ are k independent random standard normal values, then

$$X^2 = \sum z_i^2 \qquad i = 1, 2, 3, \cdots, k$$

is a random sample from a chi-square distribution with k degrees of freedom. For example, an S-function that produces n chi-square distributed random values with df degrees of freedom is

```
ranchi2<- function(n,df) {
  mtemp<- matrix(rnorm(n*df)^2,n,df)
  apply(mtemp,1,sum)
}
> x<- ranchi2(10000,4)
> # expectation = df = 4 and variance = 2df = 8
> mean(x)
[1] 3.968192
> var(x)
[1] 7.965049.
```

Of course, the S-function $rchisq(n, df)$ achieves the same results (Table 1.4).

Student's t-distribution

If Z is a random value from a standard normal distribution and X^2 is an independent random value from a chi-square distribution with df degrees of freedom, then

$$T = \frac{Z}{\sqrt{X^2/df}}$$

is a random value from a t-distribution with df degrees of freedom. As noted (Table 1.4), $rt(n, df)$ produces n random values of a t-distributed variable with df degrees of freedom.

F-distribution

If X_1^2 is a random value from a chi-square distribution with df_1 degrees of freedom and X_2^2 is an independent random value also from a chi-square distribution with df_2 degrees of freedom, then

$$F = \frac{X_1^2/df_1}{X_2^2/df_2}$$

is a random selection from an F-distribution with df_1 and df_2 degrees of freedom. As noted (Table 1.4), $rf(n, df1, df2)$ also produces n random values of an F-distributed variable with df_1 and df_2 degrees of freedom.

Lognormal distribution

Another distribution related to the normal distribution is the lognormal distribution. To generate a random variable X with a lognormal distribution with geometric mean value represented by e^m and geometric standard deviation represented by e^s, then

$$X = e^{m+sZ}$$

where Z is a random selection from a standard normal distribution. The value $log(X)$ has a normal distribution with mean m and standard deviation s. In S-code,

```
> # random lognormal values
> n<- 1000
> geometric mean = 1.5
> m<- log(1.5)
> geometric standard deviation = 2.0
> s<- log(2)
> x<- exp(m+s*rnorm(n))
> mean(log(x))
[1] 0.4054651
> sqrt(var(log(x)))
[1] 0.7122497
> median(x)
[1] 1.502202
> mean(x)
[1] 1.936854.
```

For the S-code example, the expected mean of the logarithms of X of the lognormally distributed values is $m = log(1.5) = 0.405$ with standard deviation $= log(2.0) = 0.693$. The expected geometric mean is $e^m = 1.5$ and the geometric standard deviation is $e^s = 2.0$. The expected mean value of the log normal observations is $e^{m+\frac{1}{2}s^2} = 1.907$ (the value 1.937 was observed). The S-function $rlnorm(n, m, s)$ also produces n random values (parameters m and s).

SIMULATING MINIMUM AND MAXIMUM VALUES

It is occasionally useful to investigate the distribution of extreme values. Simulation of the minimum or maximum values from a specified distribution is a useful tool for exploring the properties of extreme values. Say the sequence of values $\{x_1, x_2, x_3, \cdots, x_n\}$ is a sample of n independent values from the same probability distribution $F(x)$. Then, let Y_1 denote the minimum and Y_n denote the maximum of these values. The cumulative distribution function of the minimum is

$$P(Y_1 \leq y) = F_{Y_1}(y) = 1 - [1 - F(y)]^n$$

and similarly the cumulative distribution function of the maximum is

$$P(Y_n \leq y) = F_{Y_n}(y) = [F(y)]^n.$$

The inverse functions of the cumulative distribution functions of the minimum and maximum allow the generation of random values of the minimum and maximum from a given probability distribution $F(x)$. Formally, for the minimum,

$$Y_1 = F^{-1}[1 - U^{1/n}]$$

and, for the maximum,

$$Y_n = F^{-1}[U^{1/n}]$$

where U is again a uniform random variable ($0 \leq U \leq 1$). When the inverse function F^{-1} is known or approximated, it is straightforward to simulate random minimum and maximum values from a sample of n observations. For example, to simulate the minimum and maximum values from a uniform distribution on the unit interval

$$y_1 = 1 - u^{1/n} \qquad \text{and} \qquad y_n = u^{1/n}$$

since $F^{-1}(u) = u$. The value n is the number of values in the sample that yields the minimum and maximum values and u is again a uniformly distributed value between 0 and 1. For the sample size $n = 2$, a random minimum value is generated by $y = 1 - \sqrt{u}$ and a random maximum value by $\sqrt{u}$ (previously discussed in the context of the positive triangular distribution).

For the standard normal distribution, the following S-code produces distributions of the random minimum (S-vector = $y1$) and maximum (S-vector = yn) values from a sample of $n = 6$ observations based on 1000 simulated samples:

```
# y1 = minimum, yn = maximum, and n = 6
> n<- 6
> u<- runif(1000)
> y1<- qnorm(1-u^(1/n))
```

```
> u<- runif(1000)
> yn<- qnorm(u^(1/n))
> round(cbind(n,mean(y1),mean(yn)),3)
        n     y1     yn
  [1,] 1000 -1.265  1.275
> round(cbind(n,var(y1),var(yn)),3)
        n     y1     yn
  [1,] 1000  0.431  0.408.
```

The expected values for the minimum and maximum from a standard normal distribution can be found in tables [3] and for $n = 6$ observations are ± 1.267 with variance $= 0.416$.

A similar pattern can be used to generate random minimum and maximum values from a variety of statistical distributions where $F^{-1}( )$ is calculated with *qroot.name*( ) convention from Table 1.4. For example,

```
> # 10 observations: the minimum of n = 4 lognormal values
> n<- 4
> nvalues<- 10
> m<- log(2.0)
> s<- log(1.5)
> rvalues<- qlnorm(1-runif(nvalues)^(1/n),m,s)
> round(rvalues,3)
  [1]  1.137 1.240 1.137 1.233 0.742 1.929 1.260 0.717 1.219 1.006
```

produces *nvalues* = 10 values of the minimum from a sample of $n = 4$ observations selected from a lognormal distribution.

BUTLER'S METHOD

Butler's method effectively generates random values for a number of continuous distributions. The key to this approach is dividing a density function into a series of simple geometric subareas. Using these subareas, where random values can be generated with relative ease, a variable is produced with a specific probability distribution.

To start, a series of ordinates for the specified probability density are calculated. For a sequence of $k + 1$ values $\{x_0, x_1, x_2, \cdots, x_k\}$ the height of the density function is found at each point or $\{f(x_0), f(x_1), f(x_2), \cdots, f(x_k)\}$. The x-values are selected so that $F(x_{i+1}) - F(x_i) = 1/k$. In Figure 3.11, $x = \{-2.5, -1.28, -0.842, -0.524, -0.253, 0, 0.253, 0.524, 0.842, 1.28, 2.5\}$ using a standard normal distribution so that $F(x_{i+1}) - F(x_i) = 0.1$ (approximately 0.1 for the first and last intervals). The heights are then *dnorm*(x) or $\{0.018, 0.175, 0.280, 0.348, 0.386, 0.399, 0.386, 0.348, 0.280, 0.175, 0.018\}$. Each area bounded by $f(x_i)$ to $f(x_{i+1})$ can be approximated by a triangle or a rectangle plus a triangle, a trapezoid. The process transforms the normal probability density into a series of triangles and rectangles (Figure 3.11; dotted lines). Notice that for the normal distribution the points x_0 and x_k are chosen

Butler's method -- Normal distribution

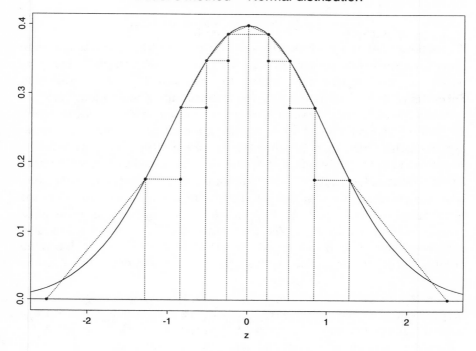

Figure 3.11

at some arbitrary but sensible value (i.e., -2.5 and 2.5 so that $f(x_0) = f(x_k) = 0.018 \approx 0$). Ideally, $f(x_0) = f(x_k) = 0$.

For each area, define

$$r_i = \frac{f(x_i) - f(x_{i-1})}{f(x_i) + f(x_{i-1})}$$

making $|r_i|$ the ratio of the triangular area to the total area of the ith subdivided region. Furthermore, the sign of r_i indicates whether the triangle slopes to the left (r_i positive) or the right (r_i negative).

To generate a random value x from $F(x)$, first one of the k intervals is randomly chosen with probability equal to $1/k$. Then, three random independent uniform random values are generated, u_1, u_2, and u_3. Calculate x for the random selected interval x_{j-1} to x_j so that

$$x = x_{j-1} + (x_j - x_{j-1})u_1$$

when $u_1 < 1 - |r_j|$; otherwise

$$x = x_{j-1} + (x_j - x_{j-1}) \times minimum(u_2, u_3)$$

if r_j is negative, or

$$x = x_{j-1} + (x_j - x_{j-1}) \times maximum(u_2, u_3)$$

if r_j is positive. For a positive triangular distribution (large values are more likely than small values—slopes to the left) the chosen variable is the maximum of two independent uniformly distributed random variables. Specifically, if u_1 and u_2 are two independent uniform random variables between 0 and 1, then maximum of u_1 and u_2 is a random selection from the positive triangular distribution. Similarly, a random variable from a negative triangular distribution (small values are more likely then large values—slopes to the right) is minimum of u_1 and u_2. The variable x is sampled from either a rectangular (uniform) distribution, a positive triangular distribution, or a negative triangular distribution. The result is a random value from the distribution approximated by the constructed triangular and rectangular regions, namely density $f(x)$. The sampling scheme, for example, produces a random value X with an approximate standard normal distribution when ordinate values are from the standard normal probability density function (Figure 3.11).

Butler's method of generating random values from a continuous distribution rests on the ability to decompose a complex distribution into a series of geometrically simple subareas. Figure 3.11 shows the standard normal distribution decomposed into triangular areas (both positive and negative) and rectangular areas (dotted lines). For some continuous distributions it is relatively easy to divide a rather complex distribution into a series of simple subareas, choose these areas with probabilities equal to their contributions to the entire area and then select random values from these subregions. The process of breaking a distribution into simple components is frequently an efficient way to produce random values from a continuous probability distribution ([1] or [4]).

RANDOM VALUES OVER A COMPLEX REGION

Acceptance/rejection sampling produces a random sample of points from a two-dimensional region. As an example, Figure 3.12 shows a polygon that could represent a county or a state or some other geographic region. It is frequently necessary to generate a distribution of random points within the region or, perhaps, simulate a distribution of some measure of association when no spatial pattern exists. To generate a distribution of random points within a specific region, bivariate random uniform values are generated for a rectangular area that completely contains the region of interest. For example, a square with dimension 15×15 contains the geographic region labeled R in

Random points in an irregular region

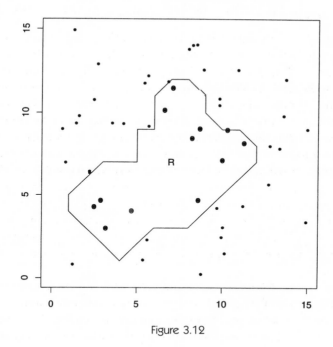

Figure 3.12

Figure 3.12. A series of random points (x_i, y_i) are generated within this square. The x-coordinates are random uniform values between 0 and 15, $x<-$ *runif*$(n, 0, 15)$. The y-coordinates are similarly independent uniform variables between 0 and 15, $y<-runif(n, 0, 15)$. Then, a point (x_i, y_i) is accepted if it falls within the boundary of the region R and rejected otherwise. The acceptance/ rejection process is repeated until the desired number of points are accepted. The accepted points are a random bivariate sample uniformly distributed over the region R, regardless of the complexity of the region.

To generate random points in this way, it must be determined whether a specific point is inside or outside the specified polygon. It is not difficult for the human mind to make this determination but it is a bit of a trick to write computer code to identify whether a point is inside or outside a defined region. One method is the following: From a given point extend a straight line in any direction so that the length is greater than the maximum dimension of region R (i.e., the endpoint of the line is guaranteed to extend outside the region). Count the number of times the line intersects a boundary. If the number is odd, the point is in the region (accept) and if the number is even, the point is outside the region (reject). Figure 3.12 shows 50 points generated at random over the 15×15 square containing the region labeled

R and each point was tested (in or out?) producing the points within the region. The 12 circled points are a random sample from a uniform distribution over the region R.

MULTIVARIATE NORMAL VARIABLES

To generate a k-dimensional observation $\{x_1, x_2, x_3, \cdots, x_k\}$ with a multivariate normal distribution requires two elements—k independent standard normal variates and a variance/covariance array. A theorem that provides the basis for simulating k-dimensional values from a multivariate normal distribution is:

the k variables $\mathbf{X} = \{x_1, x_2, x_3, \cdots, x_k\}$ are jointly normal (multivariate normal) if there exists k independent variables $\{z_1, z_2, z_3, \cdots, z_k\}$ each with a standard normal distribution ($\mu_i = 0$ and $\sigma_i = 1$) and if there exists a non-negative array $\mathbf{A}$ such that $\mathbf{X} = \mathbf{A}'\mathbf{Z} + \mu$ where μ are constant values, $\{\mu_1, \mu_2, \mu_3, \cdots, \mu_k\}$.

The quantities $\mathbf{X}$ and $\mathbf{Z}$ are vectors of values while $\mathbf{A}$ is a $k \times k$ array (note: $\mathbf{A}'$ denotes the transpose of $\mathbf{A}$). Furthermore, $\mathbf{A}$ is constructed so that $\mathbf{A}'\mathbf{A} = \mathbf{V}$, where $\mathbf{V}$ is the $k \times k$ variance/covariance array associated with the jointly normal values $\mathbf{X}$. The array $\mathbf{A}$ is sometimes referred to as the "square root" of the matrix $\mathbf{V}$ since $\mathbf{A}'\mathbf{A} = \mathbf{V}$, analogous to the square root of a single value (e.g., $a^2 = v$, then a is the square root of v).

The "square root" of a matrix is found with a Choleski decomposition that is accomplished with the S-function $chol(\ )$. The Choleski decomposition is an upper triangular matrix that has several applications in statistical analysis, one of which is the generation of multivariate normal values with a given variance/covariance structure.

To illustrate a Choleski decomposition in a simple two variable case consider $v_{11} = 9$, $v_{22} = 4$, $v_{12} = 3$ and

```
> # v = variance/covariance array
> v
      [,1] [,2]
[1,]    9    3
[2,]    3    4
> a<- chol(v)
> a
      [,1]      [,2]
[1,]    3 1.000000
[2,]    0 1.732051
attr(, "rank"):
[1] 2
> # to show a'a = v
> t(a)%*%a
```

```
      [,1] [,2]
[1,]    9    3
[2,]    3    4.
```

For this bivariate case, the elements of $\mathbf{A}$ are $a_{11} = \sqrt{v_{11}}$, $a_{21} = 0$, $a_{12} = v_{12}/\sqrt{v_{11}}$, and $a_{22} = \sqrt{v_{22} - v_{12}^2/v_{11}}$ where v_{ii} is the variance of x_i (diagonal elements of $\mathbf{V}$) and v_{12} is the covariance between x_1 and x_2. If z_1 and z_2 are two independent standard normal values, then using this 2×2 decomposition of $\mathbf{V}$ produces $\mathbf{A}$ and $\mathbf{A}'\mathbf{Z}$ produces

$$x_1 = 3z_1 \qquad \text{and} \qquad x_2 = z_1 + 1.732051z_2$$

giving x_1 a variance of 9, x_2 a variance of 4 and the covariance between x_1 and x_2 is 3 (correlation = $r_{12} = 0.5$), as required. Since the z-values are independent, random standard normal values, the x-values have a multivariate (bivariate) normal distribution with variance/covariance array $\mathbf{V}$.

A multivariate observation made up of k measurements is similarly generated. The matrix $\mathbf{A}$ is calculated from the specified variance/covariance array $\mathbf{V}$. The S-function that performs the Choleski decomposition again produces $\mathbf{A}$. Specifically, $a <- chol(v)$ where v is a $k \times k$ variance/covariance S-array. Then, k random and independent standard normal variables $\mathbf{Z} = \{z_1, z_2, z_3, \cdots, z_k\}$ are generated with the S-function $rnorm(k)$ and $\mathbf{X} = \mathbf{A}'\mathbf{Z} + \mu$ making $\mathbf{X}$ a k-dimensional random multivariate normal observation. The variance/covariance array is $\mathbf{V}$ and the expected values of the $\mathbf{X}$ variable are given by the constant values contained in the vector μ. To illustrate,

```
> # given variance/covariance array v
> v
      [,1] [,2] [,3] [,4]
[1,]   10    1    2    1
[2,]    1    4    2    1
[3,]    2    2    3    1
[4,]    1    1    1    8
> # given mean values mu
> mu<- c(1,2,3,4)
> z<- rnorm(k)
> t(chol(v))
           [,1]       [,2]       [,3]      [,4]
[1,] 3.1622777 0.0000000 0.0000000 0.000000
[2,] 0.3162278 1.9748418 0.0000000 0.000000
[3,] 0.6324555 0.9114654 1.3301243 0.000000
[4,] 0.3162278 0.4557327 0.2891575 2.758386
> x<- t(chol(v))%*%z+mu
> round(cbind(mu,x,3))
     mu     x
[1,]  1   1.993
[2,]  2   0.512
[3,]  3   3.634
[4,]  4   3.442.
```

The values labeled *mu* are the expected (population) mean values and the S-vector labeled x is a multivariate normal random observation that differs from the elements of *mu* because of the influence of random variation, described by the variance/covariance array **V**. Multivariate normal data are required for several important statistical procedures such as linear regression analysis, linear discriminant analysis, and analysis of variance. To explore issues surrounding these procedures, the simulation of multivariate normal "data" is frequently useful.

Problem set III

1. Use the Kolomogrov test to assess the "randomness" of the values generated by $a = 2^{10} + 1$, $c = 0$, and $m = 2^{20}$ (*ran1* in the chapter).

2. Chuck-a-luck is a game where one bets on the numbers 1, 2, 3, 4, 5, and 6. Three dice are rolled and if a player's number appears 1, 2, or 3 times, the pay-off is respectively 1 or 2 or 3 times the original bet (plus the player's bet). Simulate this game and estimate the player's expected gain or loss (ans: 7.9% loss [10]).

3. If a chord is selected at random from a circle with a set radius, what proportion of lengths will be smaller than the radius of the circle? Write and test a simulation program to estimate the answer to this question (ans: 1/3 [10]).

4. Which event is more likely: (i) $k = 1$ or more sixes in 6 tosses of a die or (ii) $k = 2$ or more sixes in 12 tosses of a die or (iii) $k = 3$ or more sixes in 18 tosses of a die?

   Write and test an S-program to simulate dice and answer the question: what is the probability of k or more sixes in $6k$ tosses of a die for selected values of k (ans: $k = 1, 2, 3$, and 4, then $p = 0.665, 0.619, 0.597$, and 0.584). Note: this problem is attributed to a question posed by Isaac Newton.

5. Robust linear regression: to achieve "robust" estimates of the intercept and slope of a straight line, the data are divided into three groups based on the ordered values of the independent variable x. Each group contains approximately one-third of the data (e.g., if the total number of observations is $n = 3k$, then the leftmost group has k members, the middle group has k members, and the rightmost group has k members—if the number of observations is not divisible evenly by three, then the observations are allocated as closely as possible to the ideal of $n/3$). Using these "thirds," a representative point is constructed based on the median of the x-values and the median of the y-values calculated separately from within each group. The pairs of median values

$$(x_L, y_L), (x_M, y_M), \text{ and } (x_R, y_R),$$

become the representative values of the left, middle, and right groups respectively.

   Estimates of the slope (b^*) and intercept (a^*) are then

$$\hat{b}^* = \frac{y_R - y_L}{x_R - x_L} \text{ and } \hat{a}^* = \frac{1}{3}(y_L + y_M + y_R) - \hat{b}^* \frac{1}{3}(x_L + x_M + x_R).$$

Since the estimate of the slope depends only on the median values from the left and right groups, it is almost certainly unaffected by extreme values, called a robust estimate.

   Simulate a set of "data" that conforms to the assumptions of simple linear regression—the dependent variable (y) is linearly related to the independent variable (x) and is sampled independently from a normal distribution with constant variance. Specifically,

$$y_j = a + bx_j + e_j$$

where e_j is one of series of independent and normally distributed values. Use 100 "data" sets to simulate the distribution of the "robust" estimator of the slope denoted $\hat{b}^*$. Also, compute 100 estimates of the slope b with *lsfit*( ), denoted $\hat{b}$.

Compare the variances of the two estimated values $\hat{b}^*$ and $\hat{b}$.

6.   For the positive triangular distribution, write and test four S-functions that produce the cumulative probabilities, quantiles, heights, and a random sample (e.g., *pptri*( ), *qptri*( ), *dptri*( ), and *rptri*( ) functions).

Show both theoretically and graphically that $x = max(u_1, u_2)$ has a positive triangular distribution when u_1 and u_2 are two independent values from a uniform distribution $(0,1)$.

7. Derive* the cumulative distribution and density function for a negative triangular distribution on the interval 0 to 1.

8. For the negative triangular distribution, write and test four S-functions that produce the cumulative probabilities, quantiles, heights, and a random sample (e.g., *pntri*( ), *qntri*( ), *dntri*( ), and *rntri*( ) functions).

Show both theoretically and graphically that $x = min(u_1, u_2)$ has a negative triangular distribution when u_1 and u_2 are two independent values from a uniform distribution $(0,1)$.

9. A left truncated standard normal distribution is given by the expression

$$f(z) = \frac{\frac{1}{\sqrt{2\pi}}e^{-0.5z^2}}{1 - P} \qquad \text{for } z > z_0$$

where $P = P(Z < z_0)$.

Simulate a random sample of $n = 1000$ values from this distribution when $z_0 = -1$ using two different methods.

10. Using S-code and Butler's method create an S-function that produces n random values from a chi-square distribution with df degrees of freedom. Compare the results to using *rchisq*(n, df).

11. Demonstrate that for $n > 100$ and $p < 0.05$, the binomial and Poisson distributions produce similar probabilities.

12. Demonstrate using S-functions such as *qqnorm*( ) that the Box–Muller transformation gives two independent standard normal variates from two independent and uniformly distributed random variables.

13. Plot a square with a circle inscribed within the boundaries. Generate random pairs (x, y) and determine whether these values are in the circle or not. Use the result to estimate $\pi = 3.1416$.

14. Demonstrate with an S-simulation program that the expected mean values resulting from sampling the same population with and without replacement are equal. Which sampling scheme has the smallest variance?

15. Create and test an S-function that produces n random values from a Poisson distribution using the inverse transformation method for given values of λ. Compare the results to the values generated with *rpoiss*( ).

16. The test-statistic $X^2 = (n - 1)S_x^2/\bar{x}$ has an approximate chi-square distribution with $n - 1$ degrees of freedom when the n values x_i are sampled from a Poisson distribution. Use a simulation program to verify that X^2 has an approximate chi-square distribution for $n = 100$ and $\lambda = 1.0$. Use this fact to test formally the fit of the Rutherford–Geiger data (Chapter 3) to a Poisson distribution.

*Solve theoretically and not with a computer program.

REFERENCES

1. Rubinstein, R. Y., *Simulation and the Monte Carlo Method*. John Wiley & Sons, New York, NY, 1981.
2. Conover, W. J., *Practical Nonparametric Statistics*. John Wiley & Sons, New York, NY, 1971.
3. Owen, D. B., *Handbook of Statistical Tables*. Addison-Wesley Publishing Company, Reading, MA, 1962.
4. Kennedy, W. J. and Gentle, J. E., *Statistical Computing*. Marcel Decker, New York, NY, 1980.
5. Chiang, C. L., *Introduction to Stochastic Processing Biostatistics*. John Wiley & Sons, New York, NY, 1968.
6. Johnson, N. L., and Kotz S., *Discrete Distributions*. Houghton Mifflin Company, New York, NY, 1969.
7. Moore, P. G., (1952) The estimation of the Poisson parameter from a truncated distribution. Biometrika, 39:247–251.
8. Kendall, M. G., and Stuart A., *The Advanced Theory of Statistics, Vol 1*. Charles Griffin and Company, London, 1963.
9. Hasting, C., *Approximations for Digital Computers*. Princeton University Press, NJ, 1955.
10. Mosteller, F., *Fifty Challenging Problems in Probability with Solutions*. Dover Publications, New York, NY, 1965.

4

General Linear Models

SIMPLEST CASE—UNIVARIATE LINEAR REGRESSION

The data in Table 4.1 are pairs of measurements of body weights and diastolic blood pressures recorded on 34 heavy men. Even with as few as 34 observations, it is useful to summarize the relationship between two variables. Figure 4.1 shows the results of five approaches among the numerous ways to summarize pairs of observations.

Perhaps the simplest summary arises from estimating a straight line to reflect the relationship between observed weight and blood pressure. Such a line is described by the model $y_i = a + bx_i$ where y represents the level of blood pressure (mm) and x represents an individual's body weight (pounds). The model parameters (a and b) can be estimated with the S-function *lsfit*(*weight*, *dbp*). The following S-functions create a plot (Figure 4.1) of the observed values (Table 4.1) and adds the least squares estimated line:

```
> # plot points and label axes
> plot(wt,dbp,pch="*",xlab="weight",ylab="blood pressure",
> main="Five S-function summaries of a bivariate plot of points")
```

Table 4.1. Body weight (pounds) and diastolic blood pressure (mm) recorded for heavy men (weight ≥ 230 pounds)

obs	dpb*	weight	obs	dbp*	weight	obs	dbp*	weight
1	92	240	13	94	250	25	94	240
2	98	245	14	108	255	26	90	230
3	102	235	15	96	230	27	92	230
4	88	226	16	70	235	28	84	250
5	90	265	17	116	290	29	84	227
6	108	265	18	90	228	30	88	226
7	94	244	19	112	270	31	94	230
8	90	245	20	100	230	32	90	250
9	96	240	21	80	250	33	104	245
10	98	239	22	92	232	34	88	250
11	80	320	23	78	233	–	–	–
12	86	230	24	78	235	–	–	–

* = diastolic blood pressure

Five S-function summaries of a bivariate plot of points

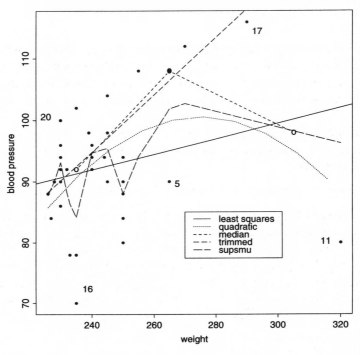

Figure 4.1

```
> # least squares estimated line y=blood pressure, x=weight
> abline(lsfit(wt,dbp))
> # estimated intercept and slope
> round(lsfit(wt,dbp)$coef,3)
   Intercept      X
      61.493    0.127
> # correlation
> round(cor(wt,dbp),3)
[1] 0.248.
```

A *t*-test to evaluate the slope (slope = 0?) of a line (not the *t.test*( )
S-function) or a test of the correlation coefficient (correlation = 0?) frequently
accompanies a least squares plot of two variables. Both tests yield identical
results. The S-function *cor.test*( ) produces one version of these two tests and
applied to the blood pressure data is

```
> cor.test(wt,dbp)

        Pearson's product-moment correlation

data: wt and dbp
t = 1.451, df = 32, p-value = 0.1565
```

```
alternative hypothesis: true coef is not equal to 0
sample estimates:
          cor
0.2484532.
```

A t-statistic of 1.451 (p-value = 0.157) indicates that the correlation between weight and blood pressure (r = 0.248) is not likely to be a result of a systematic association or, analogously, shows no strong evidence of a non-zero slope ($\hat{b}$ = 0.127) for the straight line describing the relationship of weight to blood pressure.

To evaluate the influence of selected observations on the estimation of a straight line, the interactive S-tool *identify*( ) plays an important role. The interactive command

$$identify(x, y, labels = c(``<label1>'', ``<label2>'' \cdots), \cdots)$$

assigns the listed labels to points whose coordinates are given in the argument vectors x and y when located with the mouse. This labeling is accomplished by plotting the data on the computer screen and executing the S-command *identify*( ). It is then possible to place a marker controlled by the mouse on a specific point and press the left button; the corresponding label then appears on the plot. In this fashion, points are interactively located and identified. For the systolic blood pressure data, the commands

```
> plot(wt,dpb,pch="*")
> identify(wt,dbp,labels=1:length(wt))
```

allow the data points to be identified on an xy-plot. For the example, "clicking" on the plotted point (320, 80) reveals that it is the 11th point in the *wt* and *dbp* S-vectors (several other extreme points are marked on Figure 4.1 to illustrate). To asses the impact of this point on the estimated line, two estimates of the model coefficients are compared—estimates with all data values included are compared to estimates with the point (320, 80) excluded or

```
> round(lsfit(wt,dbp)$coef,3)
 Intercept      X
    61.493  0.127
> round(lsfit(wt[-11],dbp[-11])$coef,3)
 Intercept        X
     1.119      0.379.
```

The contrast directly shows the importance of the selected point. The degree to which a single point influences the line describing the relationship between two variables is called leverage. The point (320, 80) has considerable leverage.

It is entirely possible that the association between body weight and blood pressure is more effectively described by a more complicated relationship. Perhaps a linear model including a "squared" term better represents the data where blood pressure levels are represented by a quadratic function of weight, $y_i = a + bx_i + cx_i^2$. A linear model is a sum of a series of components each multiplied by a coefficient. However, the components themselves need not be linear functions of the measured variables (*x*-values). The linear model parameters (*a*, *b*, and *c*) estimated with *lsfit*( ) produce the least squares estimated line shown in Figure 4.1. Specifically,

```
> # quadratic term added
> b<- lsfit(cbind(wt,wt^2),dbp)$coef
> x<- seq(min(wt),max(wt),10)
> lines(x,b[1]+b[2]*x+b[3]*x^2,lty=2).
```

A summary of a relationship between two variables insensitive to extreme values (frequently called a robust procedure) is a type of "band" estimate. The data are divided into series of categories based on the *x*-variable and pairs of median values are estimated to represent each category. A line connecting the median values produces a summary of the *xy*-relationship largely unaffected by extreme observations. For example, high leverage points such as the point (320, 80) in the example data have typically no effect on the estimated *xy*-relationship. Specifically,

```
> # robust band type estimate
> x<- tapply(wt,cut(wt,3),median)
> y<- tapply(dbp,cut(wt,3),median)
> lines(x,y,type="b",pch="o",lty=3)
```

and the resulting line is displayed in Figure 4.1.

A "modern" regression technique also essentially unaffected by extreme values is applied using the least trimmed squares S-function *ltsreg*( ). This method of estimating a straight line to represent the relationship between *xy*-pairs operates by estimating the model parameters *a* and *b* using only data that produce non-extreme residual values (small differences between estimated and observed values). Observations that produce large residuals are "trimmed" from the analysis. For the S-function *ltsreg*( ), the estimated regression line is based on only those data values that produce the smallest half of the residual values. The S-functions that estimate and add a "trimmed" regression line to the current plot are

```
> # least trimmed squares (lts) regression
> b<- ltsreg(wt,dbp,intercept=T)$coef
> lines(x,b[1]+b[2]*x,lty=4)
```

and again the result is displayed in Figure 4.1.

Another model-free representation of the association between blood pressure and weight is achieved by considering the data as a deviation from some relationship estimated by smoothing the observations (a number of smoothing procedures are available—Chapter 2). A specific choice is a "super smooth" estimate, which is another "modern" regression technique.

The S-command

```
> lines(supsmu(wt,dbp,lty=5))
```

creates a smooth line representing the relationship between weight and blood pressure and adds the estimated line to the current plot (Figure 4.1). The S-function *supsmu*( ) applies a complicated scheme based on nearest neighbors, cross validation and linear least squares to estimate local regression lines.

These five approaches give rather different pictures of the relationship of weight and diastolic blood pressure. The "robust" estimates (trimmed and band estimates) produce the strongest weight/blood pressure relationship since these two approaches are essentially unaffected by extreme values (e.g., *weight* = 320 and *dbp* = 80, which attenuates the association). The other three techniques (linear, quadratic, and "super smooth" estimated lines) are influenced by all observed values, where extreme values have potentially disproportional impact. Even this simple case illustrates that it is certainly important to consider carefully the analytic approach chosen to describe a relationship of one variable to another.

MULTIVARIABLE CASE

A number of different kinds of linear models are available to explore multivariable data. The S-function *glm*( ) ("glm" for general linear model) provides a natural environment to analyze data using specific linear models. The form of this general linear model S-function is

S.object<– *glm (independent variable ~ formula, family = <statistical distribution>,* · · · *)*.

The execution of this command produces estimates of the model parameters and the components necessary to evaluate the model as a representation of the data. These components include:

coefficients residual values degrees of freedom   predicted values
summaries   deviances   estimates   statistical tests.

These components are explained and illustrated in the following. Five specific applications (linear, logistic, Poisson, loglinear (Chapter 6), and analysis of variance (Chapter 7) models) provide the details of applying this command to sample data.

MULTIVARIABLE LINEAR MODEL

A natural of extension of a single variable regression equation is a linear model containing more than one explanatory variable known as a multivariable linear model. A multivariable linear model is represented by

$$y_i = a + b_1 x_{i1} + b_2 x_{i2} + b_3 x_{i3} + \cdots + b_k x_{ik} + e_i \qquad i = 1, 2, 3, \cdots, n$$

where the y_i-value and the x_{ij}-values are measurements from the ith observation. The symbol y_i represents a continuous dependent variable, the values x_{ij} denote continuous or discrete independent variables (sometimes called predictor or explanatory variables) and e_i represents a stochastic error term. The symbol k denotes the number of independent variables in the regression equation and n the total number of observations sampled. The model coefficients b_j are weights reflecting the contribution of each independent variable to the variability in the dependent variable Y. The parameter a is a constant or intercept term. The error terms e_i, providing the statistical component to the model, are generally assumed to be uncorrelated random variables with normal distributions (mean zero and constant variance). Thus, the outcome value Y is envisioned as made up of two components: a deterministic parametric component $(a + \sum b_j x_{ij})$ and a stochastic component (e_i).

Estimation of the model parameters does not require knowledge or assumptions about the population sampled. However, to make inferences (assign significance probabilities) requires a specific population structure. The dependent variable must have normal distributions, which is the same as requiring the error term to have normal distributions. These normal distributions are further required to have the same variance at all values of the independent variables. That is, the variance is the same regardless of the values of the x-variables. Finally, the observations must be sampled independently. The phrase "sampled independently" has nothing to do with the term independent variables—unfortunately the same word is used to indicate rather different features of the linear model. When these three requirements (normality, equal variance, and independence) hold or at least approximately reflect the underlying data structure, rigorous statistical inferences based on the properties of the estimated linear model provide a valuable tool for summarizing and understanding relationships within multivariate data. The process of estimating the model parameters and assessing the value of the estimated linear model as a summary of the relationships within a data set is usually called regression analysis.

To use a linear model to estimate and assess the relationships between the x-values and the dependent variable, a sample of n independent sets of $k + 1$ measurements is collected. Independence in this context means that the selection of one observation in no way influences the selection of any other observation.

The ith observed value is denoted as $\{y_i, x_{i1}, x_{i2}, x_{i3}, \cdots, x_{ik}\}$ where $i = 1, 2, 3, \cdots, n$. The data for a linear regression analysis are naturally formed into a vector of dependent variables (n values of y_j) and an array with n rows (observations) and k columns of independent variables.

For example, data collected to study the birth weight (kilograms) of newborn infants and the relationship to mother's height (centimeters), self-reported prepregnancy weight (kilograms), and the amount of weight gained (kilograms) during pregnancy are displayed in Table 4.2. The dependent variable is the birth weight of the infant (y) while maternal height (x_1), weight (x_2), and amount gained (x_3) are the independent variables. The total weight gained is the net maternal gain after the infant's birth weight has been subtracted (gain = last measured prenatal weight − prepregnancy weight − infant's birth weight). A sample of $n = 232$ observations with $k = 3$ independent variables was collected, one observation for each mother and her newborn birth or $\{y_i, x_{i1}, x_{i2}, x_{i3}\} = \{bwt_i, ht_i, wt_i, gain_i\}$ (Table 4.2).

The analysis begins with estimates of the $k + 1$ model parameters (the a- and b_j-values). The S-function $glm(\ )$ produces an S-object containing these estimates and a variety of other useful quantities. For the birth weight data (Table 4.2),

```
> otemp<- glm(bwt~ht+wt+gain, family=gaussian)
```

implements the model $y_i = a + b_1 x_{i1} + b_2 x_{i2} + b_3 x_{i3} + e_i$. The term "object" is part of modern computer language. An S-object is, in this context, the stored results created by $glm(\ )$ or any other S-function and is given a single name (e.g., *otemp*, in the example). The S-object labeled *otemp* contains a variety of results from the linear regression analysis using the birth weight data and the model described by the formula in the $glm(\ )$ command.

The term *gaussian* is an alternative word for a normal distribution and identifies the statistical distribution associated with the dependent variable. If the *family* option is omitted, the statistical distribution is assumed to be normal (gaussian). Other possible families are: Bernoulli, binomial, Poisson, and gamma.

The general linear model S-function is efficiently applied in conjunction with reading the input data from an exterior file with the S-function *read.table(\ )*. The S-function

interior.name<− read.table("exterior.file", header = <T or F>, ⋯)

does what the name suggests. It reads a table of data contained in an exterior file into a specialized S-program. If the birth weight data are contained in an exterior file named *bwt.data*, then *dframe<− read.table("bwt.data", header=T)* reads these data into an S-file and labels it with the symbol *dframe*. The option *header = T* indicates that the first line of the exterior file contains the variable names to be employed in the S-analysis. For example, the exterior file *bwt.data* looks like

Table 4.2. Birth weight of newborn infants and three maternal measurements

bwt	ht	wt	gain	bwt	ht	wt	gain	bwt	ht	wt	gain	bwt	ht	wt	gain
3.860	167.5	56.8	12.8	3.640	157.5	50.9	18.1	3.190	152.4	48.0	13.5	3.100	170.2	65.0	2.5
3.560	157.5	58.2	13.6	3.280	151.5	42.5	18.2	3.060	167.0	47.7	8.1	3.280	160.0	68.0	14.0
3.480	167.0	59.0	8.0	4.200	171.5	63.8	19.9	3.240	144.7	68.1	10.6	3.420	167.6	63.6	16.1
4.190	170.2	70.0	18.5	3.240	157.5	44.0	14.1	3.840	162.6	59.1	20.9	3.120	166.4	59.5	17.1
4.050	172.7	53.6	17.4	3.140	154.9	53.6	15.7	4.300	173.0	122.2	14.0	3.310	171.5	59.1	21.9
4.410	160.0	50.9	17.9	3.380	158.5	54.5	11.6	2.400	159.0	56.8	11.8	4.040	160.0	54.5	14.4
3.660	157.5	52.3	15.7	4.320	153.0	59.1	9.9	4.005	177.8	72.7	29.8	3.540	157.5	56.8	14.2
3.160	160.0	52.3	14.3	3.400	160.0	54.5	24.4	3.380	160.0	61.4	7.7	3.640	160.0	55.0	11.0
3.540	165.0	60.0	15.1	1.000	154.0	49.0	19.0	3.850	182.9	72.7	20.8	3.260	166.4	57.0	10.3
3.840	165.1	52.3	14.0	3.820	160.0	56.4	16.4	2.800	144.7	52.3	9.7	3.220	165.1	52.3	12.2
4.260	160.0	52.0	8.3	4.020	161.0	56.8	20.7	3.540	165.1	54.5	18.1	3.350	165.0	48.0	22.0
2.160	172.0	56.0	6.0	3.320	165.1	50.0	16.8	3.400	163.9	50.0	25.5	4.160	165.1	61.4	18.9
3.100	170.2	53.2	12.2	3.720	162.6	74.1	26.7	2.390	166.4	54.5	9.7	3.540	157.0	59.0	20.0
2.920	157.5	54.5	9.3	4.200	182.9	88.2	15.8	3.700	158.8	53.8	19.3	3.100	170.2	61.4	18.3
3.340	160.0	50.0	26.1	3.580	165.1	65.9	15.7	2.790	160.0	44.5	9.5	3.860	160.0	50.0	23.9
3.620	162.6	60.5	16.4	3.340	172.0	62.3	6.9	3.690	158.8	52.3	10.7	2.680	157.5	50.9	11.1
2.420	177.8	55.9	11.3	3.420	170.2	62.7	11.2	3.840	170.2	68.0	14.9	3.350	167.6	49.1	13.5
3.340	157.5	70.0	11.6	3.970	166.4	47.7	19.7	3.280	162.6	80.9	7.5	3.280	166.4	56.8	18.7
3.065	168.0	52.0	21.0	3.720	152.4	56.4	12.7	2.900	165.1	49.5	9.8	3.280	165.0	68.0	20.0
3.140	172.7	59.1	17.8	3.760	160.0	54.5	11.0	3.460	165.1	52.3	19.5	3.120	170.0	50.0	8.5
2.980	158.0	45.5	12.0	2.400	162.0	66.0	9.7	3.030	149.8	45.5	15.7	3.600	167.6	52.3	27.7
2.840	152.4	47.3	14.8	4.260	175.3	72.7	17.3	3.890	167.6	63.5	25.5	3.600	157.5	47.7	13.5
2.700	165.1	54.5	14.5	3.000	154.0	50.0	13.1	3.850	167.6	61.0	17.0	.710	178.0	50.0	5.0
3.840	162.0	72.0	18.0	4.200	175.3	65.5	18.4	3.620	165.1	61.4	20.1	3.160	162.6	50.0	14.9
1.400	157.5	56.8	-1.2	3.718	157.5	88.6	13.6	3.030	165.1	56.8	7.4	2.640	160.0	50.0	19.2
3.340	157.5	53.6	10.7	3.720	157.5	50.0	17.9	3.810	165.1	93.0	16.9	3.380	160.0	54.1	16.9
2.760	148.0	56.0	14.0	3.300	154.9	52.3	16.9	3.300	167.6	65.0	14.0	1.180	157.2	40.9	6.1
3.700	160.0	95.4	5.1	3.030	160.0	52.3	18.3	1.960	149.8	41.8	7.7	2.780	150.0	52.0	10.0
3.100	177.8	63.0	12.9	2.920	172.7	77.4	7.1	2.960	160.0	50.0	17.1	3.480	155.0	54.0	9.6
4.060	157.5	50.0	20.6	3.240	165.1	65.9	19.7	3.680	165.1	51.8	16.0	3.320	162.6	56.8	12.2
3.560	163.0	54.0	16.5	3.420	170.2	95.4	13.3	3.360	175.0	58.0	17.0	3.595	157.0	48.0	11.0
3.100	157.5	50.0	11.8	3.400	157.5	47.3	20.3	3.900	152.0	59.0	16.4	2.880	158.8	47.7	19.1
4.020	170.2	56.8	12.7	3.710	177.0	62.0	14.0	3.440	172.7	53.0	21.3	3.580	157.5	72.7	6.2
3.090	154.9	56.0	17.9	3.160	163.9	59.0	19.8	3.655	174.0	59.1	16.6	3.670	160.0	50.9	16.1
3.500	167.6	56.0	16.0	4.060	165.1	61.4	16.9	2.800	152.0	45.0	12.0	3.350	167.6	59.1	16.4
4.000	165.0	60.0	19.0	3.100	162.0	55.0	13.8	3.740	162.6	77.3	18.0	3.790	159.0	40.9	27.1
3.140	161.0	45.0	13.0	3.800	167.6	44.2	19.5	3.620	162.6	52.3	14.4	4.055	165.1	49.1	17.1
2.980	160.0	56.8	12.4	2.860	156.2	44.4	22.6	3.220	165.0	57.0	14.4	4.610	162.6	52.7	24.2
2.820	166.4	50.0	10.5	3.420	158.8	52.3	21.1	3.750	154.9	53.2	26.5	1.960	167.6	54.5	19.1
3.220	165.1	57.0	11.2	2.930	167.6	65.9	17.9	2.640	166.4	47.7	11.3	2.140	160.0	72.0	10.3
4.280	162.6	54.5	15.5	4.300	152.4	70.5	27.5	3.590	162.6	64.9	14.5	2.980	165.1	68.0	13.4
3.500	167.6	57.7	19.8	3.740	168.0	94.5	19.0	2.920	157.5	45.0	17.0	2.675	171.5	56.8	17.5
4.210	166.4	68.0	25.5	3.320	160.0	59.1	3.2	1.460	155.9	50.0	4.0	3.550	172.7	101.0	15.5
3.860	167.6	54.5	13.8	3.560	162.6	56.8	9.3	3.560	160.0	54.1	14.0	3.140	161.3	50.5	10.5
3.300	167.6	86.8	16.2	3.640	157.0	56.8	28.9	3.560	157.0	62.0	18.0	3.835	161.3	53.2	16.3
3.460	162.6	52.7	19.6	3.360	167.6	61.4	11.5	3.400	161.3	53.6	12.4	3.315	160.0	52.3	17.4
3.060	165.1	52.3	16.4	3.850	166.4	56.5	20.3	3.300	152.4	53.2	16.7	3.575	168.9	72.7	29.0
3.900	154.9	50.0	25.0	3.620	157.0	74.0	17.0	2.950	160.0	47.7	9.3	3.450	154.9	54.5	19.5
3.120	168.9	54.5	32.6	3.385	157.5	47.7	16.8	3.300	170.0	68.0	28.5	3.815	182.9	91.0	20.4
4.060	167.6	49.1	10.9	3.260	152.4	50.0	33.4	4.280	168.0	57.0	16.0	3.520	172.7	54.5	150.0
4.480	168.9	104.0	14.4	3.790	160.0	61.8	15.9	3.580	167.6	56.8	21.7	3.060	158.8	50.1	13.6

Table 4.2. Continued

bwt	ht	wt	gain	bwt	ht	wt	gain	bwt	ht	wt	gain	bwt	ht	wt	gain
3.820	154.9	52.3	20.4	3.180	152.4	49.1	12.7	3.640	150.0	42.0	17.0	1.420	182.9	75.0	18.2
3.540	165.5	59.0	12.5	2.970	168.9	59.1	2.4	3.980	170.2	63.6	22.7	3.500	168.9	52.3	11.7
4.080	163.5	61.4	24.5	3.000	158.8	47.7	12.6	3.070	172.7	63.6	6.1	1.930	167.6	91.0	13.5
2.030	175.3	72.0	25.5	3.420	160.0	56.0	20.0	3.620	159.0	52.3	24.5	2.570	156.2	59.5	9.1
2.760	168.0	50.0	18.7	3.140	197.0	66.0	26.0	2.280	154.0	65.0	5.0	.670	154.9	44.5	6.9
4.780	157.5	51.4	16.2	3.400	161.0	53.2	24.5	3.450	157.0	52.0	22.5	2.850	172.7	61.4	12.0
3.480	163.6	75.0	20.4	3.580	157.0	65.0	15.0	2.660	167.0	54.0	10.0	1.860	172.7	56.8	8.3

```
  bwt      ht     wt   gain
3.860  167.5  56.8  12.8
3.560  157.5  58.2  13.6
3.480  167.0  59.0   8.0
4.190  170.2  70.0  18.5
4.050  172.7  53.6  17.4
4.140  160.0  50.9  17.9
3.660  157.5  52.3  15.7
  .        .     .      .
  .        .     .      .
  .        .     .      .
1.860  172.7  56.8   8.3
```

and the S-function *read.table*(*bwt.data*, *header* = T) produces a data structure (n = 232 by k + 1 = 4) labeled *dframe*. The names *bwt*, *ht*, *wt*, and *gain* relate the corresponding data to these variable names (columns of the "table") and are used by the *glm*-function and other S-functions to identify input and label output. The command *attach*( ) communicates such a data structure, called a data frame, to the *glm*( ) command. Therefore, after reading an exterior file with *read.table*( ), the command *attach*(*data.frame*) is issued making the data and variable names available to the general linear model S-function. The command *attach*( ) is also used in connection with extracting data from an S-library [1] and, in general, adds the argument (enclosed by the parentheses) to the list of objects available to the SPLUS program. Data frames formed by *read.table*( ) or other specialized commands contain the data with specified variable labels which are then available to a variety of S-functions.

For the birth weight example, executing the three commands

```
>dframe<- read.table("bwt.data",header=T)
>attach(dframe)
>otemp<- glm(bwt~ht+wt+gain,family=gaussian)
```

creates a linear regression analysis S-object from the birth weight data, labeled *otemp* ("otemp" for temporary object file—but most any name can be used). A minimal summary of the results is displayed by executing the S-object name as a command or

```
> otemp

Call: glm(formula = bwt~ht+wt+gain, family = gaussian)

Coefficients:
  (Intercept)           ht            wt          gain
     2.915538  -0.006040597    0.01251983    0.04275235

Degrees of Freedom: 232 Total; 228 Residual
Residual Deviance: 76.12054.
```

Issuing the command *summary(object.name)* produces an expanded summary of the analytic results generated by the *glm*-function and for the birth weight example

```
> summary(otemp,correlation=F)
```

produces

```
Call: glm(formula = bwt~ht+wt+gain, family = gaussian)
Deviance Residuals:
        Min         1Q      Median         3Q        Max
  -2.411053 -0.2569752  0.03002075  0.339125   1.479748

Coefficients:
                    Value   Std. Error    t value
(Intercept)    2.915538218  0.857479083   3.400128
         ht   -0.006040597  0.005646488  -1.069797
         wt    0.012519832  0.003503077   3.573953
       gain    0.042752345  0.006601654   6.476005

(Dispersion Parameter for Gaussian family taken to be 0.333862)
Null Deviance: 94.38865 on 231 degrees of freedom
Residual Deviance: 76.12054 on 228 degrees of freedom

1pc3>Number of Fisher Scoring Iterations: 1.
```

The option *correlation* = *F* suppresses a correlation array associated with the linear model parameter estimates, which is only rarely important. This correlation array does not contain the pairwise correlations between sampled variables. The command *cor( )* produces the Pearson product–moment correlations between all possible pairs of variables when applied to a data frame. For the birth weight data frame, *cor(dframe)* gives the six pairwise correlations and

```
> round(cor(dframe),3)
        bwt     ht     wt   gain
 bwt  1.000  0.062  0.211  0.385
  ht  0.062  1.000  0.395  0.104
  wt  0.211  0.395  1.000  0.019
gain  0.385  0.104  0.019  1.000.
```

An S-function parallel to the *glm( )* command that also provides estimates of the model parameters and creates an S-object is *lm( )* ("lm" for linear model). This function produces the same parameter estimates as *glm* but has several features that apply only to multivariable linear models. Applying *lm( )* to the same birth weight data (Table 4.2) and model gives

```
> otemp0<- lm(bwtht+wt+gain)
> summary(otemp0)

Call: lm(formula = bwt ~ ht + wt + gain)
Residuals:
    Min       1Q    Median       3Q      Max
 -2.411   -0.257   0.03002   0.3391     1.48

Coefficients:
               Value Std. Error  t value Pr(>|t|)
(Intercept)   2.9155    0.8575    3.4001  0.0008
         ht  -0.0060    0.0056   -1.0698  0.2858
         wt   0.0125    0.0035    3.5740  0.0004
       gain   0.0428    0.0066    6.4760  0.0000

Residual standard error: 0.5778 on 228 degrees of freedom
Multiple R-Squared: 0.1935
F-statistic: 18.24 on 3 and 228 degrees of freedom,
   the p-value is 1.213e-10

Correlation of Coefficients:
          (Intercept)       ht      wt
     ht     -0.9678
     wt      0.1835   -0.3955
   gain     -0.0136   -0.1052  0.0242.
```

Both S-functions estimate the regression coefficients by a process called ordinary least squares (discussed in detail in Chapter 5). The name derives from the property that the estimated values $\hat{a}$, $\hat{b}_1$, $\hat{b}_2$, $\hat{b}_3$, $\cdots$, $\hat{b}_k$ are exactly those values that make the sum of squared differences between observed and estimated values as small as possible. That is, $\sum(y_i - \hat{y}_i)^2$ is as small as possible where the expression

$$\hat{y}_i = \hat{a} + \hat{b}_1 x_{i1} + \hat{b}_2 x_{i2} + \hat{b}_3 x_{i3} + \cdots + \hat{b}_k x_{ik}$$

is an estimate of the ith observation based on these least squares estimates. The "hat" or circumflex indicates values estimated from the data. The estimates of the regression coefficients $\hat{b}_j$ are labeled "Value" by the *summary*( ) command. Any other choices of the $k + 1$ parameter values produce a larger sum of squared differences between the data and estimates. The least squares estimates of the coefficients produce an estimated model that is as "close" as possible to the observed data.

Occasionally observations within a data set are not complete. One or more values of the independent variables are missing (i.e., *NA*) making the observation unusable by *glm*( ) or *lm*( ). If the *NA*-values are not removed, the execution of the S-function stops and an error message is produced. To eliminate these incomplete observations from a particular application of *glm*( ) or *lm*( ), the *na.omit* option is available (see *?na.omit*).

When it is useful to reduce a regression analysis data set to only those values with complete measurements, then

```
> for(j in 1:ncol(x)) {
  y<- y[!is.na(x[,j])]
  x<- x[!is.na(x[,j]),]
  }
```

produces a new array x with all rows containing an "NA" value removed. Also the corresponding dependent values contained in the y-vector are removed. Using the reduced x and y input data, all applications of the $glm(\ )$ or $lm(\ )$ functions will have the same number of observations, given by $nrow(x)$ or $length(y)$. For some applications (discussed later), it is important that all analyses are based on exactly the same number of complete observations.

Three important properties of a linear model should be noted at this point. Consider the difference between two model values of Y. The difference between two independent values y_i and y_j is

$$y_i - y_j = b_1(x_{i1} - x_{j1}) + b_2(x_{i2} - x_{j2}) + b_3(x_{i3} - x_{j3}) + \ldots + b_k(x_{ik} - x_{jk})$$

disregarding for the moment the influence of the error term (random variation). This difference (a natural measure for a linear model) depends only on the differences $(x_{im} - x_{jm})$ and not the absolute magnitude of the values themselves. For example, the difference between two estimated birth weights is equally affected by two mothers who differ by 10 kilograms in prepregnancy weight whether they weigh 50 and 60 kilograms or 100 and 110 kilograms. The influence is estimated as $\hat{b}_2 \times 10$ regardless of the mother's prepregnancy weight. The fact that the difference between two independent variables has the same impact on the dependent variable regardless of the magnitude of the variables compared is a property of a linear model in general and is potentially unrealistic for certain applied situations.

Independent variables have separate effects when described by an additive linear model. Another way of stating this fact is: the influences from the k independent variables are said to be additive when the effect on the dependent variable from any specific independent variable is not influenced by the values of the other independent variables in the model. For example, the impact of maternal weight gain on an infant's birth weight is the same regardless of the mother's height or prepregnancy weight. The estimated impact is $\hat{b}_3 x_3$ whether the mother is tall or short (x_1) or whether she is heavy or light (x_2).

The expression for the difference between two values from an additive linear model gives rise to an important interpretation of the linear model coefficients. Envision two dependent values where all independent variables are identical except for one pair of variables that differ by one unit. The difference between these two values of the dependent variable is then equal to the regression coefficient. Specifically, if $k - 1$ of the x-values are equal ($x_{il} = x_{jl}$) and one specific pair differs by one unit ($x_{im} = x_{jm} + 1$), then $y_i - y_j = b_m$. A regression coefficient, therefore, indicates the amount of response in the dependent variable from a one unit increase in a specific independent variable while the other $k - 1$ variables are held constant. The ability to assess the isolated influence of one variable "adjusted" for the influences of the other independent variables is the essence of the additive linear model. The estimated regression coefficient associated with weight gain is $\hat{b}_3 = 0.043$, which means that a one kilogram increase in weight gained during pregnancy produces an estimated 0.043 kilogram increase in the infant's birth weight while accounting for the influences of maternal height and prepregnancy weight. Of course, this interpretation is useful only when the additive linear model adequately represents the relationships within the data set.

Assessing the adequacy or the goodness-of-fit of a linear model is a critical part of a linear regression analysis. Just because an estimated model is "closest" to the observed data does not guarantee that the estimated values reflect the relationships among the independent variables. Least squares estimates produce the "closest" model but the "closest" model may fall short of being useful.

A number of quantities calculated from a regression analysis reflect on the worth of the estimated model. A natural measure is the comparison of the observed dependent variables y_i to the corresponding values estimated from the model $\hat{y}_i$. The usual summary measure of the correspondence is

$$residual\ deviance = \sum (y_i - \hat{y}_i)^2 \qquad i = 1, 2, 3, \cdots, n.$$

The residual deviance (in a linear model context, typically called the residual sums of squares) plays a key role in the analysis and is displayed by the *summary( )* command or extracted from the regression analysis S-object by the expression *object.name\$deviance*. The residual deviance calculated from the birth weight analysis is 76.121 or

```
> rdev<- otemp$deviance
> rdev
[1] 76.12054
> df0<- otemp$df.residual
> df0
[1] 228.
```

The difference $y_i - \hat{y}_i$ directly measures the lack of fit of the model and is called the residual value for the ith observation. The n residual values (one for each observation) are extracted from the *glm*-object by the S-expression *object.name\$residuals*. Specifically, *otemp\$residuals* is a vector of $n = 232$ residual values $y_i - \hat{y}_i$. The residual deviance is then *sum(object.name\$residuals^2)*. The "Dispersion Parameter" from the *summary( )* command is the residual deviance divided by its associated degrees of freedom, $n - (k + 1)$. This quantity is an estimate of the constant "background" variability intrinsic in the dependent variable Y (i.e., the variance of e_i). The "Dispersion Parameter" for the birth weight data is $otemp\$deviance/otemp\$df.residual = 76.121/228 = 0.334$ (denoted $S^2_{Y|x_1,\cdots,x_k}$). The estimated standard error is $S_{Y|x_1,\cdots,x_k} = \sqrt{0.334} = 0.578$ and is directly calculated by the $lm()$ command (labeled "Residual standard error"). Again, this estimate of the "background" variation is only useful if the linear model accurately reflects the relationship among the sampled variables.

The magnitude of the residual deviance is frequently compared to a baseline value where it is assumed that the x-values have absolutely no relationship to the response value Y. The null deviance measures this conjecture of no relationship where

$$null\ deviance = \sum (y_i - \bar{y})^2 \qquad i = 1, 2, 3, \cdots, n$$

when $\bar{y}$ is the mean of the n dependent variables. The null deviance is displayed by the $summary()$ command or extracted from the S-object by $object.name\$null.deviance$. These two quantities (residual and null deviances) can be formally compared with an F-test—to be described. For the birth weight data, the null deviance is 94.389 from the S-function $summary(otemp)$. The difference between the null deviance and the residual deviance directly measures the impact of using $\hat{y}_i$ rather than $\bar{y}$ as an estimate of an infant's birth weight. In other words, the difference results from including the independent variables as part of the description of the dependent variable.

Another measure of the correspondence between the observed values and the values based solely on the model is the correlation between these two quantities, $correlation(y, \hat{y})$. This correlation is called the multiple correlation coefficient (denoted R) when applied to estimates from a linear regression analysis. The S-function $predict()$ extracts n estimated values $\hat{y}_i$ from the glm or lm object named between the parentheses. The estimated values $\hat{y}_i$ are produced by $predict(object.name)$ and, for the example birth weight data, $predict(otemp)$ produces $n = 232$ estimated birth weights and the correlation with the corresponding observed values is

```
> R<- cor(bwt,predict(otemp))
> R
[1] 0.4399334
> R^2
[1] 0.1935414.
```

The multiple correlation coefficient indicates the degree of linear association between the observed birth weights and the values estimated from the regression model. A correlation $R = 1$ means that the observed and the estimated values are identical. A correlation $R = 0$ means that the independent variables have absolutely no linear relationship to the estimated values.

The squared multiple correlation coefficient is frequently defined in terms of the null and residual deviances where

$$R^2 = 1 - \frac{residual\ deviance}{null\ deviance}.$$

Specifically, for the birth weight data

```
> 1-otemp$deviance/otemp$null.deviance
  [1] 0.1935414.
```

In this context, R^2 estimates the proportion of variation in Y "explained" by the x-values and, conversely, $1 - R^2$ is the proportion of "unexplained" variation in Y. For example, if $\sum(y_i - \hat{y}_i)^2 = 0$, then $R^2 = 1$ and if $\sum(y_i - \hat{y}_i)^2 = \sum(y_i - \bar{y})^2$, then $R^2 = 0$. Values of R^2 between these two extremes measure the explanatory worth of the independent variables (in a linear model!).

The 232 observed and the model estimated birth weights are plotted in Figure 4.2, created by

```
> plot(bwt,predict(otemp),pch="x",xlab="birth weight",
    ylab="predicted birth weights",
    main="Additive model -- predicted plotted against
    observed values")
> text(1.5,3.8,paste("multiple correlation coefficient =",
    round(R,3)))
```

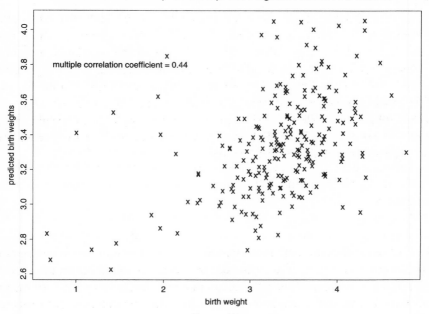

Additive model -- predicted plotted against observed values

multiple correlation coefficient = 0.44

Figure 4.2

The *text*( ) and *paste*( ) S-functions produce the insert in the upper left of Figure 4.2.

Comparisons among the k estimated regression coefficients are a basic tool in evaluating the relative roles of the independent variables in the observed variability of the dependent variable. However, the values of the coefficients cannot be directly compared when they are measured in differing units. Different results emerge, for example, depending on whether maternal height is measured in inches or centimeters. To usefully contrast the estimated regression coefficients, they need to be expressed in the same units. One way to make regression coefficients commensurate is to multiply each estimated value by the estimated standard deviation of its associated independent variable giving $\hat{B}_j = b_j \times sd(x_j)$. Standardized coefficients $\hat{B}_j$ from the birth weight example are calculated by

```
> # standardized regression coefficients
> b<- otemp$coefficients
> sd<- sqrt(diag(var(dframe)))
> bstd<- b[-1]*sd[-1]
> bstd
>          ht         wt       gain
 -0.04452282 0.1479587 0.247617.
```

The ability to extract results from one S-calculation and use them in other computations is a major strength of the S-language. The command *otemp$coefficients* extracts the estimated coefficients from the S-object and the S-vector *sd* contains the standard deviations associated with the maternal variables *ht*, *wt*, and *gain* which result from applying three S-functions, namely *var*( ), *diag*( ), and *sqrt*( ). Combining these S-functions yields standardized estimated coefficients. These commensurate coefficients measure the estimated response of Y per standard deviation of x_j, indicating the relative contributions of the variables height, weight, and gain to the variability of infant birth weight. For example, two mothers who differ by one standard deviation in weight gained during pregnancy would be expected to have infants who differ by 0.248 kilograms in birth weight while mothers who differ in height by one standard deviation would be expected to have infants who differ in birth weight by 0.045 kilograms. The comparison shows a considerably stronger influence of weight gain on an infant's birth weight.

To calculate the significance levels associated with the estimated coefficients (p-values) a similar pattern of commands is utilized. The value $t = \hat{b}_j / S_{\hat{b}_j}$ has a t-distribution ($S_{\hat{b}_j}$ is the standard error of the estimate $\hat{b}_j$—labeled "Std. Error" by the *summary*( ) command) with degrees of freedom $n - (k + 1)$ when the independent variable x_j is unrelated to the dependent variable (i.e., $b_j = 0$) For the example data, the following produces the "two-tail" p-values for the birth weight data:

```
> estimates<- otemp$coefficients
> df<- otemp$df.residual
> tvalues<- summary(otemp)$coefficients[,3]
> # "two-tailed" p-value
> pvalues<- 2*(1-pt(abs(tvalues),df))
> round(cbind(estimates,tvalues,pvalues),4)

            estimates tvalues  pvalues
(Intercept)    2.9155  3.4001   0.0008
        ht    -0.0060 -1.0698   0.2858
        wt     0.0125  3.5740   0.0004
      gain     0.0428  6.4760   0.0000.
```

The command *summary(otemp)$coefficients*[, 3] extracts the third column of the array of values displayed by the *summary(otemp)* command, labeled "t value" in the output. These *p*-values are also directly displayed using the *lm*( )-object.

The most important tool for evaluating the influence of the independent variables involves comparing residual deviance values. The residual deviance is the sum of the squared residual values, as noted. A comparison is made between the residual deviance computed from a specific model and a second residual deviance computed from a model created by deleting one or more independent variables from the first model. The difference in fit measured by these two summaries reflects the impact of the deleted variables. Say, a model with k independent variables produces a residual deviance represented by SS_k (degrees of freedom $n - [k + 1]$) and second model with q of these variables deleted produces a residual deviance represented by SS_{k-q} (degrees of freedom $n - [k - q + 1]$). The difference $SS_{k-q} - SS_k$ measures the influence of the q deleted variables plus random variation. If the dependent variable has a normal distribution and the deleted variables have no relevance to Y, then the values SS_k and $SS_{k-q} - SS_k$ have independent chi-square distributions. The test-statistic

$$F = \frac{(SS_{k-q} - SS_k)/q}{SS_k/(n - [k + 1])}$$

then has an F-distribution with q and $n - (k + 1)$ degrees of freedom when the q deleted variables play no role in the linear model describing Y. An F-statistic provides a formal assessment of the differences between sums of squares induced by deleting specific variables from a linear model. Therefore, large values of F reflect an unlikely event or indicate a systematic influence associated with the deleted independent variables.

For example, to evaluate the joint influence of maternal height and weight ("size" of the mother) on the birth weight of an infant, the model containing three variables (*ht*, *wt*, and *gain*) is compared to the model with only *gain* included (two variables, *ht* and *wt* deleted—$q = 2$) or

```
> ss1<- otemp$deviance
> ss1
[1] 76.12054
```

```
> df1<- otemp$df.residual
> otemp0<- glm(bwt~gain,family=gaussian)
> ss0<- otemp0$deviance
> ss0
[1] 80.43175
> df0<- otemp0$df.residual
> q<- df0-df1
> Fstat<- ((ss0-ss1)/q)/(ss1/df1)
> pvalue<- 1-pf(Fstat,q,df1)
> round(cbind(Fstat,q,df1,pvalue),3)
      Fstat   q    df1    pvalue
[1,]  6.457   2    228    0.002.
```

The two measures of fit are SS_1 = 76.121 (degrees of freedom = $232 - 4$ = 228) and SS_0 = 80.432 (degrees of freedom = $232 - 2 = 230$ since q = 2). The large value of F = 6.457 (small level of significance = 0.002) indicates that the deleted variables (*wt* and *ht*) likely play an important role in predicting an infant's birth weight. This analytic process is sometimes referred to as the "F-to-remove" test. Less complicated linear models (fewer parameters) will always describe the data less well. The question is: is the reduction in fit due to chance or due to the fact that the variables removed play an important role? The "F-to-remove" approach is a major step toward an answer.

To evaluate the simultaneous influences of all k independent variables, the $q = k$ independent variables are deleted from the model making $SS_{k-q} = SS_0$ the null deviance. An F-test formally compares the null deviance (no x-values in the model) to the residual deviance (all measured x-variables in the model). For the birth weight data, F = 18.24 with 3 and 228 degrees of freedom yielding a p-value < 0.001 (given in the *lm*( ) summary output—labeled "F-statistic:"). This F-test is equivalent to comparing the observed squared multiple correlation coefficient to zero (is the observed value of R^2 a random deviation from 0?).

The comparison of residual deviances does not address the question of the overall "correctness" of a model. The differences between SS_{k-q} and SS_k can be large or small but the model may not adequately represent the relationships within the data, making comparisons of deviances relatively worthless for assessing the importance of the independent variables. The evaluation of a linear model as a description of the relationships within the data is complicated and many approaches exist (e.g., [2] or [3]). To begin to get some idea of the adequacy of the linear model, a plot of the residual values is frequently valuable. If the assumptions underlying the model (linearity, normality, equal variance, and independence) hold, then the residual values $(y_i - \hat{y}_i)$ have a normal distribution. Since residual values always have a mean of zero, the issue becomes one of whether the residual values are randomly distributed about the line *residual* = 0 or whether some sort of systematic pattern exists.

To display and analyze residual values they are usually normalize. One way to normalize residual values is by dividing by the estimated standard deviation of the dependent variable ($S_{Y|x_1,\cdots,x_k}$ = "Residual standard error" from the *lm*( ) S-function). Other divisors exist, producing alternative standardized residual values that occasionally provide a more sensitive measure of "fit" (next section). A plot of the residual values for the birth weight data is achieved by

```
> se<- sqrt(otemp$deviance/otemp$df.residual)
> rvalues<- otemp$residuals/se
> plot(rvalues,ylim=c(-3,3),ylab="residual values",xlab="index",
    main="Plot of consecutive residuals")
> abline(h=0)
```

Residuals from the birth weight data are shown in Figure 4.3. It is important to keep in mind that a plot of the residual values depends on the ordering of the data (i.e., the residual value from the first observation is plotted furthest the left, the residual value from the second observation is plotted next, and so on). The potential exists that different orderings might reveal different patterns among the plotted residual values.

Inspection of the birth weight residual plot shows perhaps an excess of positive values. If the residual values are random, about half should be positive and half negative. There are 127 positive values out of the 232 calculated birth

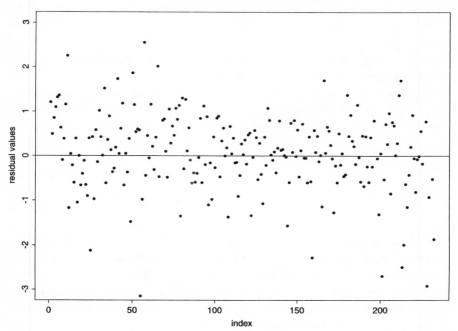

Figure 4.3

weight residual values. A statistical evaluation is accomplished with a binomial test or

```
> n<- length(otemp$residuals)
> # count the positive residual values
> test<- sum(ifelse(otemp$residuals>0,1,0))
> binom.test(test,n)
            Exact binomial test
data: test out of n
number of successes = 127, n = 232, p-value = 0.1678
alternative hypothesis: true p is not equal to 0.5.
```

Other tests for randomness (e.g., the run test, Kolmogorov test, or autocorrelation discussed in Chapter 3) can be applied to evaluate formally observed patterns of residual values [4].

It might be tempting to plot the residual values against the observed values. However, these two quantities are related (i.e., $correlation(y_i - \hat{y}_i, y_i) = \sqrt{1 - R^2}$). Small values of R produce a strong correlation between the residual and observed values. Incidentally, the correlation between the residual values and the estimated values is zero (i.e., $correlation(y_i - \hat{y}_i, \hat{y}_i) = 0$) making any pattern in the residual values "unexplained" by the linear model.

The distribution of the residual values can be assessed (are they normal?) with the quantile plot produced by $qqnorm( )$. Continuing the birth weight example, the S-command

```
> qqnorm(sort(rvalues),type = "l",
    main="qqnorm(additive model) -- 20 random qqnorm plots")
```

yields an approximate straight line when the residual values have a normal or at least an approximate normal distribution.

To judge the magnitude of the deviations of the plotted points from the straight line expected when the data are normally distributed, 20 "data" sets of $n = 232$ simulated standard random normal values are also plotted on the qqnorm plot by

```
> n<- 232
> for (i in 1:20) {
    par(new=T)
    qqnorm(rnorm(n),pch=".",ylab="",yaxt="n")
}
```

The "data" (Figure 4.4—second column) show the behavior of 232 random normally distributed values. These values exactly conform to the underlying requirement that the residual values be normally distributed with mean = 0, and variance = 1, giving a picture of the impact of random variation on the qqnorm plot. As before, $par(new=T)$ causes the simulated values to be placed on the current plot and the options $ylab=$"" and $yaxt=$"n" suppress the repeated labeling of the y-axes.

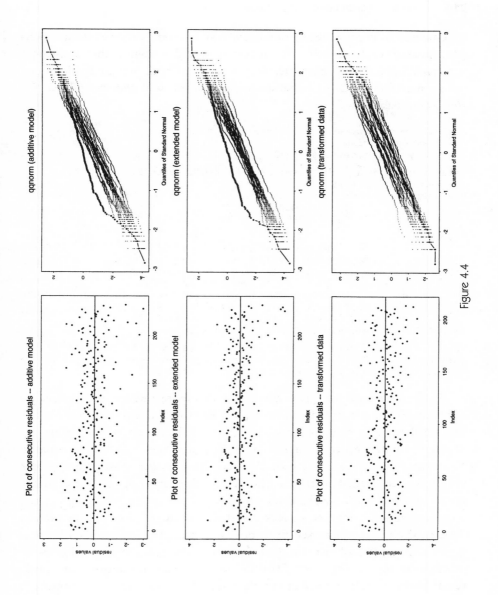

Figure 4.4

One way to improve the fit of a linear regression model is to add independent variables to the analysis. Adding variables and evaluating their influences
is straightforward. For example, to evaluate the birth weight model when
the squared influences of maternal height, weight, and gain are added, the
glm( )-command gives

```
> otemp1<- glm(bwt~wt+wt^2+ht+ht2+gain+gain^2,
    family=gaussian)
> summary(otemp1,correlation=F)

Call: glm(formula = bwt~wt+wt^2+ht+ht^2+gain+gain^2,
    family = gaussian)
Deviance Residuals:
      Min         1Q      Median         3Q        Max
 -2.403279 -0.2250031 0.02957368 0.3309177 1.390099

Coefficients:
                  Value    Std. Error     t value
(Intercept) -2.510269e+01 1.033871e+01 -2.428030
         wt  3.335288e-02 2.041119e-02  1.634049
    I(wt^2) -1.448722e-04 1.417937e-04 -1.021711
         ht  3.174884e-01 1.252077e-01  2.535694
    I(ht^2) -9.813029e-04 3.783207e-04 -2.593839
       gain  1.410204e-01 2.445551e-02  5.766406
  I(gain^2)  -2.993065e-03 7.236076e-04 -4.136310

(Dispersion Parameter for Gaussian family taken to be 0.302588)
Null Deviance: 94.38865 on 231 degrees of freedom
Residual Deviance: 68.0823 on 225 degrees of freedom.
```

The residual and the qqplot plots from this more sophisticated model are
shown in Figure 4.4 (middle row). A more extensive model necessarily better
fits the data. The residual deviance is always decreased by increasing the
number of independent variables (i.e., SS_{k+m} is always less than or equal to
SS_k when m variables are added). A direct consequence is that the multiple
correlation coefficient increases when additional terms are included in the
model. For the birth weight data, $new - R = 0.528$ when the three squared
terms are added compared to $R = 0.440$ without these terms. An important
issue is whether the increased fit is more than would be expected by chance.
Again comparison of two residual deviances addresses the question as to
whether or not the improved fit of the model containing more terms likely
results from capitalizing on random variation. An F-statistic ("F-to-remove")
along the lines previously described yields $F = 8.855$ with an extremely small
significance probability (p-value < 0.001). The large F (a small p-value) indicates that the decrease in the residual deviance (76.121 to 68.082) caused by
adding squared terms to the model is likely due to systematic ("real") influences associated with the added variables. Despite the improved fit, the residual values do not appear to be a random sample of 232 normally distributed
values (middle row, Figure 4.4). The line plotted by *qqnorm*( ) lies mostly
outside the range described by the 20 simulated random normal samples.

To improve the normality of the data, low birth weight infants were eliminated (birth weight < 2.5 kilograms) and the remaining birth weights were transformed to produce a more symmetric distribution. There are a variety of ways to select optimum transformations [4]. For the variable birth weight, the logarithm of the dependent variable was chosen (i.e., new-$y = log[bwt]$). A linear regression analysis based on the three independent variables wt, ht, and $gain$, using the truncated data ($n = 213$ birth weights greater than 2.5 kilograms) and a transformed dependent variable produces residual and quantile plots also shown in Figure 4.4 (bottom row). Although a model based on a subset of the birth weight data and a transformed dependent variable does not fit the data as well as the untransformed model with squared terms (multiple correlation coefficient 0.462 versus 0.528), the restricted model better fulfills the underlying requirements of a linear regression model and, therefore, allows more valid statistical inferences.

A CLOSER LOOK AT RESIDUAL VALUES

The simple residual value $y_i - \hat{y}_i$ measures the deviation of the estimated value from the corresponding observed value. Directly measured residual values depend on the scale used to measure the y-variable. The difference $20 - 10$ is not likely comparable to $220 - 210$ or a value with a variance of 2 is not comparable to a value with a variance of 20. To statistically test or visually describe residual values, it is important to make comparisons free of the influences of scale. One way to essentially eliminate the influence of scale is to divide by an associated standard deviation. The "new" residual values are unitless and have approximately constant variance, namely = 1.0. The mean of the n residual values is always (mathematically) equal to 0.0. Once transformed, the descriptions "large" and "small" take on a somewhat arbitrary but useful meaning. For example, "large" residual values can be defined as greater than 1.6 and "small" residual values as less than -1.6, regardless of the original measurement units.

First, a presentation of some relevant standard errors is necessary before describing three common ways to express residual values. The estimated standard error of the dependent variable Y, as before, is

$$S_{Y|x_1,\ldots,x_k} = \sqrt{\frac{\sum(y_i - \hat{y}_i)^2}{n - (k + 1)}}$$

and in terms of S-functions

```
> otemp<- glm(y~x,family=gaussian)
> s<- sqrt(otemp$deviance/otemp$df.residual)
```

where y is an S-vector of n dependent variables and x is a $n \times k$ array of independent variables.

All observations are not equally important in determining the estimated value $\hat{y}_i$. Some observations have small influences, some have large influences and some can have extremely disproportional effects (outliers). To identify the importance of each observation, a first step is a measure of each observation's influence on the estimated value $\hat{y}_i$. One such measure is called leverage, as mentioned. Leverage measures the degree of conformity of a single observation to the linear pattern established by the other $n - 1$ observations. Leverage addresses the question: is y_i usual? If the answer is no, the leverage value will be large and possibly close to 1.0 and if the answer is yes, the leverage value will be close to $1/n$. The diagonal elements of the "hat" matrix measure leverage. In matrix algebra terms, the "hat" matrix is $\mathbf{X}(\mathbf{X}'\mathbf{X})^{-1}\mathbf{X}'$ and the diagonal elements are the leverage values (h_i) or, in symbols,

$$h_i = diagonal(\mathbf{X}(\mathbf{X}'\mathbf{X})^{-1}\mathbf{X}') = [\mathbf{X}(\mathbf{X}'\mathbf{X})^{-1}\mathbf{X}']_{ii}.$$

The symbol $\mathbf{X}$ represents an array that contains the independent variables and is defined specifically in Chapter 5. In terms of S-functions, either

```
> h<- lm.influence(lm(y~x))$hat
```

or

```
> h<- ls.diag(lsfit(x,y))$hat
```

produces the n leverage values. The h_i-values (one for each observation) theoretically range from $1/n$ to 1. Large values are those that exceed $2k/n$ ([3] or [5]). A value of h_i in the neighborhood of one indicates that the ith observation almost completely determines the regression equation. A value near $1/n$ indicates an observation with no unusual impact on the estimate of the dependent variable. For a regression model with one independent variable, the leverage associated with the specific observation (x_m, y_m) is

$$leverage \ of \ the \ m^{th} \ observation = h_m = \frac{1}{n} + \frac{(x_m - \bar{x})^2}{\sum(x_i - \bar{x})^2}.$$

To illustrate leverage for a linear regression model with more than one independent variable, the birth weight data produce

```
> h<- lm.influence(lm(bwt~cbind(wt,ht,gain)))$hat
> hord<- order(h)
> n<- length(h)
> m<- hord[n:(n-4)]
> m
[1] 121 114 28 51 217
> cbind(round(h[m],3),bwt[m],wt[m],ht[m],gain[m])
        [,1] [,2]   [,3]  [,4] [,5]
  121 0.134 4.30 122.2 173.0 14.0
  114 0.109 3.14  66.0 197.0 26.0
```

```
 28 0.074 3.70  95.4 160.0  5.1
 51 0.072 4.48 104.0 168.9 14.4
217 0.061 3.55 101.0 172.7 15.5.
```

which are the five observations with the greatest leverage values (k, h, bwt, wt, ht, and $gain$, respectively columns 1–6). More complete descriptions of leverage values and their properties are found elsewhere ([2] or [3]).

The main issue here is that leverage values play a role in the variances associated with linear model residuals. The estimated standard error of the ith residual value $y_i - \hat{y}_i$ is

$$S_{y_i - \hat{y}_i} = S_{Y|x_1, \cdots, x_k} \sqrt{1 - h_i}.$$

The standard deviation of a residual value takes into account two sources of variability—the variability from the estimated value plus the variability associated with the observed value.

Another measure of variability important in using residual values to diagnose problems in a regression analysis is the estimated standard error of Y when the ith observation is removed from the computation, or

$$S_{y_{(i)}} = \sqrt{\frac{\sum (y_i - \hat{y}_{(i)})^2}{(n-1) - (k+1)}}.$$

The symbol $\hat{y}_{(i)}$ represents the estimated dependent variable based on $n - 1$ observations (i^{th} observation removed). This estimate of variability is the usual estimate of the standard deviation of the dependent variable Y from a regression equation but based on one less observation ($n - 1$). In terms of S-functions, the n standard deviations (one for each observation removed) are estimated by

```
> se<- NULL
> for (i in 1:nrow(x)) {
  otemp<- glm(y[-i]~x[-i,],family=gaussian)
  se[i]<- sqrt(otemp$deviance/otemp$df.residual)
> }
```

or using a short-cut formula [3] that is considerably faster when n is large ($n > 30$ or so)

$$S_{y_{(i)}}^2 = \frac{S_{Y|x_1,x_2,\cdots,x_k}^2 (n-k) - (y_i - \hat{y}_i)^2/(1 - h_i)}{n - (k+1)}.$$

Three ways to transform simple residual values are:

1. normalized residual values

$$resnorm_i = \frac{y_i - \hat{y}_i}{S_{Y|x_1,\cdots,x_k}},$$

2. standardized residual values

$$resstd_i = \frac{y_i - \hat{y}_i}{S_{y_i - \hat{y}_i}} = \frac{y_i - \hat{y}_i}{S_{y_i}\sqrt{1 - h_i}},$$

3. and Studentized residual values

$$resstud_i = \frac{y_i - \hat{y}_i}{S_{y_{(i)}}\sqrt{1 - h_i}}.$$

The three residual values calculated with S-functions again from the birth weight data are

```
> # n=observations, k=variables and h=leverage values
> res<- otemp$residuals
> resnorm<- res/s
> resstd<- res/(s*sqrt(1-h))
> se0<- sqrt((n-k)*s^2/(n-k-1)-res^2/((n-k-1)*(1-h)))
> resstud<- res/(se0*sqrt(1-h))
```

Normalized residual values are simple but have only approximately constant variance. However, the variance is close to 1.0 for most regression analyses. Standardized residuals are a more typical statistical measure, that is, a statistical quantity divided by its standard error. Standardized residual values are essentially scale free (variance = 1.0) but suffer from the flaw that the numerator and denominator are related. Extreme values of the standard error $S_{y_i - \hat{y}_i}$ tend to occur when the residual value $y_i - \hat{y}_i$ is itself extreme, making it difficult to use these two estimates in a formal test-statistic. Studentized residual values (sometimes called jackknife residuals— Chapter 5) are a bit complicated but are close to scale free and have t-distributions. The statistic $resstud_i$ has an approximate t-distribution with $n - (k + 1)$ degrees of freedom when the difference $y_i - \hat{y}_i$ represents only random variation. Studentized residuals, therefore, make it possible to use a formal statistical test as part of the analysis of residual values if desired, which is not usually the case.

The distinction among the three types of transformed residual values is frequently more theoretical than practical since the h_i-values tend to be small (i.e., $\sqrt{1 - h_i} \approx 1$), producing transformed residual values that are more or less equal. For example, a few of the 232 residual values from the regression analysis of birth weight with independent variables maternal weight, height, and weight gain (Table 4.2) are:

```
> round(cbind(bwt,predict(otemp),res,resnorm,resstd,resstud),3)
       y    yhat     res normres resstd resstud
 1  3.860  3.162   0.698   1.208  1.213   1.214
 2  3.560  3.274   0.286   0.495  0.496   0.496
 3  3.480  2.987   0.493   0.852  0.858   0.858
 4  4.190  3.555   0.635   1.099  1.105   1.106
 5  4.050  3.287   0.763   1.320  1.331   1.333
 6  4.140  3.352   0.788   1.365  1.369   1.372
 7  3.660  3.290   0.370   0.640  0.642   0.642
 8  3.160  3.215  -0.055  -0.096 -0.096  -0.096
 9  3.540  3.316   0.224   0.388  0.389   0.389
10  3.840  3.172   0.668   1.157  1.161   1.162
11  4.260  2.955   1.305   2.259  2.273   2.294
```

```
  .       .        .       .       .       .       .
  .       .        .       .       .       .       .
  .       .        .       .       .       .       .
  .       .        .       .       .       .       .
224 3.520  3.196  0.324    0.561  0.565    0.564
225 3.060  3.165 -0.105   -0.182 -0.182   -0.182
226 1.420  3.528 -2.108   -3.648 -3.715   -3.824
227 3.500  3.050  0.450    0.778  0.783    0.783
228 1.930  3.620 -1.690   -2.924 -2.983   -3.036
229 2.570  3.106 -0.536   -0.928 -0.934   -0.934
230 0.670  2.832 -2.162   -3.742 -3.782   -3.898
231 2.850  3.154 -0.304   -0.526 -0.530   -0.529
232 1.860  2.938 -1.078   -1.866 -1.888   -1.898.
```

PREDICT—POINTWISE CONFIDENCE INTERVALS

The S-function *predict*($S.object$) produces estimated values from an application of the *glm*( ) or *lm*( ) functions, as noted. For the birth weight data, *predict*(*otemp*) produces $n = 232$ estimated values $\hat{y}_i$ estimated from the regression model

$$\hat{y}_i = b\hat{w}t_i = 2.915 - 0.006ht_i + 0.013wt_i + 0.043gain_i$$

and the 232 observed sets of the independent variables $\{ht_i, wt_i,$ and $gain_i\}$.

The *predict*( ) function also can be used to estimate values from the regression model based on any specified values of the independent variables. The independent variables are communicated to the *predict*( ) function by way of a data frame. The S-function *data.frame*( ) is used to create a data frame containing the input values. For the birth weight data, say it is of interest to estimate the birth weights of infants whose mothers gain 12, 15, or 18 kilograms during pregnancy and have heights 163 centimeters (mean) and weights 58 kilograms (mean). A data frame is created by

```
> d.gain<- data.frame(ht=c(163,163,163),wt=c(58,58,58),
    gain=c(12,15,18))
```

Using this specially constructed data frame, then

```
> yhat<- predict(otemp,d.gain)
> yhat
        1          2          3
 3.170099   3.298356   3.426613
```

calculates the desired predicted birth weights. The standard errors associated with these estimates are also available as an option associated with the *predict*( ) function or

```
> se<- predict(otemp,d.gain,se=T)$se.fit
> se
         1            2            3
 0.04511388   0.03823817   0.04090875.
```

Estimated standard errors of the predicted values are used to construct point-wise $(1 - \alpha)\%$ confidence intervals. For $1 - \alpha = 0.95$, then

```
> df<- otemp$df.residual
> # lower 95% bound
> yhat-qt(0.975,df)*se
         1           2           3
  3.081206    3.223011    3.346006
> # upper 95% bound
> yhat+qt(0.975,df)*se
         1           2           3
  3.258993    3.373702    3.507221
```

are the lower and upper bounds of a 95% confidence interval based on the estimated birth weights and their standard errors. The S-function *pointwise*( ) produces the identical confidence intervals. For example,

```
> pointwise(predict(otemp,d.gain,se=T),coverage=0.95)$lower
         1           2           3
  3.081206    3.223011    3.346006
> pointwise(predict(otemp,d.gain,se=T),coverage=0.95)$upper
         1           2           3
  3.258993    3.373702    3.507221
```

are the same lower and upper bounds based on the values estimated from the independent variables described by the data frame *d.gain*. The value estimated by $\hat{y}_i$ has a pointwise probability of 0.95 of lying between the two confidence interval bounds. Specifically, for mothers with average height and weight who gain 12 kilograms during their pregnancy, the likely range (95%) for their infant's birth weight is 3.081 to 3.260 kilograms.

For a simple linear regression analysis (one independent variable), these pointwise confidence intervals are sometimes confused with a confidence band. A confidence band is constructed so that the probability is $1 - \alpha$ that the "true" regression line lies between two bounds. A pointwise confidence interval is constructed so that the probability is $1 - \alpha$ that the "true" dependent value lies between two bounds. Occasionally, the end points of a series of pointwise intervals are connected and incorrectly interpreted as a confidence band. The correct confidence band is larger [6].

FORMULAS FOR *glm*( )

The S-language allows a number of ways a linear model can be communicated to an S-function. Without going into detail the following are nine examples employing two independent variables:

1. $y \sim x_1 + x_2$ y equals the sum of x_1 and x_2 $(y_i = a + bx_{i1} + cx_{i2})$
2. $y \sim x_1 + x_2 + x_1 * x_2$ y equals the sum of x_1 and x_2 with an interaction term
3. $y \sim (x_1 + x_2)^2$ equivalent to 2

4. $y^\sim x_1 * x_2$ equivalent to 2
5. $y^\sim x_2 + x_1/x_2$ variable x_2 is nested within x_1 (Chapter 6)
6. $y^\sim x_1/x_2$ equivalent to 5
7. $y^\sim x_2\%in\%x_1$ equivalent to 5
8. $y^\sim -1 + x_1 + x_1$ y equals the sum of x_1 and x_2 with origin equal zero
9. $y^\sim poly(x, 2)$ y equals a second degree polynomial ($y_i = a + bx_i + cx_i^2$).

Inserting a "-1" into the *glm*( ) formula makes the origin zero ($a = 0$). For example, the expression $y \sim -1 + x$ is the S-formula for the model $y_i = bx_i$ and not the model $y_i = -1 + bx_i$. The S-formulas with more than two independent variables have analogous forms.

POLYNOMIAL REGRESSION

The *glm*( )-function readily applies to estimating the components of a linear model based on a polynomial function of an independent variable. A polynomial expression

$$a + b_1 x + b_2 x^2 + b_3 x^3 + \cdots + b_k x^k$$

can be represented by the S-convention *poly*(x, k) and the *glm*-function used to estimate the coefficients. For example,

```
> b<- glm(y~poly(x,4))$coefficients
```

estimates the five regression coefficients necessary to describe the data contained in the vector y by a fourth degree polynomial based on the measurements x. The S-language has a shorthand notation for polynomials, as illustrated, that allows a polynomial expression to be communicated to the *glm* function with the syntax *poly*(*independent variable, degree*). In fact, the S-function *poly*( ) produces a set of orthogonal polynomials that are the basis for a polynomial regression analysis. Note again that a polynomial function produces a polynomial (linear) model. The independent variables are not linear functions but the sum (linear combination) of the each of these variables makes up a linear model describing the dependent variable Y.

To illustrate a polynomial regression and at the same time introduce an important transformation, data on perinatal mortality (fetal deaths plus deaths within the first month of life) and birth weight for black and white racial classifications are analyzed (Table 4.3). A comparison of the black perinatal mortality probability $\hat{p}_{black} = 0.024$ to the white value $\hat{p}_{white} = 0.011$ shows a greater than twofold increase in risk associated with black infants ($\hat{p} = deaths/births$). However, the black infants have, by and large, lower birth weights and smaller infants have higher mortality regardless of race. To assess differences in mortality experience associated with race, comparisons must

Table 4.3. Perinatal mortality for black and white infants born in California classified by 37 birth weight (grams) categories, 1988

weight	black			white		
	deaths	births*	probability × 1000	deaths	births*	probability × 1000
<800	533	618	862.5	1 585	1 759	901.1
801–900	65	131	496.2	173	322	537.3
901–1000	40	122	327.9	148	337	439.2
1001–1100	30	131	229.0	134	398	336.7
1101–1200	29	137	211.7	106	381	278.2
1201–1300	21	143	146.9	103	444	232.0
1301–1400	19	143	132.9	86	427	201.4
1401–1500	19	165	115.2	108	597	180.9
1501–1600	20	167	119.8	85	560	151.8
1601–1700	24	219	109.6	84	682	123.2
1701–1800	12	194	61.9	86	722	119.1
1801–1900	26	298	87.2	100	935	107.0
1901–2000	15	299	50.2	81	978	82.8
2001–2100	21	420	50.0	74	1589	46.6
2101–2200	10	453	22.1	87	1 714	50.8
2201–2300	14	603	23.2	82	2 322	27.7
2301–2400	12	763	15.7	80	2 885	27.7
2401–2500	13	977	13.3	80	4 149	19.3
2501–2600	14	1 189	11.8	77	4 916	15.7
2601–2700	10	1 654	6.0	93	7 455	12.5
2701–2800	17	1 796	9.5	93	8 855	10.5
2801–2900	11	2 545	4.3	100	14 197	7.0
2901–3000	9	2 947	3.1	86	17 903	4.8
3001–3100	12	2 851	4.2	92	19 969	4.6
3101–3200	9	3 557	2.5	90	27 068	3.3
3201–3300	9	3 324	2.7	96	29 107	3.3
3301–3400	11	3 577	3.1	79	35 627	2.2
3401–3500	1	3 119	0.3	67	32 926	2.0
3501–3600	9	2 952	3.0	69	36 360	1.9
3601–3700	7	2 250	3.1	58	30 612	1.9
3701–3800	2	2 176	0.9	59	32 119	1.8
3801–3900	3	1 573	1.9	40	24 004	1.7
3901–4000	1	1 348	0.7	35	23 217	1.5
4001–4100	3	909	3.3	30	16 232	1.8
4101–4200	1	735	1.4	19	14 233	1.3
4201–4300	1	489	2.0	17	9 781	1.7
>4300	57	1 163	49.0	225	25 760	8.7
total	1 110	46 137	24.1	4 707	431 542	10.9

* births = live births + fetal deaths

compensate for differing influences of birth weight. A series of comparisons within specific birth weight categories is one way of minimizing influences from differences in birth weight because each category (the rows of Table 4.3) contain infants with approximately equal birth weights. Another approach postulates a statistical model to represent the relationship between birth weight and mortality designed to provide a single summary measure of black/white mortality differences "free" of the effects from the differing birth weight distributions.

The probabilities of perinatal death $\hat{p}_i$ are plotted in Figure 4.5 (upper left) for black (solid line) and white (dotted line) infants by birth weight (grams).

Instead of directly analyzing the probabilities p_i, a transformation $y_i = log(-log(p_i))$ is used. This function of the probability p_i is called the complementary log-log transformation and applies in a variety of statistical contexts. A plot of the transformed values is displayed in Figure 4.5 (upper right). To evaluate the influence of race on mortality, an "adjusted" estimate that accounts for differences in birth weight is produced by the linear model

$$y_i = a + b_0 g + b_1 x_i + b_2 x_i^2 + b_3 x_i^3 + b_4 x_i^4$$

where y_i is the complementary log-log transformed perinatal mortality probability and x_i represents a specific birth weight. The variable g is a binary variable indicating race ($g = 1$ for black and $g = 0$ for white). The complementary log-log transformation was chosen because it produces mortality differences that are approximately constant at all birth weights (no interaction). The coefficient b_0 then measures this constant difference in perinatal mortality between black and white infants "adjusted" for birth weight. Specifically, the difference $y_{black} - y_{white}$ equals b_0 at any birth weight x. To estimate the coefficients of this polynomial model, particularly the coefficient b_0, then

```
> # p contains the mortality probabilities
> # 37 black and 37 white observations
> x0<- c(800,seq(850,4250,100),4400)
> x<- c(x0,x0)
> n<- length(x0)
> g<- c(rep(1,n),rep(0,n))
> y<- log(-log(p))
> otemp<- glm(y~g+poly(x,4))
```

giving estimates

```
> summary(otemp,correlation=F)

Call: glm(formula = y ~ g + poly(x, 4))
Deviance Residuals:
      Min        1Q      Median        3Q        Max
 -1.132475  -0.09386523  0.01372841  0.113068  0.5261284

Coefficients:
                 Value Std. Error     t value
(Intercept)   1.12352675 0.04116187  27.295326
          g   0.09371383 0.05821168   1.609880
poly(x, 4)1   5.80151250 0.25037790  23.171025
poly(x, 4)2  -2.99723576 0.25037790 -11.970848
poly(x, 4)3   0.70069884 0.25037790   2.798565
```

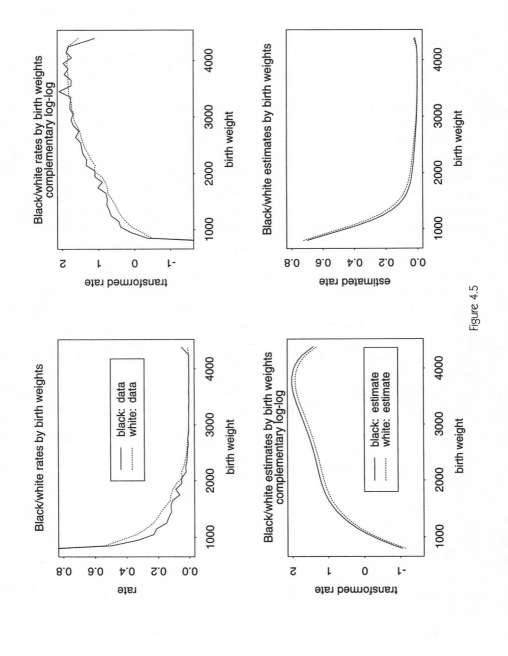

Figure 4.5

```
poly(x, 4)4 -1.37424762 0.25037790  -5.488694
```

```
(Dispersion Parameter for Gaussian family taken to be 0.0626891 )
    Null Deviance: 49.44584 on 73 degrees of freedom
Residual Deviance: 4.262858 on 68 degrees of freedom.
```

The model estimated values $\hat{y}_i$ closely correspond to the observed values y_i or

```
> cor(y,predict(otemp))
[1] 0.9559222.
```

Of particular interest is the estimate $\hat{b}_0 = 0.094$, which effectively summarizes the differences in mortality probabilities "free" of the influence of birth weight (at the same birth weight). The model represents race-specific transformed mortality probabilities by parallel lines yielding a single estimate of black/white differences at any birth weight. The estimated relationship between birth weight and the specific values y_i for black and white infants is displayed in Figure 4.5 (lower two plots). As before, the estimated curves are calculated with the S-command *predict(otemp)*. The distance between the two parallel lines $\hat{b}_0 = 0.094$ reflects the influence of race. However, a statistical evaluation shows only marginal evidence of a significant role of race in perinatal mortality after accounting for birth weight ($z = 1.610$ from *summary*( ) yields a *p*-value = 0.058).

To compare "adjusted" black/white perinatal mortality probabilities (per 1000 births) for a few selected birth weights (1000, 2000, 3000 and 4000 grams), then

```
> b<- otemp$coefficients
> pwhite<- c(337,47,5,2)/1000
> pblack<- pwhite^(exp(b[2]))
> bwt<- c(1000,2000,3000,4000)
> # probability*1000
> pwhite<- 1000*pwhite
> pblack<- 1000*pblack
> round(cbind(bwt,pblack,pwhite),2)
      bwt pblack pwhite
[1,] 1000 302.85 337.0
[2,] 2000  34.80  47.0
[3,] 3000   2.97   5.0
[4,] 4000   1.09   2.0.
```

In symbols, since $\hat{y}_{black} - \hat{y}_{white} = \hat{b}_0$, then $p_{black} = [p_{white}]^{\hat{c}}$ where $\hat{c} = e^{\hat{b}_0}$ or, specifically, $p_{black} = [p_{white}]^{1.098}$, comparing perinatal risk "free" of birth weight influences.

DISCRIMINANT ANALYSIS

Discriminant analysis is primarily designed to classify observations into two or more groups based on combining multivariate measurements into a summary score. Emphasis is on constructing these scores and using them to classify observations into a series of predefined categories. Although this statistical technique appears rather different from linear regression analysis, in fact the two approaches are essentially the same under specific conditions.

Discriminant analysis applies to data consisting of k multivariate measurements $x_1, x_2, x_3, \cdots, x_k$ made on each of n observations along with a variable indicating group membership. In the following, classification into only two groups is considered. The more general multi-group case is described elsewhere [7]. The defining characteristic of a discriminant analysis is the combining of the multivariate measurements into a score, a simple linear combination, denoted by D. These scores are weighted sums of the x-values and the members of each group are summarized by a mean discriminant score given by

$$\bar{D}_1 = a_1\bar{x}_{11} + a_2\bar{x}_{12} + a_3\bar{x}_{13} + \cdots + a_k\bar{x}_{1k} \quad \text{(group I)}$$
$$\bar{D}_2 = a_1\bar{x}_{21} + a_2\bar{x}_{22} + a_3x_{23} + \cdots + a_k\bar{x}_{2k} \quad \text{(group II)}$$

where $\bar{x}_{gj}$ is the mean of the variable j from group $g = 1$ or 2 and k represents again the number of measurements made on each of n observations.

Data (Table 4.4) were collected on $n = 48$ painted turtles [8] where the length (x_1), width (x_2), and height (x_3) of each turtle's carapace were measured ($k = 3$). The turtles were also classified by gender (group I = male and group II = female). For these measurements, the group mean values are *group I: male* = $\{\bar{x}_{11}, \bar{x}_{12}, \bar{x}_{13}\}$ = $\{113.375, 88.292, 40.708\}$ and *group II: female* = $\{\bar{x}_{21}, \bar{x}_{22}, \bar{x}_{23}\}$ = $\{136.000, 102.583, 51.958\}$.

The specific mean discriminant scores are then

$$\bar{D}_1 = a_1(113.375) + a_2(88.292) + a_3(40.708) \quad \text{(male)}$$
$$\bar{D}_2 = a_1(136.000) + a_2(102.583) + a_3(51.958) \quad \text{(female)}$$

where the $\bar{x}_{gj}$-values are the mean lengths, widths, and heights of the turtle shells within each gender group.

The fundamental question is: how should the discriminant score coefficients a_j be selected? To answer this question the data must meet two requirements. The observations must be sampled independently and the variables must have the same variances and covariances in both groups I and II. The values of the discriminant coefficients a_j are the chosen so that

$$\hat{M}^2 = \left[\frac{\bar{D}_1 - \bar{D}_2}{\text{standard deviation of } D}\right]^2$$

is maximum. The quantity $\hat{M}$ is the difference between mean discriminant scores measured in standard deviations. The coefficients based on this criter-

Table 4.4. Carapace dimensions of "painted" turtles (Chrysemys picta marginata)

Males			Females		
length	width	height	length	width	height
93	74	37	98	81	38
94	78	35	103	84	38
96	80	35	103	86	42
101	84	39	105	86	40
102	85	38	109	88	44
103	81	37	123	92	50
104	83	39	123	95	46
106	83	39	133	99	51
107	82	38	133	102	51
112	89	40	133	102	51
113	88	40	134	100	48
114	86	40	136	102	49
116	90	43	137	98	51
117	90	41	138	99	51
117	91	41	141	105	53
119	93	41	147	108	57
120	89	40	149	107	55
120	93	44	153	107	56
121	95	42	155	115	63
125	93	45	155	117	60
127	96	45	158	115	62
128	95	45	159	118	63
131	95	46	162	124	61
135	106	47	177	132	67

ion guarantee the greatest "distance" between mean discriminant scores for the analyzed data set.

The coefficients that maximize M^2 are found by applying usual least squares regression analysis using the x-measurements as independent variables and specially constructed values as the dependent variables. The dependent variables are created by:

if an observation belongs to group I, then set $\quad y_i = -\dfrac{n_2}{n_1 + n_2}\quad$ and

if an observation belongs to group II, then set $\quad y_i = \dfrac{n_1}{n_1 + n_2}$

where i indicates the ith observation ($i = 1, 2, 3, \cdots , n$ = total number of observations) with n_1 members of group I and n_2 members of group II ($n_1 + n_2 = n$). The least squares estimated regression coefficients from a multivariable linear model are then the a_j-values that maximize M^2 [7]. In fact, no unique set of discriminant coefficients maximizes M^2. A little algebra shows that if the discriminant coefficients a_j maximize M^2, then $ba_j + c$ also maximize M^2

where b and c are constant values. Different coefficients are calculated by different software systems.

Using the S-function $glm(\ )$ produces a specific set of discriminant score coefficients. A standardization (specific choice of the constants b and c) yields the discriminant scores calculated by many discriminant analysis programs. An S-language discriminant analysis function $discr(\ )$ produces a slightly different set of coefficients for linear discriminant analysis. Using a linear regression approach to discriminant analysis, the S-function $glm(\ )$ applied to the turtle data gives

```
> # x = array, cols = length (x1), width (x2) and
       height (x3) and  n = rows = 48 = observations
> # n1 = 24 males and n2 = 24 females
> # g = 0 = male and g = 1 = female
> ytemp<- ifelse(g==0,-n2/(n1+n2),n1/(n1+n2))
> otemp<- glm(ytemp~x)
> summary(otemp,correlation=F)

Call: glm(formula = ytemp ~ x)
Deviance Residuals:
          Min          1Q     Median          3Q          Max
 -0.4870349-0.2469211 -0.1002869  0.2431237  0.7861947

Coefficients:
                  Value Std. Error      t value
(Intercept) -1.14518681 0.51183612  -2.2374091
         x1 -0.02914385 0.01272524  -2.2902396
         x2 -0.01025028 0.01947690  -0.5262786
         x3  0.12425872 0.02313557   5.3708946

(Dispersion Parameter for Gaussian family taken to be 0.1112625)
Null Deviance: 12 on 47 degrees of freedom
Residual Deviance: 4.895549 on 44 degrees of freedom

> y<- predict(otemp)
> # estimated pooled within group variance of y
> v<- ((n1-1)*var(y[g==0])+(n2-1)*var(y[g==1]))/(n1+n2-2)
> # standardized discriminant scores
> d<- y/sqrt(v)
> d1<- d[g==0]
> d2<- d[g==1]
> # squared distance between mean discriminant scores
> m2dist<- (mean(d2)-mean(d1))^2
> cat(" group 1 =",round(mean(d1),4)," group 2 =",
      round(mean(d2),4),"m2dist =",round(m2dist,4),"\n")
   group 1 = -1.1793 group 2 = 1.1793 m2dist = 5.563.
```

Two mean discriminant scores are formed based on estimates calculated with $predict(\ )$, one from each group. The overall mean value of the estimated scores is zero. If S_p^2 represents the pooled estimated variance combining within group variance estimates from groups I and II of the predicted values $\hat{y}_{gj}$, then standardized values produce discriminant scores (d_{gj}) with overall mean = 0 and pooled variance = 1. In symbols, a standardized discriminant score is

$$d_{gj} = \frac{\hat{y}_{gj}}{S_p}$$

where $g = 1, 2 =$ groups and $j = 1, 2, 3, \cdots, n_g =$ observations per group.

The values $\{d_{11}, d_{12}, d_{13}, \cdots, d_{1n_1}\}$ represent the n_1 standardized discriminant scores from group I and similarly $\{d_{21}, d_{22}, d_{23} \cdots, d_{2n_2}\}$ represent the n_2 standardized discriminant scores from group II. The mean values $\bar{d}_1$ ($\sum d_{1j}/n_1$) and $\bar{d}_2$ ($\sum d_{2j}/n_2$) are the mean discriminant scores summarizing the multivariate characteristics of these two groups. The squared distance between these two means is $\hat{M}^2 = (\bar{d}_2 - \bar{d}_1)^2$ since the estimated standard deviation of D is 1.0. The quantity $\hat{M}^2$ is a measure of the multivariate distance between groups I and II based on the x-measurements. The symbol $\hat{M}^2$ stands for the estimated Mahalanobis distance, which is another term for this important summary measure of the difference between two groups. For the turtle data, $M^2 = [1.179 - (-1.179)]^2 = 5.563$. Unlike Euclidean distance, this measure of multivariate distance accounts for the interrelationships (correlations) among the k measurements that makeup the compared observations.

Once a multivariate distance is estimated, the question arises: does this distance represent a systematic difference between groups or is the observed distance likely to have occurred due to capitalizing on random variability? A statistical measure called Wilk's lambda is an often used quantitative function of the distance $\hat{M}^2$ and when it is transformed has an approximate chi-square distribution, allowing statistical assessment of an estimated multivariate distance. Wilk's statistic $\hat{\lambda}$ is defined as

$$\hat{\lambda} = \frac{within\ group\ sum\ of\ squares}{total\ sum\ of\ squares} = \frac{\sum\sum(d_{gj} - \bar{d}_g)^2}{\sum\sum(d_{gj} - \bar{d})^2} = \frac{n_1 + n_2 - 2}{\sum\sum(d_{gj} - \bar{d})^2}$$

based on the discriminant scores d_{gj}. Alternatively,

$$\hat{\lambda} = 1 - \frac{\frac{n_1 n_2}{n_1 + n_2}\hat{M}^2}{\sum\sum(d_{gj} - \bar{d})^2} \qquad g = 1, 2 \text{ and } j = 1, 2, 3, \cdots, n_g.$$

The measure $\hat{\lambda}$ reflects the "size" of the distance $\hat{M}^2$ as a number between 0 and 1 $(0 \leq \hat{\lambda} \leq 1)$. Small values of $\hat{\lambda}$ (near zero) reflect large multivariate distances and, conversely, small multivariate distances result in large values of $\hat{\lambda}$ (near one). An important feature of Wilk's lambda is that $X^2 = -(n - k/2 - 2)log(\hat{\lambda})$ has an approximate chi-square distribution with k degrees of freedom when the x-measurements are not relevant to classifying the multivariate observations into two groups. In terms of the turtle data, an assessment of the multivariate distance between males and females is

```
> # vector d contains n1 + n2 = 48 discriminant scores
> lam<- (n1+n2-2)/sum((d-mean(d))^2)
> x2<- -(n1+n2-ncol(x)/2-2)*log(lam)
```

```
> pvalue<- 1-pchisq(x2,ncol(x))
> round(cbind(lam,x2,pvalue),4)
       lam       x2     pvalue
[1,] 0.408   39.8978        0.
```

The distance $\hat{M}^2$ (5.563) or Wilk's $\hat{\lambda}$ (0.408) or the chi-square value X^2 (39.898) indicate that the multivariate difference observed between the male and female turtles is not likely to be a result of random variation (p-value < 0.001).

A more direct assessment of the effectiveness of a discriminant function (d-values) to summarize and classify multivariate values is the error associated with placing observations into their respective groups based on the estimated discriminant scores. An optimum rule for classifying a new observation D is

if observation $D \geq d_0$, then assign the observation to group II, and

if observation $D < d_0$, then assign the observation to group I .

The value d_0 is defined by the expression

$$d_0 = -\frac{1}{\hat{M}} log[\frac{P(II)}{P(I)}] + \frac{1}{2}(\bar{d}_2 + \bar{d}_1).$$

The quantities $P(I)$ and $P(II) = 1 - P(I)$ are called prior probabilities. A prior probability is the probability that an observation belongs to group I or II without considering the individual measured x-values. For example, the prior probability that a turtle is a male based only on population considerations is 0.5, prior to making any carapace measurements. The value d_0 (justified rigorously elsewhere [7]) combines prior information (P(I) and P(II) probabilities) with information from the groups ($\bar{d}_1$ and $\bar{d}_2$) to produce an optimum classification rule based on d_0. It should be noted that the rule is optimum only when the data (x-values) have a multivariate normal distribution. If $P(I) = P(II) = 0.5$ and $n_1 = n_2$, then $d_0 = 0$. For the turtle data, classification is then based on the sign of the discrimant score-values (i.e., D < 0, assign to male and D ≥ 0, assign to female group).

Using d_0, Table 4.5 is constructed from the $n_1 + n_2 = n$ discriminant scores to estimate the probability of misclassification.

Table 4.5. Discriminant scores classified by actual and predicted group

		predicted group		
		Group *I*	Group *II*	
actual group	Group *I*	a	b	n_1
	Group *II*	c	d	n_2

Table 4.6. The 48 turtles classified by actual gender and predicted gender based on their discriminant scores

		predicted group		
		Male	Female	
actual group	Male	24	0	24
	Female	5	19	24

The classification rule based on the cut-point d_0 and the estimated discriminant scores result in a classification error that is as small as possible when the independent variables have a multivariate normal distribution. Minimum classification error does not necessarily make the discriminant function a useful statistical tool. Frequently the minimum probability of misclassification remains too large to usefully classify observed values.

The discriminant scores based on turtle carapace measurements and $d_0 = 0$ yields Table 4.6.

An estimate of the classification error is

$$P(\textit{misclassification}) = \frac{b}{a+b}P(I) + \frac{c}{c+d}P(II).$$

For the turtle analysis, $P(\textit{misclassification}) = 5/48 = 0.104$ when $P(I) = P(II) = 0.5$. A fragment of S-code that makes this calculation is

```
> # set prior probability p1 = 0.5
> p1<- 0.5
> m2dist<- (mean(d1)-mean(d2))^2
> d0<- -log((1-p1)/p1)/sqrt(m2dist)+(mean(d1)+mean(d2))/2
> g0<- ifelse(d<d0,0,1)
> tab<- table(g,g0)
> tab
   0  1
0 24  0
1  5 19
> p<- p1*tab[1,2]/(tab[1,1]+tab[1,2])+(1-p1)*tab[2,1]/
    (tab[2,1]+tab[2,2])
> cat("misclassification =",round(p,3),"\n")
  misclassification = 0.104.
```

The actual discriminant scores involved in the classification are

```
> male<- round(d1,3)
> female<- round(d2,3)
> cbind(1:24,male,female)
      male female
1 -0.066 -0.437
2 -1.335 -1.140
3 -1.649  0.758
4 -0.413 -0.464
5 -1.065  0.970
6 -1.513  2.151
```

```
 7 -0.720   0.049
 8 -0.953   1.200
 9 -1.523   1.077
10 -1.399   1.077
11 -1.474  -0.442
12 -1.509  -0.261
13 -0.419   0.776
14 -1.526   0.619
15 -1.566   1.016
16 -1.880   2.177
17 -2.328   0.995
18 -0.511   1.026
19 -1.699   3.932
20 -0.597   2.365
21 -0.952   3.089
22 -1.027   3.345
23 -0.880   1.762
24 -1.299   2.664.
```

The coefficients that produce the discriminant scores are also readily displayed:

```
> a0<- otemp$coefficients
> cat("discriminant coefficients",round(a0[-1],4),"\n")
discriminant coefficients
 -0.0291     -0.0103     0.1243
> a1<- otemp$coefficients/sqrt(v)
> cat("discriminant coefficients",round(a1[-1],4),"\n")
discriminant coefficients
 -0.1161     -0.0408     0.495.
```

The magnitude of these coefficients, like all coefficients from a linear model, depend on the units of measurement. Again the standardized coefficients $a_j S_j$ have the same units (commensurate) where S_j is the estimated standard deviation associated with the distribution of the jth independent variable disregarding group membership. For the turtle data, commensurate coefficients are

```
> a2<- a1[-1]*sqrt(diag(var(x)))
> cat("standardized discriminant coefficients","\n",
      round(a2,4),"\n")
standardized discriminant coefficients
 -2.378     -0.5176     4.1547.
```

A comparison of these coefficients shows that the most important single contributor to discriminating between male and female turtles is the height of the shell (x_3).

A general approach to formally evaluating the role of a specific independent variable or a set of independent variables in the discriminant score derives from comparing different linear regression models. If a subset of independent variables is removed from the discriminant analysis, a summary sum of squares (residual deviance) again measures the impact of the removed variables. If the residual deviance associated with the discriminant score (regression model) containing k independent variables is denoted SS_k and the residual deviance associated with the discriminant score with q variables removed is denoted SS_{k-q}, then, as before, the test-statistic

$$F = \frac{(SS_{k-q} - SS_k)/q}{SS_k/(n - k - 1)}$$

has an F-distribution with q and $n - (k + 1)$ degrees of freedom when the q variables removed are unrelated to classifying the sampled observations. This F-test is the previous "F-to-remove" test and equally applies to assessing the components of a linear discriminant score. This test-statistic is identical to an F-statistic based on comparing values of $\hat{M}^2$ where

$$F = \frac{n_1 + n_2 - k - 1}{q} \frac{\hat{M}_k^2 - \hat{M}_{k-q}^2}{(n_1 + n_2 - 2)(n_1 + n_2)/n_1 n_2 + \hat{M}_{k-q}^2}.$$

The difference between multivariate distances $\hat{M}_k^2$ and $\hat{M}_{k-q}^2$ measures the influence of the q removed variables and the F-test indicates the likelihood the difference arose by chance. The expression based on $\hat{M}^2$ is typically used in the context of discriminant analysis [9] but the comparison of the sums of squares is a more direct approach easily implemented with linear regression S-tools. For example, an assessment of the individual roles in the discriminant scores based on the carapace measurements comes from deleting from the three-variable model each variable, one at a time, and evaluating the impact on the residual deviance. Specifically,

```
> labels<- c("length:","width:","height:")
> ss1<- otemp$deviance
> df1<- otemp$df.residual
> for(i in 1:ncol(x)) {
    otemp0<- glm(ytemp~x[,-i])
    ss0<- otemp0$deviance
    df0<- otemp0$df.residual
    f<- ((ss0-ss1)/(df0-df1))/(ss1/df1)
    pvalue<- 1-pf(f,df0-df1,df1)
    R2<- cor(ytemp,predict(otemp0))^2
    m2dist0<- (n1+n2-2)*(n1+n2)*R2/(n1*n2*(1-R2))
    cat(labels[i],"\n","m2dist0 =",round(m2dist0,4),"\n")
    mdiff<- m2dist-m2dist0
    print(round(cbind(mdiff,f,pvalue),4))
    }
```

with results

```
length:
 m2dist0 = 4.5621
      mdiff       f  pvalue
[1,] 1.0008 5.2452  0.0269

width:
 m2dist0 = 5.5042
      mdiff       f  pvalue
[1,] 0.0588 0.277  0.6013
```

```
height:
 m2dist0 = 1.8421
      mdiff         f    pvalue
[1,] 3.7208  28.8465        0
```

where $\hat{M}_3^2 - \hat{M}_2^2$ (*mdiff*) summarizes the impact of each variable removed ($q = 1$). Again, carapace height is the most important contributor to classifying turtles by gender ($F = 28.8$ with a p-value < 0.001). All three statistics (*mdiff*, F, and *pvalue*) produce commensurate values indicating the relative influence of each x-measurement. Also note that the squared t-statistics ("t value" from the *summary*( ) function) are identical to the F-statistics when a single variable is tested ($q = 1$) yielding the same two-tail significance probability.

The S-code uses the relationship

$$\hat{M}^2 = \frac{(n_1 + n_2 - 2)(n_1 + n_2)R^2}{n_1 n_2(1 - R^2)}$$

to compute $\hat{M}^2$ (*m2dist0*) where R^2 (*R2*) is the usual squared multiple correlation coefficient from the linear regression calculations [7]. The S-functions *cat*( ) and *print*( ) are used within a *for*-loop to display output for each value of the index variable.

It is important to note that classifying observations into two groups employs that same statistical quantities as Hotelling's T^2-test for comparing two multivariate sets of mean values (Chapter 1). Specifically, the T^2-statistic is directly related to $\hat{M}^2$ where

$$T^2 = \frac{n_1 n_2}{n_1 + n_2}\hat{M}^2$$

leading to the same F-test for both approaches for assessing distance between two multivariate means.

LINEAR LOGISTIC MODEL

The dependent variable in a linear model is required to be continuous with a normal distribution. A linear logistic model requires the dependent variable to be binary with a binomial distribution. However, these two multivariable models are otherwise similar in many respects making it possible for a logistic regression analysis to be implemented with the *glm*( ) command. Both models are special cases of a general linear model.

The logistic model is a major statistical tool employed in the analysis of data with two outcomes—diseased or not diseased, case or control, or just about any variable with two outcomes. Each multivariate observation is made up of a binary dependent variable and a series of independent variables, discrete or continuous. The ith observation is represented as $\{(0 \text{ or } 1), x_{i1}, x_{i2}, x_{i3}, \cdots, x_{ik}\}$. This is essentially the data structure underlying a discriminant analysis—the two analytic approaches are closely related [7]. The key element of a logistic analysis is a series of probabilities p_i. The symbol p_i represents the probability that the binary outcome occurs (i.e., the dependent variable = 1) in the ith group or individual. The relationship between this probability and k independent measurements is modeled by a logistic function.

In it simplest form, a logistic function is

$$f(x) = \frac{1}{1 + e^{-x}}.$$

Values of this function are always greater than zero and less than one, making it ideal for modeling probabilities $(0 < f(x) < 1)$. The linear logistic model postulates that the relationship between the independent variables x_{ij} and probability p_i is

$$p_i = \frac{1}{1 + e^{-(a + b_1 x_{i1} + b_2 x_{i2} + b_3 x_{i3} + \cdots + b_k x_{ik})}} \qquad i = 1, 2, 3, \cdots, n$$

where p_i represents the probability associated with the ith multivariate observation. The x-values are again independent variables where the strength of the relationship to p_i is determined by the coefficients b_j. As before, n is the total number of observations each with k measurements. At the heart of a logistic analysis is this function and a transformation. The transformation produces a linear relationship between the binary outcome and the independent variables where

$$y_i = \log\left[\frac{p_i}{1 - p_i}\right] = a + b_1 x_{i1} + b_2 x_{i2} + b_3 x_{i3} + \cdots + b_k x_{ik}.$$

Technically, the transformation is called a link function (i.e., that function linking a dependent variable to a linear combination of the independent variables). The transformed value y_i has a linear relationship with the independent variables x_{ij} when p_i is described by a logistic function and conversely. The S-tools designed to analyze a general linear model now apply. The quantity y_i is called the logit and is the logarithm of the odds associated with the probability p_i. The odds are the probability an outcome occurs divided by the probability the outcome does not occur (i.e., $p/[1 - p]$). Therefore, the statistical structure underlying a logistic analysis requires the probability of an event to be described by a logistic function of the independent variables or, equivalently, requires the log-odds to be described by a linear function of the independent variables.

Since the log-odds is a linear combination of the independent variables, the logistic model shares a number of properties with the multivariable linear model. The difference between two log-odds values $(y_i - y_j)$ does not depend on the magnitude of the independent variables. When a linear logistic model is additive, as before, each x-value has a separate influence on the log-odds. Also, the coefficient b_m measures the response in the log-odds for a one unit increase in the mth independent variable when the other $k - 1$ independent variables are held constant. In short, since the right-hand side of the equation relating the independent variables to the log-odds is the same as that in the linear regression case, both models have these same three basic properties.

The difference between two log-odds values is the logarithm of the odds ratio or

$$\textit{difference in log-odds} = y_i - y_j = \log\left[\frac{p_i}{1 - p_i}\right] - \log\left[\frac{p_j}{1 - p_j}\right]$$

$$= \log\left[\frac{p_i(1 - p_j)}{p_j(1 - p_i)}\right] = \log(or_{ij}),$$

where

$$\textit{odds ratio} = or_{ij} = \frac{p_i/(1 - p_i)}{p_j/(1 - p_j)}.$$

The odds ratio is a common measure of association reflecting the association between two binary variables ($or = 1$ occurs when no association exists and $or \neq 1$ measures the strength of association—details in Chapter 6).

Since the coefficient b_m measures the change in the log-odds for a one unit increase in the mth variable, the odds ratio associated with a one unit increase in the mth variable is

$$e^{y_i - y_j} = e^{b_m} = or_m$$

when the other $k - 1$ independent variables are held constant. The quantity $or_m = e^{b_m}$ measures the impact of a single variable accounting for the other $k - 1$ independent variables in the model and is referred to as an adjusted odds ratio.

For the additive logistic model, it follows that the overall odds ratio comparing the ith and the jth observation is a product of a series of adjusted odds ratios and

$$or_{ij} = or_1^{(x_{i1} - x_{j1})} \times or_2^{(x_{i2} - x_{j2})} \times or_3^{(x_{i3} - x_{j3})} \times \cdots \times or_k^{(x_{ik} - x_{jk})}.$$

When the log-odds is an additive function of the independent variables, the influences of the adjusted odds ratios are multiplicative. The separate influence of each independent variable increases or decreases the overall odds ratio by a multiplicative factor and, to repeat, the change is not influenced by the levels of the other independent variables included in the additive logistic regression model. The interpretation of the overall odds ratio as a product of adjusted odds ratios is a direct result of the property that the logit response y_i is a sum of the measured influences.

CATEGORICAL DATA—BIVARIATE LINEAR LOGISTIC MODEL

A logistic model applies to data contained in a series of categories summarizing a binary outcome. For example, the data in Table 4.7 show the case and control status (binary outcome) of individuals participating in a study of pancreatic cancer [10] where males and females are classified into categories based on the amount of coffee they consumed (0, 1–2, 3–4 and 5 or more cups per day). Case/control status is not an outcome variable in the usual sense. Case/control status does not result from the random sampling of a defined population. Cases are chosen because they have, for example, a specific disease and are not a random binary variable with a statistical distribution. Nevertheless, a logistic analysis using case/control status as the outcome variable remains an effective statistical tool for investigating the role of a series of measured independent variables [11].

There are r_i cases out of n_i total participants in each coffee/gender category ($i = 1, 2, 3, \cdots, 8$ categories). The variable x_1 reflects the amount of coffee consumed and x_2 indicates a male ($x_2 = 1$) or female ($x_2 = 0$) study participant. The symbol $\tilde{p}_i$ represents the probability of case status associated with n_i specific outcomes within the ith category (a row in Table 4.7). Furthermore, the independent variables x_1 and x_2 are assumed related to p_i by

$$p_i = \frac{1}{1 + e^{-(a + b_1 x_{i1} + b_2 x_{i2})}}$$

or

$$y_i = \log\left[\frac{p_i}{1 - p_i}\right] = a + b_1 x_{i1} + b_2 x_{i2}.$$

Table 4.7. Case-control status by gender and coffee consumption (cups/day)

coffee	gender	r_i	n_i	x_{i1}	x_{i2}	$\tilde{p}_i = r_i/n_i$
0 cups per day	male	9	41	0.0	1	0.220
1–2 cups per day	male	94	213	2.0	1	0.441
3–4 cups per day	male	53	127	4.0	1	0.417
5+ cups per day	male	60	142	5.0	1	0.423
0 cups per day	female	11	67	0.0	0	0.164
1–2 cups per day	female	59	211	2.0	0	0.280
3–4 cups per day	female	53	133	4.0	0	0.398
5+ cups per day	female	28	76	5.0	0	0.368

Specifically, the relationship between case/control status and the independent variables is modeled by an additive linear logistic equation. However, each coffee/gender category does not contribute equally to the understanding of the relationship of the independent variables to case/control status since the number of observations n_i varies from category to category. The magnitude of these unequal contributions is proportional to the sample size in each category (n_i in Table 4.7). To properly weight each category, the sample sizes are communicated to the *glm*-function with the option *weights = nsize* where *nsize* is an S-vector containing the number of observations within each category. If the option is omitted, equal category weights are assigned.

The linear logistic model

$$y_i = a + b_1 x_{i1} + b_2 x_{i2} + b_3 x_{i1} x_{i2}$$

summarizes the log-odds values associated with case/control status by two straight lines with different slopes and intercepts and

```
> # r = cases and n = total number
> r<- c(9,94,53,60,11,59,53,28)
> n<- c(41,213,127,142,67,211,133,76)
> p<- r/n
> x1<- rep(c(0,2,4,5),2)
> x2<- rep(c(1,0),c(4,4))
> otemp<- glm(p~x1+x2+x1*x2,family=binomial,weights=n)
> summary(otemp,correlation=F)
```

produces the estimates and summaries

```
Call: glm(formula = p ~ x1 + x2 + x1 * x2,
     family = binomial, weights = n)
Deviance Residuals:
      1      2       3       4       5      6      7       8
 -1.967 1.410 -0.223 -0.516 -0.596 0.274 0.733 -0.933

Coefficients:
                 Value   Std. Error     t value
(Intercept)  -1.4349257  0.21451000  -6.689319
         x1   0.2231851  0.06448328   3.461132
         x2   0.8660164  0.29513935   2.934263
      x1:x2  -0.1543696  0.08633029  -1.788127

(Dispersion Parameter for Binomial family taken to be 1)

     Null Deviance: 33.46853   on 7 degrees of freedom
Residual Deviance: 8.014666 on 4 degrees of freedom.
```

The model contains the term $x_{i1} x_{i2}$ allowing the relationship of coffee drinking and the probability of case status to differ between the two sexes (non-additivity). One straight line is estimated when $x_{i2} = 0$ (females), namely

$$\hat{y}_i = \log\left[\frac{\hat{p}_i}{1 - \hat{p}_i}\right] = \hat{a} + \hat{b}_1 x_{i1}$$

and a different straight line is estimated when $x_2 = 1$ (males), where

$$\hat{y}_i = \log\left[\frac{\hat{p}_i}{1 - \hat{p}_i}\right] = \hat{a} + \hat{b}_1 x_{i1} + \hat{b}_2 + \hat{b}_3 x_{i1} = (\hat{a} + \hat{b}_2) + (\hat{b}_1 + \hat{b}_3) x_{i1} = \hat{A} + \hat{B} x_{i1}.$$

The inclusion of the $x_1 x_2$-term produces two linear models, one for $x_2 = 0$ and one for $x_2 = 1$.

From the illustrative data, for females ($x_2 = 0$)

$$\hat{y}_i = -1.435 + 0.223 x_{i1} \qquad \text{or} \qquad \hat{p}_i = \frac{1}{1 + e^{-(-1.435 + 0.223 x_{i1})}}$$

and for males ($x_2 = 1$)

$$\hat{y}_i = -0.569 + 0.068 x_{i1} \qquad \text{or} \qquad \hat{p}_i = \frac{1}{1 + e^{-(-0.569 + 0.068 x_{i1})}}.$$

In terms of S-output, the estimated logit values $\hat{y}_i$ are produced by the S-function *predict(object)* and the corresponding estimated probabilities $\hat{p}_i$ are produced by $1/(1 + exp(-predict(object)))$. These estimated logistic probabilities are plotted in Figure 4.6 using

```
> # data plot
> plot(x1[x2==1],p[x2==1],type="b",xlab="Coffee -- cup/day",
    ylab="P(case)",ylim=c(0.1,0.5),pch="+",main="Coffee
    consumption and P(case) -- Pancreatic cancer")
```

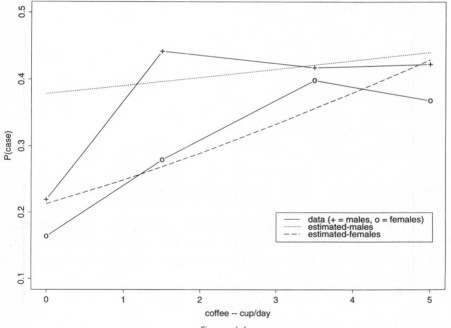

Figure 4.6

```
> points(x1[x2==0],p[x2==0],type="b",pch="o")
> # estimated values
> b<- otemp$coefficients
> x<- 0:5
> p0<- 1/(1+exp(-(b[1]+b[2]*x)))
> # logistic probabilities (male)
> lines(x,p0,lty=4)
> # logistic probabilities (female)
> p1<- 1/(1+exp(-((b[1]+b[3])+(b[2]+b[4])*x)))
> lines(x,p1,lty=2)
> legend(c(3,5),c(0.2,0.15),c("data (+ = males, o = females)",
      "estimated-males","estimated-females"),lty=c(1,2,4))
```

The plot displays two lines representing the observed proportion of cases (solid lines) and the modeled relationships (dashed almost straight lines) derived from the logistic model estimates. Visually it is clear that the estimated values are not a perfect representation of the data but some lack of fit is expected for most statistical models.

To formally assess the correspondence between the model generated values and the data, the eight observed values (r_i) are compared to the eight values estimated from the model $(n_i \hat{p}_i)$ and evaluated with a chi-square statistic as follows:

```
> # estimated model values
> ex<- n/(1+exp(-predict(otemp)))
> xtemp<- (r-ex)/sqrt(ex)
> round(cbind(r,ex,xtemp),3)
      r     ex  xtemp
 1    9 14.821 -1.512
 2   94 83.884  1.105
 3   53 54.243 -0.169
 4   60 63.052 -0.384
 5   11 12.886 -0.525
 6   59 57.223  0.235
 7   53 48.901  0.586
 8   28 31.990 -0.705
> chi2<- sum(xtemp^2)
> pvalue<- 1-pchisq(chi2,4)
> round(cbind(chi2,pvalue),3)
       chi2   pvalue
[1,]  4.855    0.303.
```

The S-vector *xtemp* contains the eight contributions to the chi-square test-statistic reflecting the fit of each estimated number of cases from the eight coffee/gender categories and shows no extreme deviations (e.g., $-1.6 < xtemp < 1.6$). The non-extreme chi-square statistic (not extremely unlikely by chance) indicates that the model is not an especially good nor an especially bad representation of the data.

MULTIVARIABLE DATA—LINEAR LOGISTIC MODEL

The coffee drinking data illustrate 1010 binary outcomes classified into a table with eight categories. A logistic analysis equally applies to a series of individual binary outcomes that are not classified into categories. Consider the data in Table 4.8 [12]. Each individual is recorded as experiencing a coronary disease event or not (the binary dependent variable {no coronary event = 0, coronary event = 1}—*chd*) over a period of about eight years. Furthermore, each individual is measured for seven risk factors. These independent risk variables are height (inches—*ht*), weight (pounds—*wt*), systolic blood pressure (mm of Hg—*sbp*), diastolic blood pressure (mm of Hg—*dbp*), cholesterol (%/100ml—*chol*), cigarette exposure (smoker = 1 and non-smoker = 0—*cigs*), and type-A/type-B behavior (A = 1 and B = 0—*ab*). These $n = 100$ observations were made on men aged 58–60. An additive logistic model (log-odds version) describing the relationship of the seven independent variables to the risk of a coronary event is

$$log\text{-}odds = y_i = a + b_1 x_{i1} + b_2 x_{i2} + b_3 x_{i3} + \cdots + b_7 x_{i7},$$

where y_i represents the log-odds measure of the risk associated with the ith individual ($i = 1, 2, 3, \cdots, 100$). The estimates and summary statistics using all seven risk variables are produced by

```
> otemp<- glm(chd~ht+wt+sbp+dbp+chol+cigs+ab,family=binomial)
> summary(otemp,correlation=F)
lpc7>Call: glm(formula = chd~ht+wt+sbp+dbp+chol+cigs+ab,
    family = binomial)
Deviance Residuals:
      Min        1Q      Median        3Q       Max
 -1.548042 -0.6043283 -0.4497987 -0.3073782 2.183636

lpc7>Coefficients:
                  Value     Std. Error      t value
(Intercept) -22.757935665  10.247938730   -2.2207330
        ht    0.217362169   0.150526862    1.4440092
        wt    0.004083124   0.016516310    0.2472177
       sbp   -0.008634463   0.027146894   -0.3180645
       dbp    0.062283567   0.053683592    1.1601975
      chol    0.004443769   0.007738806    0.5742189
      cigs   -0.165612505   0.598701195   -0.2766196
        ab    0.194241755   0.664282710    0.2924083

(Dispersion Parameter for Binomial family taken to be 1)

Null Deviance: 87.93398 on 99 degrees of freedom
Residual Deviance: 79.4893 on 92 degrees of freedom

Number of Fisher Scoring Iterations: 4.
```

Table 4.8. Coronary risk factors among men aged 58–60

	ht	wt	sbp	dpb	chol	cigs	ab	chd		ht	wt	sbp	dpb	chol	cigs	ab	chd
1	70	150	144	86	255	1	0	1	51	69	187	130	80	248	0	1	0
2	67	136	148	90	227	1	1	0	52	70	160	132	88	153	0	1	0
3	71	168	120	84	235	0	1	0	53	71	155	114	82	298	1	1	0
4	69	165	156	94	223	0	0	0	54	66	142	112	78	203	1	0	0
5	70	185	126	80	210	0	0	0	55	72	200	128	86	184	0	1	1
6	69	170	134	76	252	1	0	0	56	72	176	124	82	294	0	1	1
7	69	192	130	76	146	0	1	0	57	67	138	170	92	283	0	1	0
8	69	145	120	84	195	0	0	0	58	69	154	110	74	216	1	0	0
9	71	172	114	84	293	1	1	0	59	74	210	120	86	326	1	1	0
10	70	175	126	84	241	0	0	1	60	64	208	160	98	253	0	1	0
11	70	150	102	70	272	0	1	0	61	72	160	130	90	241	1	1	1
12	67	145	120	76	216	0	1	0	62	71	190	180	102	211	1	1	0
13	72	159	108	70	223	0	0	0	63	67	132	108	72	187	1	1	0
14	70	170	168	102	231	0	1	1	64	68	151	134	76	250	1	1	0
15	68	174	134	90	229	0	0	0	65	69	160	122	64	217	0	0	0
16	71	172	140	90	286	1	1	1	66	69	160	134	80	257	1	0	0
17	64	143	140	76	240	0	1	0	67	70	175	120	76	246	0	1	0
18	70	160	138	76	191	1	0	0	68	70	175	122	80	215	1	1	0
19	68	168	130	80	273	1	0	0	69	73	175	176	96	198	0	0	1
20	72	206	130	86	181	1	1	0	70	67	180	132	82	190	0	0	0
21	65	155	140	98	252	0	1	0	71	70	180	122	80	164	0	0	0
22	68	175	120	76	202	1	1	0	72	67	142	138	84	322	1	0	0
23	70	150	130	74	173	1	0	0	73	72	175	126	82	177	1	1	0
24	71	133	170	106	210	0	1	0	74	70	166	152	88	225	1	1	0
25	68	173	142	98	212	0	1	0	75	70	233	122	78	263	0	0	0
26	72	181	118	68	274	0	1	0	76	70	175	138	78	192	1	0	0
27	74	185	140	76	170	1	1	0	77	71	178	124	82	199	0	1	0
28	73	196	172	114	252	0	1	0	78	71	176	152	92	268	0	1	1
29	71	205	146	86	268	0	0	0	79	70	191	116	76	236	0	1	1
30	68	186	178	104	232	1	1	0	80	66	165	138	88	272	1	0	0
31	70	162	130	86	203	0	0	0	81	64	130	110	78	254	1	0	0
32	71	165	120	80	187	1	0	0	82	71	170	180	106	199	1	1	0
33	68	180	128	88	276	1	0	1	83	69	164	132	86	242	0	1	0
34	70	200	158	94	258	0	1	0	84	66	132	110	74	176	0	0	0
35	72	195	126	74	222	0	1	0	85	71	200	140	96	244	0	1	0
36	73	203	140	86	241	0	0	0	86	71	155	110	68	219	0	1	0
37	67	168	124	74	226	0	1	0	87	71	158	104	60	216	0	1	0
38	74	185	120	78	229	1	0	0	88	71	186	146	94	299	0	1	0
39	67	168	130	80	204	0	0	0	89	71	208	148	86	246	0	1	1
40	66	163	140	84	204	1	0	0	90	66	144	150	92	252	1	1	0
41	70	172	138	86	194	0	1	1	91	66	160	132	80	192	0	0	0
42	70	181	120	82	175	1	1	0	92	68	175	142	80	190	1	0	0
43	72	160	110	80	205	0	1	0	93	65	170	120	84	150	0	0	0
44	70	145	136	70	177	1	1	0	94	68	158	122	86	265	0	0	0
45	66	152	116	76	228	1	1	0	95	70	167	118	74	220	1	1	0
46	69	165	138	98	212	0	1	1	96	75	175	130	70	226	1	1	0
47	71	176	132	86	258	0	1	0	97	69	185	130	82	214	1	1	1
48	69	165	126	80	197	1	1	1	98	71	182	112	76	190	1	1	0
49	68	160	118	78	203	0	1	0	99	64	138	102	74	258	1	0	0
50	68	160	116	80	256	0	1	0	100	70	169	150	90	256	0	1	0

The estimated regression coefficients are

```
> b<- otemp$coefficients[-1]
> round(b,3)
   ht     wt     sbp    dbp   chol    cigs      ab
0.217  0.004  -0.009  0.062  0.004  -0.166  0.194
```

producing commensurate regression coefficients (standardized) as

```
> temp<- cbind(ht,wt,sbp,dbp,chol,cigs,ab)
> sd<- sqrt(diag(var(temp)))
> bstd<- b*sd
> round(abs(bstd),3)
   ht     wt     sbp    dbp    chol    cigs     ab
0.514  0.081  0.153  0.595  0.167  0.083  0.094.
```

The estimated regression coefficients converted to adjusted odds ratios (i.e., $\hat{or}_j = e^{\hat{b}_j}$) are

```
> round(exp(b),3)
   ht     wt     sbp    dbp   chol    cigs     ab
1.243  1.004  0.991  1.064  1.004  0.847  1.214.
```

Products of these adjusted odds ratios measure the joint influence of combinations of independent variables on the risk of coronary heart disease.

Statistical assessment of the influence of a variable or several variables on the risk of coronary disease follows the previous pattern of comparing residual deviances. However, in the logistic case the dependent variable is not normally distributed (it is a binary variable with a binomial distribution). Therefore, the F-test used in conjunction with the linear model is not appropriate since an F-test requires the data to be normally distributed. A result from mathematical statistics is helpful. For most distributions of the dependent variable, the residual deviance has an approximate chi-square distribution when only random variation causes the data to differ from the model. The degrees of freedom equal the sample size minus the number of parameters estimated to specify the model. Specifically, the *summary(otemp)* function shows the residual deviance from the coronary heart disease data is 79.489 with 92 degrees of freedom ($n = 100$ observations and $k = 8$ parameters estimated).

More importantly, the difference between two residual deviances calculated from two nested models has an approximate chi-square distribution. The degrees of freedom equal the difference between the degrees of freedom associated with each of the residual deviances. By nested model, it is meant that the second model is a special case of the first model. Parallel to the linear regression case, nested models result from deleting variables from the first model to form a second model. In symbols, if D_1 represents the residual deviance from the first model (degrees of freedom = df_1) and D_0 represents the residual deviance from a second reduced model (degrees of freedom = df_0), then $D_0 - D_1$ has an approximate chi-square distribution with $df_0 - df_1$

degrees of freedom when D_0 and D_1 differ by chance alone (the deleted variables have no impact on the binary outcome variable).

When data values are missing, it is possible that estimates from nested models containing different variables are based on different numbers of complete observations. A critical requirement for the comparison of residual deviances from two nested models is that the sample sizes be identical for both models. The residual deviance increases as the sample size increases. Comparison of two models will, therefore, reflect differences in sample sizes when they are based on different numbers of observations, obscuring any differences associated with the deleted variables.

To evaluate, for example, the joint influence of height and weight on the risk of coronary disease, two models are compared—the model containing all seven risk variables to the model containing five risk variables (height and weight removed). The values D_1 and df_1 for the seven-variable model (full model—all seven variables included) are extracted from the S-object *otemp* by

```
> D1<- otemp$deviance
> df1<- otemp$df.residual
```

The residual deviance for the full model is 79.489 ($D1$) with 92 degrees of freedom ($df1$), as already noted. The parallel quantities extracted from the reduced model (height and weight removed) are calculated by

```
> otemp0<- glm(chd~sbp+dbp+chol+cigs+ab,family=binomial)
> D0<- otemp0$deviance
> df0<- otemp0$df.residual
```

For the reduced model, the residual deviance is increased to 82.689 ($D0$) with 94 degrees of freedom ($df0$). Once these quantities are extracted, a chi-square statistic provides a formal assessment of the removed variables and for the coronary disease data

```
> D<- D0-D1
> df<- df0-df1
> pvalue<- 1-pchisq(D,df)
> round(cbind(D,df,pvalue),3)
            D     df      pvalue
[1,]    3.208     2       0.201.
```

A residual deviance acts as a relative measure of goodness-of-fit and an increase of 3.208 indicates that the fit of the logistic model is marginally, at best, affected by the deletion of the two variables, height and weight.

The comparison of residual deviances from nested models is once again a fundamental tool used to evaluate the components of a multivariable measurement. A basic analytic strategy consists of postulating a sequence of nested models and making comparisons among the residual deviances using an analysis of variance style approach. These comparisons are accomplished with the S-function *anova( )* where a series of S-objects is the input argument. Again, all comparisons must be based on the same number of observations. Using the coronary disease data (Table 4.8), the following compares a series of five nested models each based on $n = 100$ observations:

```
> otemp5<- glm(chd~ht+wt+sbp+dbp+chol+cigs+ab,family=binomial)
> otemp4<- glm(chd~sbp+dbp+chol+cigs+ab,family=binomial)
> otemp3<- glm(chd~chol+cigs+ab,family=binomial)
> otemp2<- glm(chd~chol+cigs,family=binomial)
> otemp1<- glm(chd~chol,family=binomial)
> anova(otemp1,otemp2,otemp3,otemp4,otemp5)

Analysis of Deviance Table

Response: chd
```

	Terms	Resid.DF	Resid.Dev	Test	Df	Deviance
1	chol	98	86.91894			
2	chol+cigs	97	86.56123	cigs	1	0.357710
3	chol+cigs+ab	96	85.59665	ab	1	0.964587
4	sbp+dbp+chol+cigs+ab	94	82.69776	sbp:dbp	2	2.898889
5	ht+wt+sbp+dbp+chol+cigs+ab	92	79.48930	ht:wt	2	3.208459

The "Deviance"-table can be viewed as displaying the results from adding variables to the regression equation (reading from top to bottom) or as displaying the results from deleting variables from a regression equation (reading from bottom to top). The column labeled "Terms" lists the independent variables included in the model. The column labeled "Resid.DF" gives the degrees of freedom associated with the corresponding residual deviance (third column—"Resid.Dev"). The next three columns relate to the change in the residual deviance from deleting (or adding) terms from the model, listed in the column labeled "Test." The "Deviance" column contains the differences in residual deviances between the model including the variables listed in the column "Terms" and the model with the variables listed in the column labeled "Test" removed. These differences have approximate chi-square distributions when the variables removed are unrelated to the dependent variable. The degrees of freedom (column "Df") equal the differences in the degrees of freedom associated with the compared residual deviances, which necessarily equals the number of terms removed from the model. For the coronary disease data, the risk factors height and weight, blood pressure, smoking, cholesterol and behavior type show no substantial impact on the outcome variable. The comparison of this sequence of nested models leads to the inference that none of the traditional risk factors for coronary disease noticeably influence the probability of a coronary event in older men (aged 58–60, observed for approximately eight years).

A direct evaluation of the simultaneous influence of all seven risk factors comes from comparing the null deviance to the residual deviance based on all seven independent variables, giving

```
> D0<- otemp$null.deviance
> D0
[1] 87.93398
> df0<- length(chd)-1
> D1<- otemp$deviance
> D1
[1] 79.4893
> df1<- otemp$df.residual
> x2<- D0-D1
> df<- df0-df1
> pvalue<- 1-pchisq(x2,df)
> round(cbind(x2,df,pvalue),3)
        x2 df pvalue
[1,] 8.445  7  0.295.
```

Again, this indicates no strong influence on coronary disease outcome exists from the seven risk factors (p-value = 0.295). A comparison of residual deviances contrasts differences in the relative fit of two models but does not address the question of the correspondence between the data and the model — goodness-of-fit in an absolute sense.

GOODNESS-OF-FIT

When a logistic regression model is applied to a sample of observations contained in a contingency table, a goodness-of-fit evaluation is based on estimating an expected frequency for each cell in the table. These values are generated using estimated logistic probabilities calculated from the estimated model (i.e., a function of the *predict*( ) command). The statistical assessment of the differences between the estimated and the observed frequencies is usually accomplished with a chi-square statistic (as in the case/control pancreatic cancer data). The situation becomes a bit more complicated when one or more of the independent variables consist of a large number of categories or are continuous.

One goodness-of-fit strategy for dealing with continuous variables involves creating a somewhat arbitrary table based on the estimated logistic probabilities.Once the table is constructed, the Pearson chi-square test-statistic applies in much the same way as the evaluation of most contingency tables. Typically, 10 groups are formed. The first group contains the 10% of the observations with the lowest estimated logistic probabilities, the second group contains the 10% with the next lowest estimated probabilities, and so forth until the tenth group contains the 10% of the observations with the highest estimated logistic probabilities. If the number of observations does not divide evenly into 10 groups, groups are formed so that each category contains approximately 10%. This process classifies the data into percentiles based on logistic probabilities, called "deciles of risk." For each decile, the mean logistic probability is estimated. If $\hat{p}_i$ represents the estimated logistic probability for the ith observation, then for a specific decile the mean value is

$$\bar{p}_j = \frac{1}{n_j}\sum \hat{p}_i \qquad i = 1, 2, 3, \cdots, n_j,$$

where n_j is as close as possible to $n/10$. The estimated value $\bar{p}_j$ is simply the mean logistic probability calculated from the n_j members of one of the 10 deciles, denoted by j. The estimated logistic probabilities $\hat{p}_i$ come from the S-function *predict( )* and

```
> p<- 1/(1+exp(-predict(object.name))
```

calculates an estimated $\hat{p}_i$ corresponding to each sampled observation using the estimated logistic model and the independent variables specific to the ith observation. Based on each of the 10 model generated logistic probabilities, the expected number of occurrences and non-occurrences of the binary outcome are estimated by $e_j = \sum \hat{p}_i = n_j\bar{p}_j$ and $n_j - e_j = n_j(1 - \bar{p}_j)$ for the jth decile of risk. This process repeated for all 10 groups produces 20 estimated cell frequencies based on the model (denoted e_j and $n_j - e_j$). These estimated values are compared to the corresponding 20 observed values derived from classifying the observed binary outcomes into exactly the same deciles of risk (denoted o_j and $n_j - o_j$). The Pearson chi-square test statistic is

$$X^2 = \sum \frac{(observed - expected)^2}{expected}$$

and for the "deciles of risk" goodness-of-fit test, the specific chi-square statistic becomes

$$X^2 = \sum \frac{(o_j - e_j)^2}{n_j\bar{p}_j(1 - \bar{p}_j)} \quad \text{where, as before, } \bar{p}_j = \frac{1}{n_j}\sum p_i \qquad j = 1, 2, 3, \cdots, 10.$$

The test-statistic X^2 has an approximate chi-square distribution with eight degrees of freedom when the logistic regression model produces expected values e_j that differ from the observed values o_j only because of chance variation (more on the goodness-of-fit of the logistic model is found in [13]). The degrees of freedom are eight, which is not intuitive or easily justified [13]. A fragment of S-code applied to the coronary heart disease data (seven-variable model) produces this "decile of risk" goodness-of-fit test:

```
> p<- 1/(1+exp(-predict(otemp5)))
> ord<- order(p)
> # vector chd = 100 (0,1) indicators of coronary disease
> chd0<- chd[ord]
> p0<- sort(p)
> # 20 observed and expected values
> o<- apply(matrix(chd0,10,10),2,sum)
> e<- apply(matrix(p0,10,10),2,sum)
```

```
> pbar<- e/10
> # chi-square statistic
> xtemp<- (o-e)/sqrt((10*pbar*(1-pbar)))
> round(cbind(pbar,o,e,xtemp),3)
          pbar   o        e    xtemp
  [1,]  0.037   0    0.370   -0.620
  [2,]  0.058   0    0.582   -0.786
  [3,]  0.077   0    0.766   -0.911
  [4,]  0.100   1    1.005   -0.005
  [5,]  0.124   1    1.240   -0.231
  [6,]  0.144   3    1.435    1.411
  [7,]  0.168   2    1.685    0.266
  [9,]  0.276   6    2.761    2.291
 [10,]  0.393   3    3.933   -0.604
> x2<- sum(xtemp^2)
> pvalue<- 1-pchisq(x2,8)
> round(cbind(x2,pvalue),3)
              x2     pvalue
  [1,]    12.421      0.133.
```

The *xtemp* column contains the 10 contributions to the chi-square statistic showing which deciles exhibit a good fit and which exhibit a poor fit of the model estimated values to the data. The seven-variable model appears to be an adequate but not a great representation of the data (moderate chi-square value).

POISSON MODEL

A linear model involves a continuous outcome and a logistic model a binary outcome. The Poisson model lies somewhere between these two extremes, focused on an outcome variable that is a count. Frequently, counts are expressed as rates classified into a table. A Poisson model is a powerful statistical tool for analyzing a table of rates. The use of a Poisson model to analyze table of counts follows in Chapter 6.

A Poisson model postulates that the logarithm of a rate is a linear function of k independent variables where the independent variables are fequently derived from categorical classifications. For example, lung cancer deaths (Table 4.9) are classified by a measure of exposure to radiation from the World War II atomic bomb explosions, age at death, gender, and the city of residence (Hiroshima or Nagasaki). These data form a table with dimensions 10 (exposure) $\times$13 (age) $\times$2 (sex)$\times$2 (city). Also recorded are the total person-years at risk for each of the $10 \times 13 \times 2 \times 2 = 520$ categories. The rate (r_i) is the number of lung cancer deaths divided by the person-years at risk for each cell in the table (justified in Chapter 8). A Poisson model relates the logarithm of a rate to k independent variables by a linear function or

$$log(r_i) = a + b_1 x_{i1} + b_2 x_{i2} + b_3 x_{i3} + \cdots + b_k x_{ik} \qquad i = 1, 2, 3, \cdots, n$$

Table 4.9. Data on lung cancer from Hiroshima and Nagaski—deaths and person-years by age and exposure

dose	2.5	7.5	12.5	17.5	22.5	27.5	32.5	37.5	42.5	47.5	52.5	57.5	70
HIROSHIMA MALES													
0	0	1	1	4	0	4	6	16	20	24	11	6	3
	35465	24336	35436	24152	7537	12832	14428	16935	16886	17186	10593	6489	5582
0.025	0	0	0	3	2	0	3	11	7	9	7	7	1
	31240	16275	12744	13245	4404	6797	7939	8560	9759	8128	5957	3458	2730
0.075	0	0	0	3	0	1	2	3	5	6	1	2	1
	6714	4304	5836	3917	1226	2150	2503	2505	2665	2877	1793	1063	1060
0.15	0	0	0	0	0	1	0	2	4	6	2	1	1
	9500	6019	4794	4009	1189	2086	2446	2772	3760	4089	2207	1292	1122
0.3	0	0	0	1	0	1	0	5	8	6	5	1	1
	10450	6314	6016	6191	1492	2707	4118	3725	4443	4303	2505	1601	1484
0.75	0	0	0	0	1	1	1	2	5	6	5	1	1
	4289	2997	3181	3408	1075	161	1385	2498	2844	2640	1732	986	804
1.5	0	0	0	1	0	0	1	2	3	0	3	0	0
	2003	1324	1522	2635	450	1236	1123	1357	1975	1229	1111	516	238
2.5	0	0	1	0	0	0	0	1	0	1	1	0	0
	717	263	708	1288	270	176	219	289	428	374	173	173	130
3.5	0	0	0	0	0	0	1	0	0	0	0	0	0
	212	141	238	476	48	35	144	149	104	113	141	22	35
5.0	0	0	0	0	0	0	1	0	0	0	0	0	0
	109	95	468	465	90	174	91	130	170	164	98	33	59
HIROSHIMA FEMALES													
0	0	0	0	1	2	2	7	6	11	8	6	2	0
	39241	22963	29393	46215	36919	30413	30490	33660	28448	23929	13366	9217	8893
0.025	1	2	0	0	3	6	10	8	12	7	3	3	1
	34065	18254	14738	26397	23274	21404	23519	22354	18172	13701	8131	5763	6151
0.075	0	0	0	0	1	1	0	2	2	3	1	2	0
	7586	4099	585	7151	5887	5649	5479	5960	4679	3442	2370	1441	1442
0.15	0	0	0	1	1	0	2	3	0	5	6	2	2
	9817	5709	4115	9460	8006	7773	7541	8284	7021	6024	2968	1911	1987

(continued)

Table 4.9. Data on lung cancer from Hiroshima and Nagaski—deaths and person-years by age and exposure—Continued

dose	2.5	7.5	12.5	17.5	22.5	27.5	32.5	37.5	42.5	47.5	52.5	57.5	70
NAGASKI	**FEMALES**												
0.3	0	0	1	0	0	1	5	5	3	7	5	2	2
	12206	6279	7267	10133	10193	8643	9251	10612	8407	6798	4240	2468	2547
0.75	0	0	0	1	0	2	0	3	3	1	0	0	0
	4423	3068	4265	6813	6219	4481	4670	5380	5205	3301	2146	1292	1057
1.5	0	0	0	0	1	0	0	2	2	2	0	0	1
	2022	1564	2039	2699	2753	2259	1895	2628	2243	1436	777	392	359
2.5	0	0	0	2	0	0	0	1	1	1	0	0	0
	836	367	1029	963	1429	719	789	720	768	509	140	108	114
3.5	0	0	0	0	0	0	1	0	0	1	4	0	0
	106	35	1030	317	209	304	240	125	175	282		0	4
5.0	0	0	0	0	0	0	0	0	1	0	0	0	0
	282	131	125	461	363	243	152	193	186	104	98	36	32
NAGASKI	**MALES**												
0	0	1	0	2	0	4	7	12	17	18	6	7	2
	30084	28059	32930	17715	4107	7371	8670	8377	10351	9614	5953	3409	2885
0.025	0	0	1	1	0	0	1	4	5	7	2	2	0
	18448	11350	11411	6014	1317	1826	1956	2012	2907	2729	2214	1520	1121
0.075	0	0	0	0	0	0	1	1	2	0	0	0	0
	2118	1767	1216	752	247	195	292	381	513	435	185	87	168
0.15	0	0	0	0	0	1	0	0	0	0	0	0	0
	1578	1586	1506	969	144	566	291	415	515	429	367	160	175
0.75	0	1	1	1	0	1	0	1	1	1	1	1	1
	2435	2342	2596	1705	511	379	508	662	538	711	421	338	185
0.3	0	0	0	1	0	1	0	0	0	1	0	1	0
	1231	1097	1129	1225	326	197	423	349	342	399	128	120	105
1.5	0	0	0	1	0	0	1	1	1	1	1	1	1
	1175	927	846	772	35	508	254	240	326	279	362	71	68
2.5	0	0	0	0	0	0	0	0	0	0	0	1	0
	338	317	361	406	71	71	71	43	66	27	0	34	3

(continued)

NAGASKI

FEMALES

Dose													
3.5	0 176	0 65	0 42	0 176	0 35	0 71	0 0	0 7	0 1	0 0	0 11	0 0	0 19
5.0	0 71	1 176	0 291	0 176	0 0	0 55	0 91	0 98	0 58	0 116	0 31	0 15	0 0
0	1 30411	0 27722	0 28272	1 29145	7 24405	3 16958	7 16243	3 16681	2 15593	3 11387	6 7664	2 4621	1 4642
0.025	0 17685	0 13598	0 15486	0 11620	4 12088	0 96930	1 9486	3 8965	5 7759	1 6767	4 4479	1 2244	1 2256
0.075	0 2268	0 1908	0 2195	1 1335	0 1142	0 987	1 844	0 1076	1 909	0 767	0 417	0 215	0 189
0.15	0 1913	0 1909	0 2344	0 1595	0 1371	0 1212	0 1316	0 1064	0 1067	1 618	0 168	0 260	0 235
0.3	0 2374	0 248	1 2565	0 3364	0 1838	0 1564	0 1913	0 1397	2 1024	0 871	0 613	0 297	0 299
0.75	0 1223	0 1551	0 2504	1 2098	0 1695	1 1049	1 606	0 938	0 750	0 726	0 333	0 194	0 193
1.5	0 860	0 701	0 1289	0 1760	2 1571	0 799	0 494	2 837	1 374	0 448	0 266	1 154	0 60
2.5	0 215	0 353	0 492	0 388	0 247	0 335	0 242	0 196	0 130	0 143	0 6	0 36	0 25
3.5	0 109	0 247	0 0	0 0	0 139	0 71	0 35	0 21	0 0	0 6	0 0	0 0	0 5
5.0	0 216	0 106	0 141	0 141	0 142	0 35	0 104	0 159	0 43	0 50	0 35	0 10	0 1

where n represents the total number of cells in the table. Since

$$log(r_i) = \log\left[\frac{d_i}{P_i}\right] = \log(d_i) - log(P_i)$$

when d_i represents the number of deaths for P_i person-years at risk from the ith cell, the Poisson model becomes

$$log(d_i) = a + b_1 x_{i1} + b_2 x_{i2} + b_3 x_{i3} + \cdots + b_k x_{ik} + \log(P_i)$$

or

$$d_i = P_i \times e^{a + b_1 x_{i1} + b_2 x_{i2} + b_3 x_{i3} + \cdots + b_k x_{ik}}.$$

The log-rate model requires the number of deaths in a specific cell to be determined by the person-years at risk multiplied by a factor that reflects the influence of the independent variables. Like the previous linear models, the influence of a specific independent variable x_j is measured by the magnitude of the associated regression coefficient b_j. The independent variables are frequently continuous quantities divided into a series of categories. For example, if reported age is used to classify individuals into a series of categories, the independent variable x_j is usually coded as the mid-point of each age interval. The statistical properties of the model depend on the knowledge or the assumption that the counted events in each cell of the table have a Poisson or at least an approximate Poisson distribution. Mortality and disease data are particularly likely to produce Poisson distributions since these data typically represent counts of rare events with approximately constant probability of occurring among large numbers of individuals. Furthermore, risk factors associated with mortality and disease are often thought to behave in a multiplicative fashion which is a primary reason for applying a Poisson model to a series of observed rates.

Analogous to the linear and logistic models, the logarithm of a rate is a linear function of the independent variables producing the previously described properties of a general linear model. The link function in this case is the logarithmic transformation of the rate. As before, differences between the logarithms of the rates do not depend on the magnitude of the independent variables, the influence of each independent variable is unaffected by the values of the other variables in the additive model and the coefficient b_m measures the isolated influence of the mth independent variable on the logarithm of a rate for a one unit increase in that specific variable when the other $k - 1$ independent variables in the model are held constant.

For the bivariate case where the rates are classified into a two-way table, the additive Poisson model is expressed as

$$\log(r_i) = a + b_1 x_{i1} + b_2 x_{i2}$$

or

$$d_i = P_i \times e^{a+b_1 x_{i1} + b_2 x_{i2}} = P_i \times e^a \times (e^{b_1})^{x_{i1}} \times (e^{b_2})^{x_{i2}} = P_i A B^{x_{i1}} C^{x_{i2}}$$

where x_1 represents quantitative levels of the row variable and x_2 represents quantitative levels of the column variable. The last expression emphasizes the multiplicative nature of the risk factors in a Poisson model.

Additivity translates into constant differences between log-rates or constant ratios between rates when either x_1 or x_2 is held constant — comparisons between table rows or columns. In symbols, for x_2 constant (e.g., same column of the table), then

$$\log(r_i) - \log(r_j) = b_1(x_{i1} - x_{j1}) \quad \text{or} \quad \frac{r_i}{r_j} = e^{b_1(x_{i1}-x_{j1})}$$

shows that the row influences (x_1) on the comparison of two rates are unaffected by the column influences (x_2). That is, the ratio is the same regardless of which column is considered. Similar expressions show that the column influences on the outcome variable are unaffected by the row variable. Geometrically, if the logarithms of the rates are perfectly additive, then a plot of the log-rates from each row of a table produces parallel lines. Similarly, a plot of the column log-rates also produces parallel lines.

To illustrate the properties of the additive Poisson model, the hypothetical data in Table 4.10 perfectly conform to an additive structure.

The rates differ by multiplicative factors and the log-rates, therefore, differ by additive constants in the hypothetical 2×5 table. For example, the difference in rates between rows 1 and 2 is three-fold (for all columns) and the difference between the log-rates is $\log(3) = 1.099$ (again, for all columns). The columns have the same property. Figure 4.7 displays these "data" (Table 4.10) in terms of both rates and log-rates (parallel lines). An "analysis" of this hypothetical data verifies the perfect fit (residual deviance $= 0$) and

```
> d<- c(4,12,3,7,18,144,252,480,756,1080)
> P<- c(1000,2000,300,500,1000,12000,14000,16000,18000,20000)
> x1<- c(rep(1,5),rep(2,5))
> x2<- rep(1:5,2)
> rate<- round(d/P,3)
> lograte<- round(log(d/P),3)
> cbind(d,P,rate,lograte,x1,x2)
           d     P  rate lograte x1 x2
 [1,]      4  1000 0.004  -5.521  1  1
 [2,]     12  2000 0.006  -5.116  1  2
 [3,]      3   300 0.010  -4.605  1  3
 [4,]      7   500 0.014  -4.269  1  4
 [5,]     18  1000 0.018  -4.017  1  5
 [6,]    144 12000 0.012  -4.423  2  1
 [7,]    252 14000 0.018  -4.017  2  2
 [8,]    480 16000 0.030  -3.507  2  3
 [9,]    756 18000 0.042  -3.170  2  4
[10,]   1080 20000 0.054  -2.919  2  5
```

Table 4.10. Hypothetical data that perfectly fit an additive Poisson model (deaths, populations at risk, rates, and log-rates)

		column 1	column 2	column 3	column 4	column 5
row 1	deaths	4	12	3	7	18
	person-years	1 000	2 000	300	500	1 000
	rate	0.004	0.006	0.01	0.014	0.018
	log-rate	−5.521	−5.116	−4.605	−4.269	−4.017
row 2	deaths	144	252	480	756	1 080
	person-years	12 000	14 000	16 000	18 000	20 000
	rate	0.012	0.018	0.03	0.042	0.054
	log-rate	−4.423	−4.017	−3.507	−3.170	−2.919

or

i	deaths	person-years	rate	log-rate	row	column
1	4	1 000	0.004	−5.521	1	1
2	12	2 000	0.006	−5.116	1	2
3	3	300	0.010	−4.605	1	3
4	7	500	0.014	−4.269	1	4
5	18	1 000	0.018	−4.017	1	5
6	144	12 000	0.012	−4.423	2	1
7	252	14 000	0.018	−4.017	2	2
8	480	16 000	0.030	−3.507	2	3
9	756	18 000	0.042	−3.170	2	4
10	1 080	20 000	0.054	−2.919	2	5

```
> otemp<- glm(d~factor(x1)+factor(x2)+offset(log(P)),
    family=poisson)
> round(otemp$deviance,4)
 [1] 0
> rate0<- exp(predict(otemp))
> rate0
     1     2     3     4     5     6     7    8    9    10
0.0040.006 0.01 0.014 0.018 0.012 0.018 0.03 0.042 0.054
> round(log(rate0[x1==2])-log(rate0[x1==1]),4)
      6      7      8      9     10
 1.0986 1.0986 1.0986 1.0986 1.0986
> rate0[x1==2]/rate0[x1==1]
 6 7 8 9 10
 3 3 3 3 3
> P*rate0
 1   2 3 4   5   6   7   8   9   10
 4 12 3 7 18 144 252 480 756 1080.
```

Since the residual deviance is zero, the estimated number of deaths is identical to the observed "deaths" (e.g., $d_i = \hat{d}_i$). The *offset*( ) option used in the Poisson model analysis is discussed in the next section.

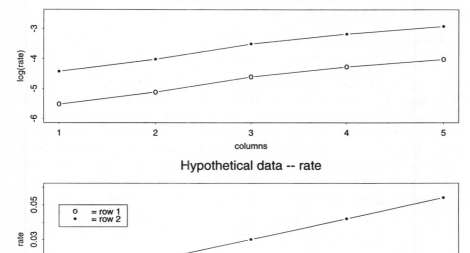

Figure 4.7

MULTIVARIABLE POISSON MODEL

Additivity of the independent variables is not always the case. Situations certainly arise where one variable influences the relationship between another variable and the outcome (non-additivity). A good place to start an investigation of a series of independent variables is to address the question of interactions.

For the Japanese lung cancer data (Table 4.9), there are a variety of ways the four independent variables (exposure (x_1), age (x_2), sex (x_3), and city (x_4)—$k = 4$) could affect the way the other variables influence the rate of lung cancer mortality. Using pairwise multiplicative terms in a linear model allows the relationships with the dependent variable to depend on combinations of independent variables. In other words, the independent variables do not have separate effects on the outcome. For example, non-additivity in the lung cancer data could mean that the relationship between radiation exposure and lung cancer risk is different for males and females. Another possible interaction might be between exposure and city, meaning that the relationship between lung cancer rates and radiation exposure is different in the two cities,

Hiroshima and Nagasaki. A Poisson model incorporating these two sources of non-additivity and four others is

$$\log(r_i) = a + b_1 x_{i1} + b_2 x_{i2} + b_3 x_{i3} + b_4 x_{i4} + b_5 x_{i1} x_{i2} + b_6 x_{i1} x_{i3} + b_7 x_{i1} x_{i4}$$
$$+ b_8 x_{i2} x_{i3} + b_9 x_{i2} x_{i4} + b_{10} x_{i3} x_{i4} \qquad i = 1, 2, 3, \cdots, 520$$

where again $n = 520$ is the total number of cells in Table 4.9. The variable indicating city is binary (*city*—Hiroshima = 0 and Nagasaki = 1). The gender variable is also binary (*sex*—male = 1 and female = 0). Ages range from 0 to over 70 years and are coded by the midpoint of 13 five-year age intervals (i.e., 2.5, 7.5, 12.5, $\cdots$, 70). Exposure was reconstructed for all participants and is coded as the midpoints of 10 exposure categories (i.e., units = mGy: 0.0, 0.025, 0.075, 0.15, 0.3, 0.75, 1.5, 2.5, 3.5, 5.0). Such a model is a bit complicated but easily implemented with the *glm*( ) command or

```
> otemp1<- glm(deaths~dose+age+sex+city+dose*age+dose*sex+
      dose*city+age*sex+age*city+sex*city+offset(log(pyears)),
      family=poisson)
> summary(otemp1,correlation=F)

Call: glm(formula = deaths ~ dose+age+sex+city+dose*age+
      dose*sex+dose*city+age*sex+age*city+sex*city+
      offset(log(pyears)), family = poisson)
Deviance Residuals:
      Min         1Q      Median          3Q        Max
 -4.226579 -0.7883404 -0.4696731 0.1981769 2.85637

Coefficients:
                  Value   Std. Error      t value
(Intercept) -9.1835751185 0.557153097 -16.4830370
       dose -0.0328222673 0.301063741  -0.1090210
        age  0.0566437225 0.009221671   6.1424576
        sex -0.3712572447 0.315228637  -1.1777396
       city  0.2450059115 0.334325586   0.7328363
   dose:age -0.0006855381 0.003313966  -0.2068633
   dose:sex  0.1981688808 0.115943080   1.7091911
  dose:city  0.0189947292 0.128146623   0.1482265
    age:sex -0.0071400968 0.004430089  -1.6117278
   age:city  0.0031455930 0.004576569   0.6873255
   sex:city -0.2039528086 0.177612859  -1.1482998

(Dispersion Parameter for Poisson family taken to be 1)
Null Deviance: 1303.939 on 507 degrees of freedom
Residual Deviance: 595.589 on 497 degrees of freedom

Number of Fisher Scoring Iterations: 4.
```

The "coefficient" in the linear model associated with the *log*(*pyears*) term is always one. Such a term is called an offset and is part of the computer implementation. The offset term has a general definition. However, in the context of a Poisson regression model the offset term is an additive effect that is not an independent variable. An offset term incorporating person-years into the model provides a weighting for each number of deaths (*log*(d_i)—dependent variable) but is not a risk or categorical variable and, therefore, not a statistical quantity to be analyzed. For the Poisson model to include person-years as a weight for the number of deaths, the logarithm of the person-years is used rather than the actual person-years measured. In short, the term *offset(variable.name)* in the *glm*-formula identifies a non-statistical part of a linear model and *offset(log(pyears))* is used when the Poisson regression dependent variable is the number of deaths (glm-input).

A basic purpose for postulating a model with all pairwise interaction terms is to contrast it to the purely additive model (all interaction terms excluded). For the Japanese lung cancer data, the additive model

$$\log(r_i) = a + b_1 x_{i1} + b_2 x_{i2} + b_3 x_{i3} + b_4 x_{i4} \qquad i = 1, 2, 3, \cdots, 520$$

is estimated and summarized by

```
> otemp0<- glm(deaths~dose+age+sex+city+offset(log(pyears)),
      family=poisson)
> summary(otemp0,correlation=F)

Call: glm(formula = deaths~dose+age+sex+city+
             offset(log(pyears)), family = poisson)
Deviance Residuals:
      Min        1Q     Median        3Q       Max
 -4.54065 -0.7911987 -0.4696079 0.2780769 2.816751

Coefficients:
                Value    Std. Error     t value
(Intercept) -8.63834378 0.194439154 -44.426977
       dose  0.24535283 0.057118437   4.295510
        age  0.05071325 0.002141267  23.683756
        sex -0.88130182 0.080305917 -10.974307
       city  0.09102392 0.086652896   1.050443

(Dispersion Parameter for Poisson family taken to be 1 )
Null Deviance: 1303.939 on 507 degrees of freedom
Residual Deviance: 603.5457 on 503 degrees of freedom

Number of Fisher Scoring Iterations: 4.
```

The process of comparing residual deviances to evaluate nested logistic models equally applies to investigating Poisson models. A formal comparison of the Poisson model with all pairwise interaction terms to the purely additive model is

```
> # non-additive model
> D1<- otemp1$deviance
> df1<- otemp1$df.residual
> # additive model
> D0<- otemp0$deviance
> df0<- otemp0$df.residual
> df<- df0-df1
> x2<- D0-D1
> pvalue<- 1-pchisq(x2,df)
> cbind(x2,df,pvalue)
           x2 df      pvalue
[1,] 7.956718  6 0.2412915.
```

The chi-square test-statistic (moderately large significance probability) indicates that the six interaction terms are not critical in describing the relationships between lung cancer deaths and radiation exposure, age, gender, and location. Assuming that the effects are additive suggests, for example, that the relationship between lung cancer mortality and radiation exposure is the same in both cities and for both sexes. Males have higher rates of lung cancer mortality than females but when an additive model describes the data, the estimated relationship between disease and radiation exposure is the same for both sexes.

The goodness-of-fit of an additive Poisson model can be assessed in several ways. Expected log-rates using *predict*( ) can be estimated and compared to the corresponding observed values. The expression *predict*(*otemp*0) produces the model derived log-rates of lung cancer. The expression *exp*(*predict*(*otemp*0)) produces the expected rates and *pyears* * *exp*(*predict*(*otemp*0)) produces the expected number of lung cancer deaths, based on the additive model. If the S-object *otemp*0 is replaced by *otemp*1, these expected values are calculated from the non-additive model. A Pearson chi-square test-statistic summarizing the correspondence between the observed number of deaths and the number of deaths estimated from the additive model is

```
> ex<- pyears*exp(predict(otemp0))
> x2<- sum((deaths-ex)^2/ex)
> pvalue<- 1-pchisq(x2,df0)
> cbind(x2,df0,pvalue)
          x2        df0             pvalue
[1,] 617.3705       503        0.0003563902.
```

The large chi-square statistic (small *p*-value) indicates that the additive Poisson model is not a good representation of the data and inferences drawn from this model are, at best, approximate. Notice that the value of the chi-square statistic is similar to the residual deviance (617.371 versus 603.546). Similarity between the two approaches is generally the case, especially for tables with large numbers of observations distributed so that no cells in the table are empty or contain only a few observations.

From considerations not shown, the lack of fit of the Japanese data is mostly due to influences from the younger and older age groups while the Poisson model effectively describes the relationships within the data for the ages 40 to 55. To get some idea of the relationships between exposure, age, and gender for two age groups (40–45 and 50–55), specific model generated lung cancer mortality rates for the Hiroshima data are

```
> rate<- function(isex,icity,iage) {
    etemp<- ex[sex==isex & city==icity & age==iage]
    ptemp<- pyears[sex==isex & city==icity & age==iage]
    base<- 100000
    base*etemp/ptemp
  }
```

```
> ex<- pyears*exp(predict(otemp0))
> r1<- rate(1,1,42.5)
> r2<- rate(2,1,42.5)
> r3<- rate(1,1,52.5)
> r4<- rate(2,1,52.5)
> r<- cbind(r1,r2,r3,r4)
> round(r,1)
          r1    r2     r3     r4
 [1,]   69.4  28.7  115.2   47.7
 [2,]   69.8  28.9  115.9   48.0
 [3,]   70.7  29.3  117.3   48.6
 [4,]   72.0  29.8  119.5   49.5
 [5,]   74.7  30.9  124.0   51.4
 [6,]   83.4  34.5  138.5   57.4
 [7,]  100.2  41.5  166.5   69.0
 [8,]  128.1  53.1  212.8   88.1
 [9,]  163.8  67.8  271.9  112.6
[10,]  236.6  98.0  392.9  162.7.
```

The output values are the model estimated lung cancer mortality rates per 100,000 person-years from the city of Hiroshima for the 10 exposure categories for two age groups and the two sexes ($r1$ = male rates, age 40–45; $r2$ = female rates, age 40–45; $r3$ = male rates, age 50–55; $r4$ = female rates, age 50–55). Plots of these estimated log-rates and rates are achieved by

```
> par(mfrow=c(2,1))
> exposure0<- c(0,0.025,0.075,0.15,0.3,0.75,1.5,2.5,3.5,5)
> matplot(exposure0,log(r),type="l",xlab="exposure",
    ylab="log(rate/base)",main="lung cancer rates
    by exposure and sex and age")
> matplot(exposure0,r,type="l",xlab="exposure",ylab="rate/base")
> legend(0,350,c("male -- age 40-45","female -- age 40-45"
    "male    -- age 50-55","female -- age 50-55"),lty=1:4)
```

and produce Figure 4.8. The S-function $matplot(x, y, \cdots)$ plots the values in vector y for each value in x. If y is an array of values, then each column of y is plotted for the values contained in x. If x and y are both two-dimensional arrays with the same dimensions, then each column of y is plotted for the values contained in each column of x producing as many plots as there are columns on a single set of axes. The S-function $matplot(\ )$ is an extension of the S-function $plot(\ )$. It combines the command $plot(\ )$ with a series of commands to plot lines or points ($lines(\ )$ or $points(\ )$ S-functions) into one S-function automatically changing the line type or character type option (lty or pch) for each column of input plotted.

Figure 4.8 geometrically displays the magnitude of the coefficients estimated from the additive Poisson model. As required, the estimated log-rates form parallel lines each representing an estimated linear dose–response relationship for a specific age/gender group. The distance between specific lines is determined by the modeled relationship and the outcome regardless of the values of the other variables (additivity). For example, the difference between log-rates for males and females is $-0.881(\hat{b}_3)$ and between age groups 40–45

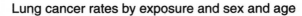

Lung cancer rates by exposure and sex and age

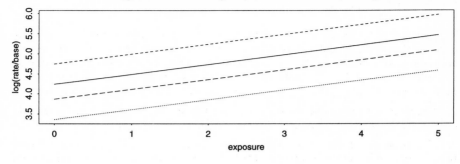

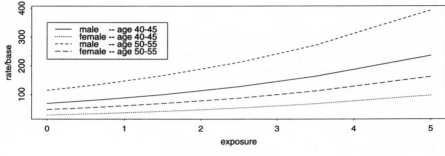

Figure 4.8

and 50–55 the difference is 0.051 ($\hat{b}_2$) for all levels of exposure (Figure 4.8). The slope of the estimated exposure response lines is the same for all four age/gender groups (again, additivity) and is 0.245 ($\hat{b}_1$) yielding an increase in log-rates of $5(0.245) = 1.227$ over the range 0 to 5 mGy for all four groups. The estimated differences in log-rates translate into multiplicative comparisons among rates. Gender differences show a female/male rate ratio of $e^{-0.881} = 0.414$, a difference in one year of age multiplies the risk of lung cancer by $e^{0.051} = 1.052$ and a $e^{5 \times 0.245} = e^{1.227} = 3.410$-fold increase in lung cancer mortality is associated with an increase in exposure of 5 mGy. Under the assumption that these variables have additive influences on the logarithm of the lung cancer mortality rates, each independent variable contributes separately to the risk of death. For example, the dose–response relationship is the same for both age groups and both sexes making the interpretation of the relationship between lung cancer and exposure easy to understand and report. The overall risk associated with several variables is simply the product of the individual risks. The presence of interactions does not allow data to be as readily summarized and interpreted.

Problem set IV

1. A measure of influence on the estimated value $\hat{y}_i$ associated with the ith independent variable x_i can be defined as $\hat{b} - \hat{b}_{(i)}$ where $\hat{b}$ is estimated from all n observations and $\hat{b}_{(i)}$ is estimated from the same data set but with the ith observation removed. Compute all such values for the diastolic blood pressure data (Table 4.1) and determine the five most influential points. Locate the five points on a plot of the data.

2. Show* that if the coefficients a_i maximize the multivariate distance M^2, then the coefficients $ba_i + c$ also maximize M^2 where b and c are constants.

3. The goodness-of-fit S-code for the logistic model in the chapter requires the number of observations to be evenly divisible by 10. Write and test an S-program for the same goodness-of-fit test but make no assumptions about the total number of observations used in the logistic regression analysis.

4. The table showing case/control status and coffee consumption (Table 4.7) is a summary of $n = 1010$ individuals where the frequencies in the table are the counts of observations with the identical values of the dependent and independent variables. For example, there are nine records (one for each person) where the outcome is a case who reports no coffee consumption ($x_1 = 0$) and is a male participant ($x_2 = 1$)—first cell in the summary table.

Using Table 4.7 reconstruct the data so that there are 1010 individual records where each record contains a 0 or 1 for case/control status as well as the corresponding values of the independent variables (x_1 and x_2).

Use these $n = 1010$ records and *glm*( ) and conduct a logistic regression analysis showing that the results are identical to the ones in the chapter where the analysis is performed directly on the tabular data using the cell frequencies as weights.

5. Consider the following data where birth weight and maternal age are recorded for three groups based on smoking exposure status:

| | non-smoker | | | quitters | | | smokers | |
	bwt	age		bwt	age		bwt	age
1	9.1	35	1	7.2	32	1	6.7	24
2	8.9	29	2	7.7	30	2	6.5	24
3	8.5	34	3	6.8	26	3	7.2	28
4	7.4	32	4	7.0	33	4	6.5	26
5	7.5	28	5	7.4	28	5	6.5	26
6	7.3	28	6	6.2	29	6	7.1	26

Using S-tools conduct a separate simple linear regression analysis for each smoking exposure group.

Use the same data and the model, $y = a + b_1 x + b_2 g_1 + b_3 g_2 + b_4 g_1 x + b_5 g_2 x$, to conduct a linear regression analysis using all 18 observations simultaneously where $y =$ birth weight (dependent variable) and $x =$ age (independent variable). The design variable g is defined as $g_1 = g_2 = 0$ for non-smokers, $g_1 = 0$, $g_2 = 1$ for quitters and $g_1 = 1$ and $g_2 = 0$ for smokers.

Demonstrate these two approaches are identical.

Formally, test the influence of the three-level smoking exposure categorical variable on birth weight.

6. The following data are deaths from lung cancer and person-years at risk, classified by age and exposure to radiation for workers at the Oak Ridge National Laboratory:

age	mSv	deaths	p-years	age	mSv	deaths	p-years	age	mSv	deaths	p-years	age	mSv	deaths	p-years
1	1	0	29901	2	3	2	2423	3	5	0	476	4	7	0	184
2	1	1	6251	3	3	1	2281	4	5	0	387	5	7	1	109
3	1	4	5251	4	3	2	1918	5	5	0	225	6	7	0	60
4	1	3	4126	5	3	0	1322	6	5	1	164	7	7	1	23
5	1	3	2778	6	3	2	723	7	5	0	150	1	8	0	2104
6	1	1	1607	7	3	3	538	1	6	0	779	2	8	0	1027
7	1	3	1358	1	4	0	2341	2	6	0	296	3	8	1	1029
1	2	1	71382	2	4	0	972	3	6	0	282	4	8	3	827
2	2	5	16705	3	4	1	958	4	6	1	251	5	8	1	555
3	2	4	13752	4	4	1	816	5	6	0	193	6	8	2	297
4	2	10	10439	5	4	0	578	6	6	0	125	7	8	2	153
5	2	11	7131	6	4	2	375	7	6	0	69				
6	2	16	4133	7	4	3	303	1	7	0	520				
7	2	11	3814	1	5	0	1363	2	7	0	188				
1	3	0	6523	2	5	0	478	3	7	0	217				

Recode age categories 1, 2, 3, 4, 5, 6, 7 into ages 45, 47.5, 52.5, 57.5, 62.5, 67.5, and 70 years. Recode exposures categories 1, 2, 3, 4, 5, 6, 7, 8 into exposures 0, 15, 30, 50, 70, 90, 110, and 120 mSv (milliseiverts).

Evaluate the exposure response in these data using a Poisson regression approach.

When the open-ended (last) interval coded at 120 mSv is recoded to 160 mSv, assess the impact on the exposure/risk relationship using a Poisson regression analysis.

Plot the impact on the dose-response relationship varying the definitions of the coded value for the last exposure group (e.g., 120, 130, 140, $\cdots$, 220).

7. Generate a sample of $n = 200$ random observations that are described by the logistic model

$$p_i = \frac{1}{1 + e^{-(a+bx_i)}}$$

where a and b are such that $or = 3.0$.

Using $glm(\ )$ and the simulated data, estimate the odds ratio.

*Solve theoretically and not with a computer program.

REFERENCES

1. Venables, W. N. and Ripley, B. D., *Modern Applied Statistics with S-Plus*. Springer-Verlag, New York, NY, 1994.
2. Belsley, D. A., Kuh, E., and Welsch, R.E., *Regression Diagnostics*. John Wiley & Sons, New York, NY, 1980.

3. Hamilton, L. C., *Regression with Graphics: A Second Course in Applied Statistics.* Brooks/Cole Publishing Company, Pacific Grove, CA, 1992.

4. Hoaglin, D. C., Mosteller, F., and Tukey, J. W., (eds) *Understanding Robust and Exploratory Data Analysis.* John Wiley & Sons, New York, NY, 1985.

5. Miller, A. J., *Subset Selection in Regression.* Chapman and Hall, New York, NY, 1990.

6. Miller, R. G., *Simultaneous Statistical Inference.* McGraw-Hill Book Company, New York, NY, 1966.

7. Lachenbruch, P. A., *Discriminant Analysis.* Hafner Press, New York, NY, 1975.

8. Atchley, W. R. and Bryant, E. D., (eds) *Multivariate Statistical Methods: Among-Group Covariation.* Dowden, Hutchinson & Ross, Inc., Stroudsburg, PA, 1975.

9. Rao, C. R., *Linear Statistical Inference and Its Applications.* John Wiley & Sons, New York, NY, 1965.

10. McMahon, B. *et al.*, (1981) Coffee consumption and pancreatic cancer. *New England Journal of Medicine*, 304:11; 630–633.

11. Schlesselman J. J., *Case-Control Studies.* Oxford University Press, New York, NY, 1982.

12. Roseman, R. H., Brand, R. J., Jenkins, C. D., *et al.*, (1975) Coronary heart disease in the Western Collaborative Group study. *Journal of the American Medical Association*, 223:872-877.

13. Hosmer, D. W. and Lemeshow, S. T., *Applied Logistic Regression.* John Wiley & Sons, New York, NY, 1985.

5

Estimation

Estimation: Maximum Likelihood

ESTIMATOR PROPERTIES

An estimate is a numerical value calculated from a sample of data. An estimator is the method or rule for finding that estimate. It is the properties of an estimator that are of concern when selecting the "best" way to estimate a summary value from data.

What are useful properties of an estimator?

An estimator should increase in accuracy as the sample size increases. More specifically, the probability an estimate differs from the value to be estimated should become smaller as the sample size increases. Such an estimator is called consistent.

If one estimator is consistent, then it is easy to create others that are also consistent. For example, if $\hat{\theta}$ is a consistent estimator, then so is $(1 - a/n)\hat{\theta}$ where a is a constant and n represents the sample size. It is, therefore, reasonable to choose a "best" estimator from among consistent estimators.

Estimators that have a distribution with an expected value equal to the value to be estimated are clearly important. This property, unlike consistency, applies to any sample size. When the mean of the distribution of the estimator is the value to be estimated, the estimator is said to be unbiased. The sample mean is an unbiased, consistent estimator of the sampled population mean. The sample median is also an unbiased, consistent estimator of the population mean when the sampled data are normally distributed.

Another desirable property of an estimator is low variability. An estimator with a low variability is distributed closely around the value to be estimated (if it is unbiased). An estimator with a small variance produces a more precise estimate than one with a larger variance. Therefore, unbiased estimators with low variability are both accurate ("on target") and precise ("tightly clustered").

The variance of the sample mean ($\bar{x}$) is

$$variance(\bar{x}) = \frac{\sigma^2}{n}$$

and the variance of the sample median ($\hat{m}$) is approximately

$$variance(\hat{m}) \approx 1.571\frac{\sigma^2}{n}$$

when n observations are randomly selected from a normal distribution with variance represented by σ^2. It appears that, at least for a sample of normally distributed data, the popularity of the sample mean over the median is justified—both are consistent and unbiased but the sample mean has a smaller variance.

Consistency, unbiased, and minimum variance are properties of an ideal estimator. Only a few estimators have all three properties. However, many estimators lacking one or more of these properties remain valuable summaries of sampled data.

MAXIMUM LIKELIHOOD ESTIMATOR

A maximum likelihood estimator has several important properties when applied to a sample made up of a relative large number of observations (called asymptotic properties): they are

1. consistency,
2. minimum variance, and
3. a normal distribution.

The maximum likelihood estimation process also produces an estimator of the variance associated with a specific estimate. Therefore, a maximum likelihood estimate not only has minimum asymptotic variance but it is possible to estimate the value of this variance from the sampled data. Additionally, functions (single valued) of maximum likelihood estimates are also maximum likelihood estimates (have properties 1, 2, and 3). If $\hat{\theta}$ is a maximum likelihood estimate, then so is $f(\hat{\theta})$. For example, if $\hat{b}$ is a maximum likelihood estimate, then such functions of $\hat{b}$ as $n\hat{b}$, $\hat{b}^2$, or $e^{\hat{b}}$ are also maximum likelihood estimates.

These "large sample properties" do not imply that a maximum likelihood estimator is superior to alternatives under all circumstances, for all sample sizes. For example, maximum likelihood estimators frequently produce biased estimates, although the bias usually diminishes as the sample size increases. Furthermore, for small samples of data there is no guarantee that a maximum likelihood estimator has either minimum variance or an approximate normal distribution. However, a maximum likelihood estimator has several optimum asymptotic properties, it is relatively easy to calculate and in many situations leads to an intuitive, useful estimate.

What is a maximum likelihood estimator?

To start, a definition of a likelihood function is necessary. A likelihood function is most easily expressed when a series of sampled observations is regarded as a function of a single parameter (the multiparameter case follows). The likelihood function is the joint probability associated with the sampled observations. A single parameter (represented by θ) likelihood function is

$$L = L(x_1, x_2, x_3, \cdots, x_n | \theta) = f(x_1 | \theta) f(x_2 | \theta) f(x_3 | \theta) \cdots f(x_n | \theta)$$

when $f(x_i | \theta)$ represents the probability of occurrence of a particular observation that depends on the parameter θ and is associated with one of a series of values $x_1, x_2, x_3, \cdots, x_n$ independently sampled from the same population. It makes no difference whether the observations x_i are continuous or discrete values. The expression represented by L is called the likelihood function because it is the probability associated with the occurrence of a specific set of observations for a given parameter value.

To illustrate, if x_i is a binary variable that depends on the parameter p and

$x_i = 0$ with probability $= f(x_i | p) = 1 - p$ and
$x_i = 1$ with probability $= f(x_i | p) = p$ $\qquad i = 1, 2, 3, \cdots, n,$

then for the sample of $n = 20$ specific values of x_i

$$\{0, 1, 0, 0, 1, 0, 0, 0, 1, 0, 0, 0, 0, 0, 0, 0, 1, 0, 0, 1\}$$

the likelihood function is

$$L = L(x_1, x_2, x_3, \cdots, x_n | p) = (1 - p)p(1 - p)(1 - p)p(1 - p) \cdots (1 - p)p$$
$$= p^5 (1 - p)^{15}$$

which is a function of the parameter p. More generally, the likelihood function for the occurrence of x values of 1 and $n - x$ of 0 is

$$L = L(x_1, x_2, x_3, \cdots, x_n | p) = K p^x (1 - p)^{n - x}$$

where $K = \binom{n}{x}$ does not involve the parameter p and, therefore, does not play a role in the estimation process. In other words, the likelihood associated with the count $X = \sum x_i$ has the binomial distribution.

The maximum likelihood estimator is that value of θ that makes the likelihood function maximum (denoted $\hat{\theta}$) or

$$L(x_1, x_2, x_3, \cdots, x_n|\hat{\theta}) > L(x_1, x_2, x_3, \cdots, x_n|\theta)$$

for all permissible values of θ. Continuing the example, the maximum likelihood estimate of p (denoted $\hat{p}$) is that value of p that makes $L = L(x_1, x_2, x_3, \cdots, x_n|p) = Kp^5(1-p)^{15}$ as large as possible. A plot of the likelihood function (Figure 5.1) shows that the maximizing value occurs at $p = 0.25$, among all permissible values of the parameter p ($0 \leq p \leq 1$). Selecting $\hat{p} = 0.25$ makes the likelihood function maximum. The data are considered as fixed and the maximizing parameter value is chosen from all permissible parameter values. The maximum likelihood estimate is the choice among all permissible parameters that causes the observed sample to be most probable. Estimation reduces to searching among the permissible parameters to find the parameter that is the the most likely "explanation" of the observed data.

A calculus argument equally produces the maximum likelihood estimator. The value that maximizes the likelihood $L = L(x_1, x_2, x_3, \cdots, x_n|\theta)$ also maximizes the logarithm of the likelihood function, $log(L) = \log[L(x_1, x_2, x_3, \cdots, x_n|\theta)]$. A log-likelihood function is generally a more mathematically tract-

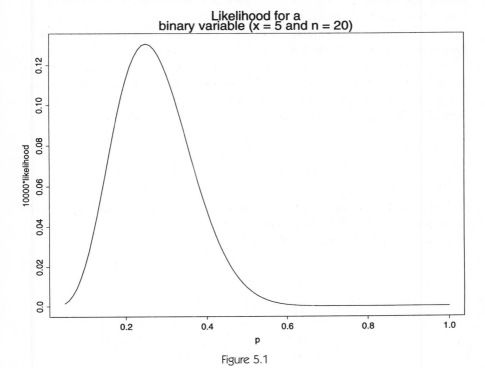

Figure 5.1

able function of the parameter θ (it is usually easier to deal with a sum than a product). The maximum likelihood estimator is then the solution to the equation

$$\frac{d}{d\theta}\log[L(x_1, x_2, x_3, \cdots, x_n|\theta)] = 0 \quad \text{or} \quad \frac{d}{d\theta}\sum \log[f(x_i|\theta)] = 0.$$

Abbreviating the notation, the solution to the equation $\frac{d}{d\theta}\log(L) = 0$ is the maximum likelihood estimate, denoted $\hat{\theta}$.

For the binary variable example,

$$\frac{d}{dp}\log(L) = \frac{d}{dp}\log[K\, p^x(1-p)^{n-x}]$$

$$= \frac{d}{dp}[\log(K) + x\log(p) + (n-x)\log(1-p)] = 0$$

therefore,

$$\frac{d}{dp}\log(L) = \frac{x}{\hat{p}} - \frac{n-x}{1-\hat{p}} = 0 \quad \text{yields} \quad \hat{p} = \frac{x}{n}.$$

Applying this estimator to the binary data example ($x = 5$ and $n = 20$) gives, as before, the maximum likelihood estimate $\hat{p} = 5/20 = 0.25$. Frequently, the maximum likelihood estimation process leads to the intuitive, "everyday" estimate often applied without statistical justification—such as $\hat{p}$, which is simply the observed proportion of the outcomes equal to one.

A valuable property of a maximum likelihood estimator emerges with a bit of further manipulation of the log-likelihood function. The resulting expression produces an estimator of the variance associated with the estimated parameter [1]. An estimator of the variance of the maximum likelihood estimate $\hat{\theta}$ is

$$variance(\hat{\theta}) = \left[-\frac{d^2}{d\theta^2}\log(L)\right]^{-1}$$

evaluated at the estimated value $\hat{\theta}$. This variance estimator is usually approximate and most useful for large sample sizes.

Continuing the binary variable example,

$$variance(\hat{p}) = \left[-\frac{d^2}{dp^2}\log[Kp^x(1-p)^{n-x}]\right]^{-1}$$

$$= \left[-\frac{d}{dp}\left(\frac{x}{p} - \frac{n-x}{1-p}\right)\right]^{-1} = \left[\frac{x}{p^2} + \frac{n-x}{(1-p)^2}\right]^{-1}$$

and evaluating this expression at the estimate $\hat{p}$ (noting that $x = n\hat{p}$) gives an estimator of the variance of the estimate $\hat{p}$ as

$$variance(\hat{p}) = \left[\frac{n}{\hat{p}} + \frac{n}{1 - \hat{p}}\right]^{-1} = \frac{\hat{p}(1 - \hat{p})}{n}.$$

Therefore, the maximum likelihood estimate $\hat{p} = x/n$ is a consistent estimator of the parameter p with an estimated minimum variance of $\hat{p}(1 - \hat{p})/n$ and has an approximate normal distribution for large samples of data. For the binary data example, the estimated variance is $variance(\hat{p}) = 0.25(0.75)/20 = 0.009$.

Statistical tests and confidence intervals based on maximum likelihood estimates are calculated using the estimated value, the estimated variance, and the fact the maximum likelihood estimate has an approximate normal distribution. In symbols, a statistical test of the hypothesis $\theta = \theta_0$ is

$$\text{test: } z = \frac{\hat{\theta} - \theta_0}{\sqrt{variance(\hat{\theta})}}$$

where z has an approximate standard normal distribution when $\theta = \theta_0$. An approximate $(1 - \alpha)\%$ confidence interval for the parameter θ is

$$\text{confidence interval: } \hat{\theta} \pm z_{1-\alpha/2}\sqrt{variance(\hat{\theta})}.$$

Consider the maximum likelihood estimate of the parameter λ from the Poisson distribution (Chapter 3) where the Poisson probability associated with a specific observation x_i is

$$f(x_i|\lambda) = \frac{e^{-\lambda}\lambda^{x_i}}{x_i!} \qquad x_i = 0, 1, 2, 3, \cdots.$$

The log-likelihood function is then

$$\log(L) = \log[f(x_1|\lambda)f(x_2|\lambda)f(x_3|\lambda)\cdots f(x_n|\lambda)]$$
$$= \log\left[\prod\frac{e^{-\lambda}\lambda^{x_i}}{x_i!}\right] = \sum\log\left[\frac{e^{-\lambda}\lambda^{x_i}}{x_i!}\right]$$

where $x_1, x_2, x_3, \cdots, x_n$ are n independently sampled observations from the same Poisson distribution. Specifically, the log-likelihood is a function of λ (the data are considered as fixed) and

$$\log(L) = -n\lambda + \log(\lambda)\sum x_i - \sum\log(x_i!) \qquad i = 1, 2, 3, \cdots, n.$$

The maximum likelihood estimator is the solution to the equation

$$\frac{d}{d\lambda}\log(L) = -n + \frac{1}{\lambda}\sum x_i = 0$$

producing an estimator $\hat{\lambda} = \bar{x}$. An estimator of the variance associated with the estimate $\hat{\lambda}$ is

$$variance(\lambda) = \left[-\frac{d^2}{d\lambda^2}\log(L)\right]^{-1} = \left[-\frac{d}{d\lambda}\left(-n + \frac{n\bar{x}}{\lambda}\right)\right]^{-1} = \left[\frac{n\bar{x}}{\hat{\lambda}^2}\right]^{-1} = \frac{\hat{\lambda}}{n}.$$

If the variable under study is continuous, the process of determining the maximum likelihood estimator is unchanged. Consider the maximum likelihood estimator of the parameter λ from the exponential distribution where x_i represents one of a series of n independent, continuous observations and

$$f(x_i|\lambda) = \lambda e^{-\lambda x_i} \qquad \lambda \text{ and } x_i \geq 0.$$

The log-likelihood function is

$$\log(L) = n\log(\lambda) - \lambda \sum x_i \qquad i = 1, 2, 3, \cdots, n$$

where $x_1, x_2, x_3, \cdots, x_n$ are n independently sampled observations from the same exponential distribution. The solution to the equation

$$\frac{d}{d\lambda}\log(L) = \frac{n}{\lambda} - \sum x_i = 0$$

produces the maximum likelihood estimator $\hat{\lambda} = \frac{1}{\bar{x}}$. An estimator of the variance of the estimate $\hat{\lambda}$ is

$$variance(\hat{\lambda}) = \left[-\frac{d^2}{d\lambda^2}\log(L)\right]^{-1} = \frac{\hat{\lambda}^2}{n}.$$

SCORING TO FIND MAXIMUM LIKELIHOOD ESTIMATES

The equation $\frac{d}{d\theta}\log(L) = 0$ is often sufficiently complex so that no closed-form solution exists. The solution $\hat{\theta}$ is then found numerically producing the maximum likelihood estimate. A simple method is based on using the slope of a straight line as an approximation for the derivative of a function. If a function is represented by $f(x)$, then

$$derivative \approx slope \quad \text{or} \quad \frac{d}{dx}f(x) \approx \frac{f(x_1) - f(x_2)}{x_1 - x_2} \qquad x_1 < x < x_2.$$

Then, to achieve an approximate solution to the equation $f(x) = 0$,

$$\frac{d}{dx}f(x) \approx \frac{f(x_1) - 0}{x_1 - x_2} \text{ and solving for } x_2 \text{ gives } x_2 \approx x_1 - \frac{f(x_1)}{\frac{d}{dx}f(x)}$$

where the derivative is evaluated at x_1. This relationship inspires the difference equation

$$x_{i+1} = x_i - \frac{f(x_i)}{\frac{d}{dx}f(x)}$$

which provides an iterative process usually leading to an accurate solution to the equation $f(x) = 0$.

An example follows: say, the solution to the equation $f(x) = x^3 + x - 12 = 0$ is desired, then

```
> f<- function(x){x^3+x-12}
> # initial starting value
> x<- 1
> for(i in 1:50){
  if(abs(f(x))<0.00001) break
  cat(" f(x) = ",round(f(x),3),"  x =",round(x,3),"\n")
  x<- x-f(x)/(3*x^2+1)
  }
  f(x) = -10          x = 1
  f(x) = 34.375       x = 3.5
  f(x) =  7.951       x = 2.589
  f(x) =  1.048       x = 2.213
  f(x) =  0.029       x = 2.146
  f(x) =  0           x = 2.144
> cat(" f(x) = 0 when  x =",round(x,3),"\n")
  f(x) = 0 when  x = 2.144.
```

The difference approach leads to the solution $f(x) = f(2.144) = 0$ where the derivative is given by

$$\textit{the derivative of } f(x) = \frac{d}{dx}f(x) = 3x^2 + 1.$$

Incidentally, the S-language supplies a function to derive derivatives. The S-function

$$D(expression(formula), \text{``argument''})$$

produces the derivative of the formula placed between the parentheses with respect to the argument placed between the quotes. For three examples,

```
> D(expression(x^3+x-12),"x")
3 * x^2 + 1
> D(expression(sin(t)),"t")
cos(t)
> D(expression(1-exp(-m*x)),"x")
exp( - m * x) * m.
```

Alternatively, an S-function *uniroot*( ) locates the roots of a univariate real-valued function between two limits given by a user-supplied *interval*. The S-function *uniroot*(*formula*, *interval* = $c(a, b)$) finds the root between the values

a and b of the function described by the formula when the formula evaluated at a and b has different signs. Continuing the polynomial example,

```
> uniroot(function(x){x^3+x-12},interval=c(0,3))$root
[1] 2.144039
> # using the S-function f previously defined
> uniroot(f,interval=c(0,3))$root
[1] 2.144039.
```

When the difference equation is applied to the equation $f(\theta) = \dfrac{d}{d\theta}\log(L) = 0$, the iterative pattern for this special case becomes

$$\hat{\theta}_{i+1} = \hat{\theta}_i - \frac{\dfrac{d}{d\theta}\log(L)}{\dfrac{d^2}{d\theta^2}\log(L)}.$$

When $f(\theta)$ represents the derivative of a likelihood function, this iterative process is called scoring to estimate a parameter. The solution $\hat{\theta}_i = \hat{\theta}$ is the maximum likelihood estimate associated with the likelihood value represented by L, when a series of iterations reduces the value of $\frac{d}{d\theta}\log(L)$ to essentially zero. The scoring process usually converges to the solution $\hat{\theta}$ when the initial starting value $\hat{\theta}_0$ is in the neighborhood of the estimate $\hat{\theta}$ (the maximum of the likelihood function).

To illustrate, situations arise where sample data are censored. A sample of n observations is said to be censored when $n - k$ observations are directly measured but all that is known about the remaining k observations is that they are above (or below) a specific value. For example, responses to a question on coffee consumption were 0, 1, and 2 cups/day but a last category was recorded as three or more cups of coffee consumed per day. It is known that individuals belonging to the three or more category consumed at least three cups per day but the actual amount of coffee consumed is not known (i.e., right censored). The following data illustrate:

cups/day	0	1	2	3 or more	total
count	x_0	x_1	x_2	x_3	n
observed	26	50	58	69	203

To estimate the mean level of coffee drinking, it is assumed that the number of cups of coffee consumed per day 0, 1, 2, 3, 4, 5, $\cdots$ by an individual has a Poisson distribution and the data represent $n = 203$ independent observations from a specific Poisson distribution. For these data, where $x_3 = 69$ observations are right censored, the likelihood function is

$$L = f(x_0|\lambda)f(x_1|\lambda)f(x_2|\lambda)f(x_3|\lambda) = [e^{-\lambda}]^{x_0} \times [\lambda e^{-\lambda}]^{x_1} \times \left[\frac{\lambda^2}{2!}e^{-\lambda}\right]^{x_2} \times P^{x_3}.$$

The symbol P represents the probability of consuming three or more cups per day and equals

$$P = \frac{\lambda^3}{3!}e^{-\lambda} + \frac{\lambda^4}{4!}e^{-\lambda} + \frac{\lambda^5}{5!}e^{-\lambda} + \cdots = 1 - (e^{-\lambda} + \lambda e^{-\lambda} + \frac{\lambda^2}{2!}e^{-\lambda}).$$

An S-function that generates log-likelihood values from a right censored Poisson distribution is

```
> # log-likelihood S-function -- Poisson distribution
> like<- function(lam,n,k,m,x)
  {-(n-k)*lam+log(lam)*sum(x[x<m])+k*log(1-ppois(m-1,lam))}
```

where x = data vector, n = number of observations, k = number censored observations, m = the value at which censoring occurs and lam = Poisson parameter. Using this S-function, a plot of the log-likelihood function is produced by

```
> # produce a data vector x (length=n=203)
> x<- rep(0:3,c(26,50,58,69))
> n<- length(x)
> table(x)
>    0  1  2  3
    26 50 58 69
> # number of censored values
> k<- 69
> # censored at m
> m<- 3
> # plot the log-likelihood function
> ltemp<- seq(0.1,10,0.1)
> lhood<- like(ltemp,n,k,m,x)
> plot(ltemp,lhood,type="l",xlab="parameter values ",
      ylab="log-likelihood", main="Log-likelihood
      function of the censored Poisson distribution")
```

The plot of the log-likelihood function for the censored Poisson data is displayed in Figure 5.2. The following S-code produces the maximum likelihood estimate of the parameter value λ using the iterative scoring process

```
> # initial value
> est<- mean(x)
> dp<- 0.001
> for(i in 1:10) {
  d1<- (like(est+dp,n,k,m,x)-like(est,n,k,m,x))/dp
  d2<- (like(est+2*dp,n,k,m,x)-2*like(est+dp,n,k,m,x)+
     like(est,n,k,m,x))/dp^2
  est<- est-d1/d2
  if(abs(d1)<0.0001) break
  }
> se<- sqrt(-1/d2)
> cat("est = ",round(est,3),"  se = ",round(se,4),"\n")
> est =   2.078   se =  0.1098.
```

The expression of the form $[like(x, \theta + \delta) - like(x, \theta)]/\delta$ in the S-program is a numerical approximation of the first derivative with respect to θ of the log-likelihood function where δ is set to a small value (e.g., $\delta = 0.001$). The

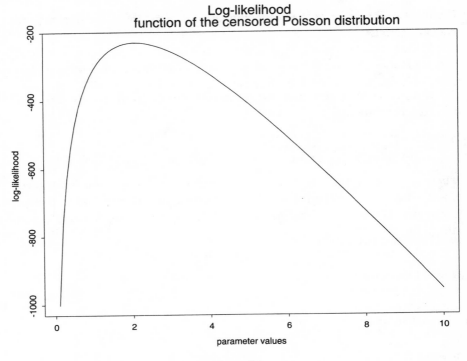

Figure 5.2

expression $[like(x, \theta + 2\delta) - 2like(x, \theta + \delta) + like(x, \theta)]/\delta^2$ is a similar numerical approximation of the second derivative of the log-likelihood function. These approximate expressions follow from a direct application of the definition of a derivative, which is

$$\frac{d}{d\theta} f(\theta) = \frac{f(\theta + \delta) - f(\theta)}{\delta}$$

as δ goes to zero.

The estimation of the Poisson parameter λ starts with the initial value $\bar{x}$ ($mean(x)$ returns 1.834) which is biased (downward) since values greater than three are treated as three. However, $\lambda_0 = \bar{x}$ provides an initial value sufficiently close to the maximum likelihood estimate to so that the iterative process quickly converges. The estimated expected level of coffee drinking is $\hat{\lambda} = 2.078$ cups per day with an estimated standard error of $\hat{se} = 0.110$. An estimate of the variance is found by evaluating the expression $\left[-\frac{d^2}{d\theta^2} \log(L) \right]^{-1}$ at the estimated value $\hat{\theta}$. Since the estimation process involves evaluating the second derivative of the likelihood function, a final value is easily extracted from the

S-code. For the coffee consumption example, $se <- sqrt(-1/d2)$ where $d2$ is the S-expression for the second derivative and $se = 0.110$.

Taking the derivative directly of the log-likelihood function and using the S-function *uniroot*( ) gives the same maximum likelihood estimate. An S-function yielding the derivative of the likelihood function is

```
dlike<- function(lam,n,k,m,x)
  {-(n-k)+sum(x[x<m])/lam+k*dpois(m-1,lam)/(1-ppois(m-1,lam))}
```

and

```
> uniroot(dlike,interval=c(1,3),n=203,k=69,m=3,x=x,
keep.xy=T)$root
[1] 2.078342.
```

MULTIPARAMETER ESTIMATION

The maximum likelihood estimate of k parameters $\theta_1, \theta_2, \theta_3, \cdots, \theta_k$ requires again finding that likelihood value that is maximum for a given set of data values or, when

$$L(x_1, x_2, x_3, \cdots, x_n|\hat{\theta}_1, \hat{\theta}_2, \hat{\theta}_3, \cdots, \hat{\theta}_k) > L(x_1, x_2, x_3, \cdots, x_n|\theta_1, \theta_2, \theta_3, \cdots, \theta_k)$$

among all permissible sets of the parameters $\{\theta_1, \theta_2, \theta_3, \cdots, \theta_k\}$, then $\{\hat{\theta}_1, \hat{\theta}_2, \hat{\theta}_3, \cdots, \hat{\theta}_k\}$ is the maximum likelihood estimate. The symbol L represents again a likelihood function based on a sample of n independently sampled observations for the same population and is a function of k parameter values. To find the maximum likelihood estimates of the k parameters, k equations must be solved where the ith equation is

$$\frac{\partial}{\partial \theta_i} \log[L(x_1, x_2, x_3, \cdots, x_n|\theta_1, \theta_2, \theta_3, \cdots, \theta_k)] = 0 \qquad i = 1, 2, 3, \cdots, k.$$

Parallel to the single parameter case, these k equations are sometimes solved directly but more often require numerical solutions. A generalization of the scoring method is one numerical approach.

The second partial derivatives of the multiparameter likelihood function are related to the variances and covariances of the maximum likelihood estimates of the k parameters [1]. Specifically, when k^2 second partial derivatives (all possible pairs)

$$g_{ij} = \frac{\partial}{\partial \theta_i} \frac{\partial}{\partial \theta_j} \log[L(x_1, x_2, x_3, \cdots, x_n|\theta_1, \theta_2, \theta_3, \cdots, \theta_k)] \qquad i, j = 1, 2, 3, \cdots, k$$

are the elements of a $k \times k$ matrix $\mathbf{G}$, the variance/covariance array associated with the k maximum likelihood estimates is related to $-\mathbf{G}^{-1}$ (the inverse of the matrix $\mathbf{G}$ multiplied by -1). The diagonal elements of $-\mathbf{G}^{-1}$ provide the estimated variances and the off-diagonal elements provide the estimated covariances.

The two parameter normal distribution, as before, is described by the probability density function

$$f(x_i|\theta_1, \theta_2) = \frac{1}{\sqrt{2\pi\theta_2}} e^{-\frac{1}{2}(x_i-\theta_1)^2/\theta_2} \qquad -\infty < x_i < \infty.$$

The logarithm of the two parameter likelihood function for a sample of n independent observations $x_1, x_2, x_3, \cdots, x_n$ from the same normal distribution is

$$\log(L|\theta_1, \theta_2) = -\frac{n}{2}\log(2\pi) - \frac{n}{2}\log(\theta_2) - \frac{1}{2\theta_2}\sum(x_i - \theta_1)^2.$$

The parameter θ_1 represents the mean of a normal distribution and θ_2 the variance (denoted previously as μ and σ^2). The two equations ($k = 2$) that yield maximum likelihood estimates are

$$\frac{\partial}{\partial\theta_1}\log(L) = \frac{1}{\hat{\theta}_2}\sum(x_i - \hat{\theta}_1) = 0$$

$$\frac{\partial}{\partial\theta_2}\log(L) = -\frac{n}{2\hat{\theta}_2} + \frac{1}{2\hat{\theta}_2^2}\sum(x_i - \hat{\theta}_1)^2 = 0 \qquad i = 1, 2, 3, \cdots, n.$$

The maximum likelihood estimates of the mean θ_1 and the variance θ_2 are then the solutions

$$\hat{\theta}_1 = \bar{x} \quad \text{and} \quad \hat{\theta}_2 = \frac{1}{n}\sum(x_i - \bar{x})^2.$$

The estimate $\hat{\theta}_2$ is biased; the unbiased estimate of θ_2 is $n\hat{\theta}_2/(n-1)$. Estimates of the variances and covariance of $\hat{\theta}_1$ and $\hat{\theta}_2$ are related to the second partial derivatives or

$$g_{11} = \frac{\partial^2}{\partial\theta_1^2}\log(L|\theta_1, \theta_2) = -\frac{n}{\hat{\theta}_2}$$

$$g_{12} = g_{21} = \frac{\partial}{\partial\theta_1}\frac{\partial}{\partial\theta_2}\log(L|\theta_1, \theta_2) = 0$$

$$g_{22} = \frac{\partial^2}{\partial\theta_2^2}\log(L|\theta_1, \theta_2) = -\frac{n}{2\hat{\theta}_2^2}.$$

Therefore, the elements of $-\mathbf{G}^{-1}$ give the estimators

$$\hat{v}_{11} = variance(\hat{\theta}_1) = \frac{\hat{\theta}_2}{n}, \hat{v}_{22} = variance(\hat{\theta}_2) = \frac{2\hat{\theta}_2^2}{n},$$

$$\text{and} \quad \hat{v}_{12} = covariance(\hat{\theta}_1, \hat{\theta}_2) = 0.$$

GENERALIZED SCORING

Two types of twins are born, monozygotic (identical) and dizygotic (fraternal). The frequency of these two types of twins can be estimated from observing three types of twin pairs with respect to gender. There are male–male pairs, male–female pairs and female–female pairs. The following model and data relate zygosity and gender:

pair type	model	symbols	observed number
male–male	$P(mm\|mz)P(mz) + P(mm\|dz)P(dz)$	$pm + p^2 d$	32
male–female	$2P(mf\|dz)P(dz)$	$2pqd$	41
female–female	$P(ff\|mz)P(mz) + P(ff\|dz)P(dz)$	$qm + q^2 d$	36

The symbol $d = 1 - m$ represents the probability of dizygotic twins and $p = 1 - q$ represents the probability of a male twin. The parameter estimation by scoring applied to these data produces maximum likelihood estimates of the two model parameters d and p. The maximum of the likelihood function (Figure 5.3) is found by numerical methods.

The generalized scoring approach is most easily described in terms of matrix notation. Let Θ_0 be a vector containing k initial parameter values $\{\theta_1^0, \theta_2^0, \theta_3^0, \cdots, \theta_k^0\}$ and $\mathbf{B}_0$ be a vector of the k first partial derivatives of the log-likelihood function evaluated at the initial parameter values where

Likelihood for twin parameter estimation

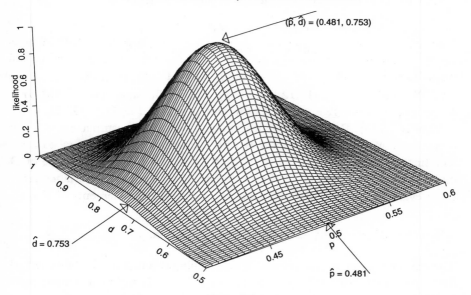

Figure 5.3

$$\mathbf{B}_0 = \left[\frac{\partial}{\partial \theta_1} \log(L), \frac{\partial}{\partial \theta_2} \log(L), \frac{\partial}{\partial \theta_3} \log(L), \cdots, \frac{\partial}{\partial \theta_k} \log(L) \right].$$

Again, L represents the multiparameter likelihood function of a sample of observations independently selected from the same population. Initial parameter values are developed from prior knowledge, plotting the likelihood functions, marginal distributions, or sometimes mathematical manipulations, but are essentially "ad hoc" starting points that are hoped to be sufficiently close to the maximum likelihood estimates to allow the estimation process to converge. Furthermore, let $\mathbf{G}_0$ represent the previously described $k \times k$ array of all possible second derivatives also evaluated at initial parameter values contained in Θ_0. A new set of parameters estimates, denoted Θ_1, becomes

$$\hat{\Theta}_1 = \hat{\Theta}_0 - \mathbf{G}^{-1}\mathbf{B}_0.$$

The process is repeated using the difference equation

$$\hat{\Theta}_{i+1} = \hat{\Theta}_i - \mathbf{G}^{-1}\mathbf{B}_i$$

and typically converges to the maximum likelihood estimates of the k parameters $\hat{\Theta} = \{\hat{\theta}_1, \hat{\theta}_2, \hat{\theta}_3, \cdots, \hat{\theta}_k\}$ when the initial value Θ_0 is in the neighborhood of the maximum value of the likelihood function. Specifically, the elements of $\mathbf{B}_i$ become essentially zero ($\mathbf{B} \approx 0$) yielding $\hat{\Theta}_i = \hat{\Theta}$. For $k = 1$, the multivariate parameter estimation process is identical to the previously described scoring approach for estimating a single parameter.

For the twin data example, the log-likelihood function is

$$\log(L) = 32 \log[p(1-d) + p^2 d] + 41\ log[2p(1-p)d]$$
$$+ 36 \log[(1-p)(1-d) + (1-p)^2 d].$$

When Θ_0 is set at $\Theta_0 = \{\theta_1^0, \theta_2^0\} = \{p_0, d_0\} = \{0.4, 0.6\}$, then $\mathbf{B}_0 = \{55.386, 19.310\}$ and $g_{11} = -719.128$, $g_{12} = g_{21} = 15.716$, and $g_{22} = -151.671$. These initial values give updated estimates of p and d as $\hat{\Theta}_0 - \mathbf{G}^{-1}\mathbf{B}_0 = \hat{\Theta}_1 = \{0.481, 0.753\}$. Repeating the process with "updated" estimates and a few more iterations produces a vector $\mathbf{B}$ with elements essentially equal to zero. The final estimates are then $\hat{\Theta} = \{\hat{p}, d\} = \{0.481, 0.753\}$. The inverse of $\hat{\mathbf{G}}$ multiplied by -1 ($\hat{\mathbf{V}} = -\mathbf{G}^{-1}$) is an estimate of the variance/covariance array when evaluated at the estimated value $\hat{\Theta}$; specifically the elements of $\hat{\mathbf{V}}$ are

$$\hat{v}_{11} = 0.00143 \qquad \hat{v}_{12} = -0.00031$$
$$\hat{v}_{21} = -0.00031 \qquad \hat{v}_{22} = 0.00863.$$

The parameter values that maximize the likelihood function for the observed data (male–male pairs $= 32$, female–female pairs $= 41$, and male–female pairs $= 36$) are $\hat{p} = 0.481$ and $\hat{d} = 0.753$ (noted in Figure 5.3) with $variance(\hat{p}) =$

0.00143 and $variance(\hat{d}) = 0.00863$. An S-program to perform the maximum likelihood estimation of these two parameters is:

```
> #twin.s - - estimation of p and d from twin data
> mm<- 32
> mf<- 41
> ff<- 36
> x<- c(mm,mf,ff)

> # log-likelihood function
> like<- function(x,p,d){
  m<- 1-d
  q<- 1-p
  x[1]*log(p*m+p^2*d)+x[2]*log(2*p*q*d)+x[3]*log(q*m+q^2*d)
  }

> dx<- 0.001
> # initial values
> d<- 0.6
> p<- 0.4
> etemp<- NULL
> for (i in 1:10) {
  f0<- like(x,p,d)
  # approximate first partial derivatives
  f1<- like(x,p+dx,d)
  f2<- like(x,p,d+dx)
  b1<- (f1-f0)/dx
  b2<- (f2-f0)/dx
  # approximate second partial derivatives
  f11<- like(x,p+2*dx,d)
  f22<- like(x,p,d+2*dx)
  f12<- like(x,p+dx,d+dx)
  g11<- (f11-2*f1+f0)/dx^2
  g22<- (f22-2*f2+f0)/dx^2
  g12<- (f12-f1-f2+f0)/dx^2
  est<- rbind(p,d)
  b<- cbind(b1,b2)
  g<- cbind(c(g11,g12),c(g12,g22))
  etemp<- est-solve(g)%*%t(b)
  p<- etemp[1]
  d<- etemp[2]
  if(sum(abs(b))<0.000001) break
  }
> cat("p = ",round(p,3),"d = ",round(d,3),"\n")
>  p =   0.481   d =   0.753.
"variance/covariance";round(gtemp,6)
> [1] "variance/covariance"
>              [,1]        [,2]
[1,]   0.001428 -0.000031
[2,]  -0.000031  0.008628.
```

To further explore the method of scoring to estimate parameters, the maximum likelihood estimation of the mean and variance is illustrated from data sampled from a normal distribution. As discussed, expressions for the maximum likelihood estimators can be derived directly but it is instructive to apply the scoring approach to achieve the same results. The following generates $n = 50$ observations from a normal distribution with mean $\mu = 4$ and standard deviation $\sigma = 2$:

```
> mu<- 4
> sd<- 2
> n<- 50
> x<- rnorm(n,mu,sd)
> round(mean(x),3)
[1] 4.155
> # maximum likelihood estimated standard deviation
> round(sqrt(((n-1)/n)*var(x)),3)
[1] 2.400.
```

The log-likelihood function was given earlier for estimating the mean and the variance from normally distributed data. An S-function to calculate values from the log-likelihood function from normally distributed data contained in the S-vector x is

```
like<- function(x,m,s){-n*log(s)-0.5*sum(((x-m)/s)^2)}
```

where m represents the mean of the sampled population and s represents the standard deviation (previously denoted θ_1 and $\sqrt{\theta_2}$). This S-function and the same "*for*-loop" from the twin data example produce maximum likelihood estimates. The intermediate results from each iteration show the convergence to the closed-form estimated mean and standard deviation or

i	$\hat{\Theta}_i$	$\mathbf{B}_i$	g_{11}	$g_{12} = g_{21}$	g_{22}	$\hat{\Theta}_{i+1}$
0	{3.000, 1.000}	{57.749, 304.388}	−50.000	−115.324	−1010.538	{3.883, 1.546}
1	{3.883, 1.546}	{17.529, 121.607}	−33.053	−28.426	−361.935	{4.034, 1.890}
2	{4.034, 1.890}	{5.691, 46.629}	−20.931	−7.357	−132.127	{4.117, 2.190}
3	{4.117, 2.190}	{1.695, 16.301}	−13.996	−1.792	−53.779	{4.149, 2.359}
4	{4.149, 2.359}	{0.401, 4.483}	−10.421	−0.366	−27.078	{4.155, 2.389}
5	{4.155, 2.398}	{0.053, 0.739}	−8.983	−0.045	−18.878	{4.155, 2.400}
6	{4.155, 2.400}	{0.002, 0.029}	−8.692	−0.001	−17.395	{4.155, 2.400}
7	{4.155, 2.400}	{0.000, 0.000}	−8.680	0.000	−17.335	{4.155, 2.400}

Starting with initial estimates $\mu_0 = 3.0$ and $\sigma_0 = 1.0$ (i.e., $\hat{\Theta}_0 = \{3.0, 1.0\}$), estimates from the iterative process are $\hat{\mu} = \hat{\theta}_1 = 4.155$ and $\hat{\sigma} = \sqrt{\hat{\theta}_2} = 2.400$ (i.e., $\hat{\Theta} = \{4.155, 2.400\}$), which agree with the maximum likelihood estimates of the mean and the standard deviation calculated directly. The estimate of the variance/covariance array follows:

```
> gtemp<- -solve(g)
> "variance/covariance"
> round(gtemp,3)

[1] "variance/covariance"
        [,1]    [,2]
[1,]   0.115   0.000
[2,]   0.000   0.058.
```

The directly estimated variance of the mean is $\hat{\sigma}^2/n = 2.40^2/50 = 0.115$, as expected.

Estimation: Bootstrap

BACKGROUND

Central to statistical analysis is the assessment of the precision of estimated summary values calculated from sampled data. When the entire population is not sampled, different samples contain different observations causing variation from sample to sample in calculated values. Without an assessment of this sampling variability, it is difficult and many times impossible to effectively use a summary quantity as part of understanding collected data, since the estimates alone do not communicate a sense of precision.

Only a few sample estimators, such as the sample mean, have exact formulas to estimate their associated sampling variability. Other useful statistical estimates have approximate estimates of their precision. Almost always both exact and approximate expressions for estimating variability depend on knowing or postulating specific properties of the sampled population. Maximum likelihood estimation, for example, often requires sometimes tricky mathematics but, more importantly, requires a specific model to obtain estimates and their standard errors. Situations inevitably arise where new or complicated summary values are necessary. The development of variance formulas for these estimates usually requires statistical theory, mathematical approximations, restrictive assumptions and, in some cases, nevertheless are impossible to derive.

A bootstrap estimation approach utilizes computer-based methods to provide estimates and measures of precision (principally standard errors and confidence intervals) without theoretical models, extensive mathematics, or restrictive assumptions about the structure of the sampled population. A model-free process based on repeated sampling of the observed data allows one "to pull oneself up by the bootstraps" to estimate and assess statistical quantities of interest. Estimates based on sophisticated statistical theory are replaced by a computer intensive process producing estimates and their standard errors. Furthermore, the bootstrap process is simple and remains simple regardless of the complexity of the estimator and its variance. Many of the following ideas are due to Bradley Ephron and can be found more fully explained in the book *An Introduction to the Bootstrap* [2].

GENERAL OUTLINE

For a sample of n independent observations $\{x_1, x_2, x_3, \cdots, x_n\}$ selected from the same population distribution, an estimator is a function of the sampled data denoted as $\hat{\theta} = s(\mathbf{x})^*$ where $\mathbf{x}$ represents some or all of the n sampled observations. For example,

$s(\mathbf{x})$ could be the sample mean, $\hat{\theta} = \frac{1}{n}\sum x_i$,

$s(\mathbf{x})$ could be the sample standard deviation, $\hat{\theta} = \sqrt{\dfrac{1}{n-1}\sum(x_i - \bar{x})^2}$,

$s(\mathbf{x})$ could be the sample range, $\hat{\theta} = largest(x_i) - smallest(x_i)$, or

$s(\mathbf{x})$ could be the sample harmonic mean, $\hat{\theta} = \dfrac{n}{\sum\dfrac{1}{x_i}}$.

In fact, $s(\mathbf{x})$ represents any simple or complex function of the sampled observations.

To calculate a bootstrap estimate of the parameter θ, a series of k bootstrap replicates is created. Each bootstrap value is obtained by selecting one observation at random from the collected data. A set of n such values sampled with replacement from the original sampled data constitutes a bootstrap replicate. If a sample of five observations is represented by $\{x_1, x_2, x_3, x_4, x_5\}$, then

$$\mathbf{x}_{[1]} = \{x_3, x_5, x_2, x_2, x_1\}$$
$$\mathbf{x}_{[2]} = \{x_4, x_2, x_4, x_1, x_3\}$$
$$\mathbf{x}_{[3]} = \{x_2, x_5, x_5, x_3, x_2\}$$
$$\mathbf{x}_{[4]} = \{x_1, x_1, x_3, x_5, x_1\}$$
$$\vdots$$
$$\mathbf{x}_{[k]} = \{x_3, x_2, x_1, x_4, x_5\}$$

illustrate k possible bootstrap replicates. The S-function *sample*( ) selects a bootstrap replicate or, specifically,

```
> repx<- sample(x,length(x),replace=T)
```

produces n values sampled with replacement from the original sample of observations contained in the S-vector x and places the result in the S-vector *repx*. A slight saving is achieved by the "default" command

```
> repx<- sample(x,replace=T)
```

$^\star s(\mathbf{x}) = s(x_1, x_2, x_3, \cdots, x_n)$ where the vector $\mathbf{X}$ represents a sample of observations. The symbol s stands for the estimation process applied to the vector of observations.

to produce a bootstrap replicate. For example, six bootstrap replicates are:

```
> x<- c(5,8,14,6,2)
> x
 [1]  5  8 14  6  2
> sample(x,replace=T)
 [1] 2 2 5 6 6
> sample(x,replace=T)
 [1] 14  2  2 14 14
> sample(x,replace=T)
 [1]  8  8  2 14  2
> sample(x,replace=T)
 [1]  8 14 14  5  5
> sample(x,replace=T)
 [1] 8 8 6 6 2
> sample(x,replace=T)
 [1] 14 14  2  5  6.
```

Each bootstrap replicate produces an estimate denoted $\hat{\theta}_{[i]} = s(\mathbf{x}_{[i]})$. The bootstrap estimator of the statistical summary θ is the mean of these k estimated values, denoted $\hat{\theta}_{[.]}$, or

$$\hat{\theta}_{[.]} = \frac{1}{k}\sum \hat{\theta}_{[i]} \qquad i = 1, 2, 3, \cdots, k.$$

Additionally, the bootstrap estimate of the standard error of the estimate $\hat{\theta}_{[.]}$ derived from the k estimated values $\hat{\theta}_{[i]}$ is

$$\hat{se}_{[.]} = \sqrt{\frac{1}{k-1}\sum (\hat{\theta}_{[i]} - \hat{\theta}_{[.]})^2}.$$

The processes that produces the estimate $\hat{\theta} = s(\mathbf{x})$ based on the n original observations is applied to each of the k replicates producing k bootstrap estimates $\hat{\theta}_{[1]}, \hat{\theta}_{[2]}, \hat{\theta}_{[3]}, \cdots, \hat{\theta}_{[k]}$. Differences among these estimates are due to sampling variations. The mean of these k values yields a bootstrap estimate of θ as well a bootstrap estimate of the standard error (i.e., $\hat{\theta}_{[.]}$ and $\hat{se}_{[.]}$) without statistical theory or formidable mathematics. The individual bootstrap estimates $\hat{\theta}_{[i]}$ are treated as if they were based on k different samples of size n selected from the same population. In other words, the distribution of the bootstrap estimates provides a picture of the distribution of the estimator $\hat{\theta}$.

SAMPLE MEAN FROM A NORMAL POPULATION

A mean value estimated from n independently sampled values (x_i) from the same normal distribution is certainly a situation where an alternative estimation process has nothing to offer. The estimate $\bar{x} = \sum x_i/n$ is simple, and has a normal distribution with a known standard error $(\sigma/\sqrt{n}$ where σ^2 represents the variance of the sampled population). The standard error is easily estimated by $S/\sqrt{n}$ where $S^2 = \sum (x_i - \bar{x})^2/(n-1)$. An estimated $(1-\alpha)$-level confidence interval is equally easy to construct (i.e., $\bar{x} \pm t_{1-\alpha/2}S/\sqrt{n}$ where $t_{1-\alpha/2}$ is the $(1 - \alpha/2)$-percentile of a t-distribution with $n - 1$ degrees of freedom). However, bootstrap estimation applied to this fundamental case illustrates the properties and features of the bootstrap approach.

To apply bootstrap estimation to normally distributed data,

```
> n<- 30
> x<- rnorm(n)
> se<- sqrt(var(x)/n)
> cat(" mean = ",round(mean(x),3)," variance = ",
      round(var(x),3)," se =",round(se,3),"\n")
  mean =  0.009  variance =  0.989  se = 0.0.180
```

produces a random sample of $n = 30$ normally distributed observations. The estimated mean and variance ($\bar{x} = 0.009$ and $S^2 = 0.989$), as expected, are close to the values used to generate the random sample ($\mu = 0$ and $\sigma^2 = 1.0$). More to the point, the estimated standard error of $\bar{x}$ is 0.180; again close to the value expected ($\sigma/\sqrt{n} = 1/\sqrt{30} = 0.183$).

A bootstrap sample of k replicates can be generated with SPLUS in two equivalent ways; using either *runif*( ) or *sample*( ) to sample the selected observations without replacement. Two sets of $k = 5000$ bootstrap replicates illustrate:

```
> # x contains n = 30 random standard normal values
> iter<- 5000
> x1<- NULL
> for (i in 1:iter) {x1[i]<- mean(x[ceiling(n*runif(n))])}
> cat("mean = ",round(mean(x1),4),"standard error = ",
    round(sqrt(var(x1)),4),"\n")
> mean =  0.0113 standard error =  0.1788

> xtemp<- matrix(sample(x,n*iter,replace=T),n,iter)
> x2<- apply(xtemp,2,mean)
> cat("mean = ",round(mean(x2),4),"standard error = ",
    round(sqrt(var(x2)),4),"\n")
> mean =  0.0098 standard error =  0.1803.
```

Figure 5.4 displays the theoretical normal distribution of the mean $\bar{x}$ ($\mu = 0$ and standard deviation $\sigma/\sqrt{n} = 0.183$) and a histogram of the 5000 bootstrap estimated mean values $\bar{x}_{[i]}$, each based on bootstrap replicate sample of 30 observations. The correspondence between these two plots indicates that the resampling process creates an accurate estimate to the distribution of $\bar{x}$. Properties based on the 5000 bootstrap estimates $\bar{x}_{[i]}$, therefore, provide estimates of the properties of $\bar{x}$ itself. For example, the 2.5^{th} and 97.5^{th} percentiles of the bootstrap distribution (*quantile*$(x2, c(0.025, 0.975))$ returns -0.350 and 0.355) are similar to the theory-based estimated 95% confidence limits (lower bound $= -0.362$ and upper bound $= 0.380$). The expected 95% confidence interval limits are $(-0.373, 0.373)$.

Histogram of bootstrap sample -- theoretical normal distribution

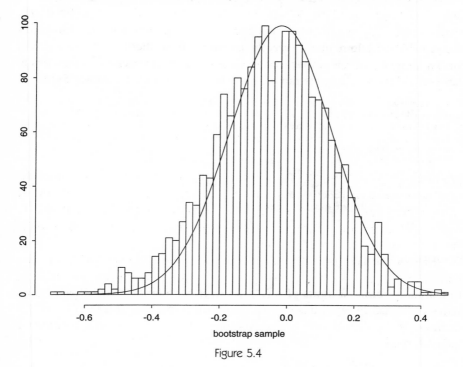

bootstrap sample

Figure 5.4

The bootstrap estimation of the sample mean and standard error indicates a general pattern. For an estimator described by an S-function (denoted by *fcn*( ), for example),

```
> # x contains the n sampled data values
> temp<- matrix(sample(x,n*iter,replace=T),n,iter)
> boot<- apply(temp,2,fcn)
> cat("mean = ",round(mean(boot),4),"standard error = ",
    round(sqrt(var(boot)),4),"\n")
```

produces an estimate and its estimated standard error based on *n* observations contained in the S-vector *x* and *iter* bootstrap replicates.

To illustrate the general bootstrap estimation pattern, consider the harmonic mean. It has been suggested that a harmonic mean is a sensitive measure of clustering in spatial data [3]. Distances of $n = 9$ cases of oral/pharyngeal cancer in females from a point source of pollution [4] are

$$d = \{43.64, 50.67, 33.56, 27.75, 43.35, 29.56, 38.83, 35.95, 20.01\}.$$

The estimated harmonic mean distance is

$$\bar{h} = \frac{n}{\sum \frac{1}{d_i}} \qquad i = 1, 2, 3, \cdots, n$$

and $\bar{h} = 33.467$ kilometers is directly calculated from the data. An expression for an estimate of the variance of this estimated distance is not as easily achieved. However, a bootstrap estimate and its estimated variance follow:

```
> # the S-vector d contains the n=9 sample distances
> d<- c(43.64,50.67,33.56,27.75,43.35,29.56,38.83,35.95,20.01)
> fcn<- function(x){length(x)/sum(1/x)}
> iter<- 2000
> n<- length(x)
> temp<- matrix(sample(d,n*iter,replace=T),n,iter)
> boot<- apply(temp,2,fcn)
> cat("mean = ",round(mean(boot),4),"standard error = ",
    round(sqrt(var(boot)),4),"\n")
 mean =   34.2836 standard error =   5.6049.
```

CONFIDENCE LIMITS

In general, estimated limits of a $(1 - \alpha)$-level confidence interval based on a series of bootstrap replicates consist of the $(\alpha/2)$-quantile and the $(1 - \alpha/2)$-quantile of the distribution of the $\hat{\theta}_{[i]}$-values. For a $(1 - \alpha)$-level confidence interval, then

$$\hat{\theta}_{lower} = [k(\alpha/2)]^{th} \text{ value of } \hat{\theta}_{[i]} \quad \text{and} \quad \hat{\theta}_{upper} = [k(1 - \alpha/2)]^{th} \text{ value of } \hat{\theta}_{[i]}$$

where the k bootstrap estimates are ordered from low to high. It is assumed that $k(\alpha/2)$ and $k(1 - \alpha/2)$ are integers which is generally the case since k is typically a large integer value. Confidence limits can also be estimated with the S-function *quantile(bootstrap.estimates, $c(\alpha/2, 1 - \alpha/2)$)*. Exploration of the properties of the bootstrap confidence interval suggests that a sample of 200 replicates ($k = 200$) produces reasonably accurate confidence limits for many situations [2]. However, most computer systems operate at speeds that make bootstrap estimates based on thousands of replicates possible. More sophisticated and more accurate methods to create confidence intervals are available [2] but not presented here.

Continuing the harmonic mean example,

```
> quantile(boot)
     0%       25%       50%       75%  100%
  20.01 30.10147 34.32056 38.11902 50.67
> quantile(boot,c(0.025,0.975))
     2.5%      97.5%
  24.38666 45.64935.
```

The estimated 95% confidence interval based on 2000 bootstrap replicates is (24.387, 45.649).

AN EXAMPLE—RELATIVE RISK

A confidence interval created from the quantiles of the bootstrap distribution estimates is not necessarily symmetric about the estimated value. When sampled values come from an asymmetric parent distribution, a bootstrap confidence interval usually reflects the asymmetry in the confidence limits. An approximate procedure based on the symmetric normal distribution would be expected to work less well under these circumstances.

Relative risk is a common epidemiologic summary measure of disease risk and has an asymmetric distribution. The $P(disease \mid risk\ factor\ present)$ is contrasted to $P(disease \mid risk\ factor\ absent)$ where the relative risk is defined as the ratio of these two probabilities. Table 5.1 shows the number of coronary events (CHD) among type-A and type-B individuals for a sample of 3154 men observed for about eight years [5].

Relative risk of a coronary disease event is defined as

$$relative\ risk = rr = \frac{P(chd \mid type - A)}{P(chd \mid type - B)}$$

and directly estimated by

$$\hat{rr} = \frac{178/1589}{79/1565} = 2.219.$$

It is somewhat difficult to estimate the standard error associated with this estimate. However, theoretical considerations lead to a normal distribution based approximate confidence interval [6]. For the coronary heart disease data in Table 5.1, such an approximation yields a 95% confidence interval based on $\hat{rr} = 2.219$ of (1.704, 2.890). The bootstrap estimate and its standard error follow the same pattern as the bootstrap estimation of the mean and readily produce a confidence interval without statistical theory or assumptions about the properties of the sampled population:

```
> # bootstrap estimates and standard error for relative risk
> a<- 178
> b<- 79
> na<- 1589
> nb<- 1565
> # x = type-A, y = type-B, 0 = no chd and 1 = chd
> x<- c(rep(1,a),rep(0,na-a))
```

Table 5.1. Counts of coronary events for type-A and type-B individuals

	CHD	no CHD	total
type-A	178	1411	1589
type-B	79	1486	1565

```
> y<- c(rep(1,b),rep(0,nb-b))
> iter<- 2000
> rr<- NULL
> for(i in 1:iter) {
  tempx<- x[ceiling(na*runif(na))]
  tempy<- y[ceiling(nb*runif(nb))]
  rr[i]<- (sum(tempx)/na)/(sum(tempy)/nb)
 }
> mean(rr)
[1] 2.22345
> # 95% confidence intervals
> quantile(rr,c(0.025,0.975))
     2.5%      97.5%
 1.757939   2.877773.
```

The 95% confidence bounds derived from 2000 bootstrap replicates are 1.758 and 2.878. The lower bound of the normal-based confidence limits is a bit smaller (1.704). This difference is partially due to the asymmetry in the distribution of estimated relative risk $\hat{r}r$ which is less accurately reflected by an approximation based on the symmetric normal distribution.

MEDIAN

A median (50th percentile) and associated standard error estimated from $n = 25$ random observations from a standard normal population and the corresponding median bootstrap estimates are given by

```
> # parametric estimate
> n<- 25
> x<- rnorm(n)
> median(x)
[1] -0.099666187
> # estimated variance
> sqrt(1.571/n)
[1] 0.2506628
> # bootstrap estimate
> iter<- 5000
> d<- matrix(sample(x,n*iter,replace=T),n,iter)
> xx<- apply(d,2,median)
> cat("median = ",round(mean(xx),4),"standard error = ",
    round(sqrt(var(xx)),4),"\n")
> median =   -0.3882 standard error =   0.1786.
```

The approximate value for the standard error of the estimated median derived from theoretical considerations is $\hat{s}e = \sqrt{1.571/n}$ when a sample of n independent observations is selected from a standard normal distribution [1].

The bootstrap estimated median and standard error substantially differ from the parametric estimates (median: -0.388 versus -0.010 and standard error: 0.179 versus 0.251). The primary reason for the difference lies in the fact that the bootstrap estimated distribution is not "smooth." A distribution is "smooth" when small changes in the bootstrap replicates cause small

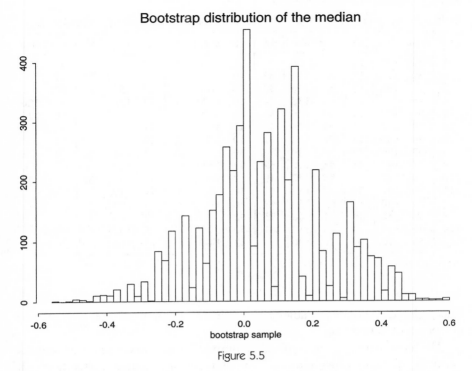

Figure 5.5

changes in the estimated value. The bootstrap process works most reliably when the distribution of $\hat{\theta}_{[i]}$-values is "smooth." This is not the case for the bootstrap estimated median. Many median estimates based on bootstrap replicates are the same estimated value. Different sampled replicates do not smoothly change estimates of the median. A plot (Figure 5.5) of 5000 estimates $\hat{\theta}_{[i]}$ (bootstrap medians) show that the bootstrap replicates produce only a few distinct values. This lack of "smoothness" means that the bootstrap estimates do not accurately reflect the distribution of the estimated median values and, therefore, do not provide accurate estimates of the median, standard error, or confidence limits.

SIMPLE LINEAR REGRESSION

A slightly more complicated application of the bootstrap method involves the estimation of the parameters of a simple linear regression model. A simple linear regression model is

$$y_i = a + bx_i + e_i$$

Table 5.2. Age and systolic blood pressure levels for 80 individuals; men aged 39–59

id	age	sbp	id	age	sbp	id	age	sbp	id	age	sbp	id	age	sbp
1	54	122	16	57	128	31	52	128	56	47	146	71	49	130
2	40	110	17	55	110	32	49	130	57	39	130	72	41	164
3	49	138	18	56	156	33	40	130	58	58	152	73	52	112
4	48	136	19	43	138	34	39	124	59	59	116	74	47	126
5	51	190	20	52	126	35	40	112	60	39	140	75	56	142
6	59	168	21	59	128	36	41	160	61	48	146	76	53	130
7	50	138	22	58	124	37	40	130	62	49	142	77	52	120
8	53	170	23	55	140	38	39	110	63	54	144	78	49	126
9	57	142	24	45	110	39	43	154	64	40	130	79	48	170
10	50	128	25	55	152	40	52	130	65	58	148	80	44	104
11	56	142	26	47	112	41	40	120	66	53	140			
12	56	140	27	43	130	42	56	190	67	55	200			
13	58	138	28	51	168	43	42	124	68	49	146			
14	59	138	29	49	112	44	50	156	69	51	132			
15	56	170	30	46	120	45	43	144	70	53	110			

where the dependent variable y_i is a linear function of the level of the independent variable x_i.

The error terms e_i are typically assumed to be uncorrelated as well as normally distributed with mean = 0 and constant variance (Chapter 4). Systolic blood pressure measurements and the corresponding reported ages of $n = 80$ middle-aged men (39–59 years old) are used to illustrate (Table 5.2). The least squares estimated line $(abline(lsfit(age, sbp)\$coef)$ S-command) and the data are displayed in Figure 5.6. The estimated intercept $\hat{a} = 94.195$ and the estimated regression coefficient $\hat{b} = 0.868$ produce the estimated line

$$\hat{y}_i = \hat{a} + \hat{b}x_i = 94.195 + 0.868x_i$$

where $x = age$ = the independent variable and $y = systolic\ blood\ pressure = sbp$ = dependent variable.

The bootstrap estimates of linear regression parameters a and b as well as the level of blood pressure at age 50 are achieved with the example S-code:

```
> n<- length(age)
> iter<- 2000
> age0<- 50
> est1<- NULL
> est2<- NULL
> est3<- NULL
> for(i in 1:iter) {
  v<- ceiling(n*runif(n))
  xtemp<- age[v]
  ytemp<- sbp[v]
  b<- lsfit(xtemp,ytemp)$coef
```

Blood pressure by age -- regression line

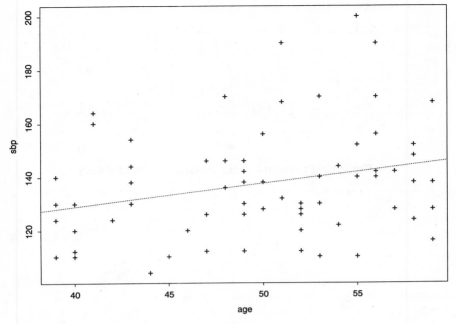

Figure 5.6

```
      est1[i]<- b[1]
      est2[i]<- b[2]
      est3[i]<- b[1]+b[2]*age0
      }
  > se1<- sqrt(var(est1))
  > cat("intercept =",round(mean(est1),3)," se1 = ",
        round(se1,3),"\n")
  > intercept = 93.726    se1 =   17.136
  > se2<- sqrt(var(est2))
  > cat("slope =",round(mean(est2),3)," se2 = ",
        round(se2,3),"\n")
  > slope = 0.878    se2 =   0.354
  > se3<- sqrt(var(est3))
  > cat("y=sbp at age 50 =",round(mean(est3),3)," se3 = ",
        round(se3,3),"\n")
  > y=sbp at age 50 = 137.602    se3 =   2.320.
```

The bootstrap procedure produces an estimated intercept, an estimated slope, and an estimated level of the systolic blood pressure for individuals 50 years old (*est1*: $\hat{a}_{[.]} = 93.726$, *est2*: $\hat{b}_{[.]} = 0.878$, and *est3*: $\hat{y}'_{[.]} = 137.602$).

The bootstrap estimated regression coefficient $\hat{b}_{[.]} = 0.878$, closely corresponds to the least squares estimate $\hat{b} = 0.868$. Both estimation procedures produce estimated standard errors that differ slightly (the bootstrap estimate is $\hat{se}_{[.]} = 0.354$ and least squares estimate is $\hat{se} = 0.379$). Figure 5.7 compares the

Estimate regression coefficient -- bootstrap sample

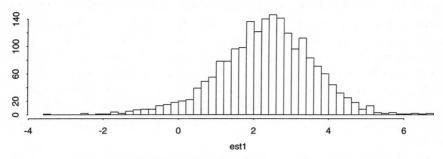

Estimated regression coefficient -- normal theory

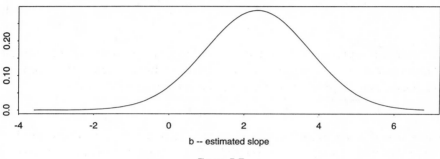

Figure 5.7

distribution of the bootstrap estimated values $\hat{b}_{[i]}$ to the theoretical distribution expected when the assumptions underlying the linear regression model hold over the range of x (independence, constant variance and normally distributed y-values—Chapter 4).

The close correspondence between estimates $\hat{b}$ and $\hat{b}_{[.]}$ can be viewed as evidence for either of two more or less equivalent points of view. The bootstrap estimates accurately reflect the distribution of the ordinary least squares estimated value. Or, the least squares estimation is insensitive to deviations from the postulated model and usually produces estimated regression coefficients with approximately normal distributions.

The estimated intercepts from both approaches are also similar (least squares: $\hat{a} = 94.195$ and bootstrap: $\hat{a}_{[.]} = 93.726$). The estimated blood pressure for individuals 50 years old is $\hat{y}'_{[.]} = 137.602$ from the bootstrap replicates with a standard error of $s\hat{e}_{[.]} = 2.320$. The least squares estimate is 137.595 ($\hat{y}_{50} = 94.195 + 0.868(50) = 137.595$) and the estimated standard error calculated from an explicit formula [7] is $\hat{se} = 2.369$.

A basic difference exists between the least squares and bootstrap approaches (at least on the conceptual level). The properties of the least squares estimator are conditional on the observed values of the independent variable x. The independent variables (e.g., *age*) are considered fixed. Treating the independent variable as fixed is not the most realistic assumption in many situations. Bootstrap replicates consist of randomly selected pairs; no assumption is made about the independent variable except that pairs of observations are independently sampled. However, as illustrated, the results of the two analytic approaches are not very different. This lack of difference is generally observed.

A different approach to estimating the regression coefficient and its standard error demonstrates the flexibility of the bootstrap estimation process. Rearranging the simple linear regression model yields

$$e_i = y_i - (a + bx_i) \qquad i = 1, 2, 3, \cdots, n.$$

The values e_i represent the influence of random variation associated with the ith observation. A bootstrap sample can be created by resampling the estimated e_i-values. Each observation x_i generates an estimated residual value

$$\hat{e}_i = y_i - (\hat{a} + \hat{b}x_i)$$

where $\hat{a}$ and $\hat{b}$ are based on the n original sampled values. These residual values are then sampled with replacement creating bootstrap replicates of the dependent variable. In symbols, a series of the n bootstrap residuals $\hat{e}_{[i]}$ produces a series of n bootstrap y-values $\hat{y}_{[i]}$ or

$$\hat{y}_{[i]} = (\hat{a} + \hat{b}x_i) + \hat{e}_{[i]}.$$

In turn, the bootstrap "data" generate a series of estimated parameters $a_{[i]}$ and $b_{[i]}$. As before, the bootstrap estimates $\hat{a}_{[.]}$ and $\hat{b}_{[.]}$ are the means of these estimates but, more importantly, the process produces an estimate of the variability associated with each of these estimates.

Estimation of the distribution of the estimated regression parameters from the age/blood pressure data based on "bootstrapping the residuals" follows:

```
> # estimation of the residuals
> otemp<- glm(sbp~age)
> b<- otemp$coefficients
> e<- sbp-(b[1]+b[2]*age)
> # bootstrap estimates of the slope
> iter<- 2000
> bb<- NULL
> for(i in 1:iter) {
  v<- ceiling(n*runif(n))
  yy<- b[1]+b[2]*age+e[v]
  bb[i]<- lsfit(age,yy)$coef[2]
  }
```

```
> mean(bb)
[1] 0.8810882
> sqrt(var(bb))
[1] 0.4064512.
```

The estimate of the regression coefficient based on the bootstrap residuals is $\hat{b}'_{[.]} = 0.881$. Comparison of the two kinds of bootstrap estimates ($\hat{b}'_{[.]}$ and $\hat{b}_{[.]}$) shows little difference (0.881 versus 0.878). The standard errors are also similar (0.406 and 0.354). The bootstrap estimate based on pairs is generally less sensitive to the assumptions underlying the typical linear regression model when compared to the resampling of the residual values. Perhaps the important point is that the bootstrap approach is not a uniquely defined method that can be applied unequivocally.

Both pair sampling and residual sampling approaches can be used with minor modifications to estimate and assess estimates from a regression model with more than one independent variable. To illustrate bootstrap estimation in a multivariable situation, the following describes estimation of the squared multiple correlation coefficient (R^2) and its standard error from a multivariable linear regression analysis. The squared multiple correlation coefficient can be estimated and evaluated, as described (Chapter 4), under the assumptions of a linear regression model (linearity, independence, normality, and constant variance). To statistically assess the least squares estimate, the value R^2 is transformed to have an F-distribution. Under the null hypothesis that the dependent variable is entirely unrelated to the independent variables (expected $R^2 = 0$?), the estimated value R^2 is evaluated using an F-test [8] (from the S-function $lm(\ )$, the test labeled "F-statistic:"—see page 205). However, the null hypothesis that all measured independent variables are unrelated to the dependent variable is rarely of much interest. It is more to the point to estimate the standard error of R^2 and construct a confidence interval to describe the impact of random variation on this estimate. A bootstrap procedure produces estimates of both quantities. Consider once again the data on birth weight and measurements of maternal height, prepregnancy weight, and weight gained during pregnancy from Table 4.2, then

```
> # bootstrap estimate and 95% confidence interval for R^2
> # read data from exterior file bwt.data
> dframe<- read.table("bwt.data",header=T)
> attach(dframe)
> x<- cbind(ht,wt,gain)
> y<- bwt
> otemp<- glm(y~x,family=gaussian)
> r2<- cor(predict(otemp),y)^2
> cat("squared multiple correlation coefficient =",
      round(r2,4),"\n")
squared multiple correlation coefficient = 0.1838
> # bootstrap estimation
> iter<- 1000
> r<- NULL
```

```
> for (i in 1:iter){
v<- ceiling(nrow(x)*runif(nrow(x)))
xtemp<- x[v,]
ytemp<- y[v]
otemp<- glm(ytemp~xtemp,family=gaussian)
r[i]<- cor(predict(otemp),ytemp)^2
}
> rbar<- mean(r)
> se<- sqrt(var(r))
> cat(" bootstrap R-squared = ",round(rbar,4)," se = ",
    round(se,4),"\n")
 bootstrap R-squared =  0.1863   se =  0.0224
> # quantile: 95% limits
> round(quantile(r,c(0.025,0.975)),4)
   2.5%  97.5%
 0.1436 0.2301
> #normal based 95% confidence limits
> lower<- rbar-1.96*se
> upper<- rbar+1.96*se
> cat("lower = ",round(lower,4)," upper = ",
    round(upper,4),"\n")
lower =  0.1424    upper =  0.2301.
```

Sampling with replacement from the vector of dependent observations y and the corresponding independent observations from array x to form bootstrap replicates (labeled in the S-code as *ytemp* and *xtemp*) produces a bootstrap estimate of the distribution of the squared multiple correlation coefficient. Using these estimates, the bootstrap estimated value is $R^2_{[\cdot]} = 0.186$ with a standard error of 0.022. The estimated 95% confidence limits are *lower* = 0.144 and *upper* = 0.230. The 95% confidence limits based on using a normal distribution as an approximation to the bootstrap distribution of R^2 are almost identical (0.142 and 0.230).

JACKKNIFE ESTIMATION

Another computer-intensive resampling strategy, much like the bootstrap approach, is called jackknife estimation. The term "jackknife" is used because the estimation process applies to a large number of situations (it is handy, like a jackknife).

A jackknife replicate is created by deleting one observation from a sample of n observations producing a truncated sample of $n - 1$ values. There are n possible different jackknife replicates, each denoted $\mathbf{x}_{(i)}$, where the ith observation is deleted (i.e., $\mathbf{x}_{(i)} = \{x_1, x_2, \cdots, x_{i-1}, x_{i+1}, \cdots, x_n\}$). If five original observations are represented by $\{x_1, x_2, x_3, x_4, x_5\}$, then

$$\mathbf{x}_{(1)} = \{x_2, x_3, x_4, x_5\}$$
$$\mathbf{x}_{(2)} = \{x_1, x_3, x_4, x_5\}$$
$$\mathbf{x}_{(3)} = \{x_1, x_2, x_4, x_5\}$$
$$\mathbf{x}_{(4)} = \{x_1, x_2, x_3, x_5\}$$
$$\mathbf{x}_{(5)} = \{x_1, x_2, x_3, x_4\}$$

is the complete set of jackknife replicates (*n* observations produce *n* replicates). When an estimator $\hat{\theta} = s(\mathbf{x})$ is considered, then *n* jackknife estimates $\hat{\theta}_{(i)} = s(\mathbf{x}_{(i)})$ are created and averaged to estimate θ or, like the bootstrap estimator,

$$\hat{\theta}_{(.)} = \frac{1}{n} \sum \hat{\theta}_{(i)}$$

and the estimated standard error is

$$\hat{se}_{(.)} = \sqrt{\frac{n-1}{n} \sum (\hat{\theta}_{(i)} - \hat{\theta}_{(.)})^2} \qquad i = 1, 2, 3, \cdots, n.$$

The specially designed S-function *jack( )* produces an array containing the *n* jackknife replicates from a sample of *n* observations. The *n* columns are different jackknife replicates and

```
> # input data contained in x0
> jack<- function(x0,n) {
 x<- matrix(rep(x0,length(x0)),n,n)
 matrix(x[row(x)!=col(x)],n-1,n)
}
```

The syntax *row(x) != col(x)* is an S-logical statement producing true (T) when the row and column indexes of array *x* are not equal and false (F) otherwise. A few other examples are

```
> # test array = a
> a<- matrix(16:1,4,4)
> a
      [,1] [,2] [,3] [,4]
 [1,]  16   12    8    4
 [2,]  15   11    7    3
 [3,]  14   10    6    2
 [4,]  13    9    5    1
> row(a)==col(a) # diagonal elements
      [,1] [,2] [,3] [,4]
 [1,]    T    F    F    F
 [2,]    F    T    F    F
 [3,]    F    F    T    F
 [4,]    F    F    F    T
> a[row(a)==col(a)]
[1] 16 11  6  1
> row(a)!=col(a) # off-diagonal elements
      [,1] [,2] [,3] [,4]
 [1,]    F    T    T    T
 [2,]    T    F    T    T
 [3,]    T    T    F    T
 [4,]    T    T    T    F
> a[row(a)!=col(a)]
[1] 15 14 13 12 10  9  8  7  5  4  3  2
> row(a)>col(a) # lower triangle elements
      [,1] [,2] [,3] [,4]
 [1,]    F    F    F    F
 [2,]    T    F    F    F
 [3,]    T    T    F    F
 [4,]    T    T    T    F
```

```
> a[row(a)>col(a)]
[1]  15  14  13  10   9   5.
```

To illustrate, the jackknife estimated mean and variance are calculated from a sample of 10 observations from a normal distribution with mean = 4 and variance = 4 where

```
> n<- 10
> x0<- rnorm(n,4,2)
> jdata<- jack(x0,n)
> round(x0,2)
[1]  10.02  1.71  4.42  3.78  3.38  2.66  1.57  1.02  6.91  2.25
> round(jdata,2)
        [,1]   [,2]   [,3]   [,4]   [,5]   [,6]   [,7]   [,8]   [,9]  [,10]
[1,]    1.71  10.02  10.02  10.02  10.02  10.02  10.02  10.02  10.02  10.02
[2,]    4.42   4.42   1.71   1.71   1.71   1.71   1.71   1.71   1.71   1.71
[3,]    3.78   3.78   3.78   4.42   4.42   4.42   4.42   4.42   4.42   4.42
[4,]    3.38   3.38   3.38   3.38   3.78   3.78   3.78   3.78   3.78   3.78
[5,]    2.66   2.66   2.66   2.66   2.66   3.38   3.38   3.38   3.38   3.38
[6,]    1.57   1.57   1.57   1.57   1.57   1.57   2.66   2.66   2.66   2.66
[7,]    1.02   1.02   1.02   1.02   1.02   1.02   1.02   1.57   1.57   1.57
[8,]    6.91   6.91   6.91   6.91   6.91   6.91   6.91   6.91   1.02   1.02
[9,]    2.25   2.25   2.25   2.25   2.25   2.25   2.25   2.25   2.25   6.91

> jmean<- apply(jdata,2,mean)
> cat("mean(jack)=",round(mean(jmean),3),
    "mean =",round(mean(x0),3),"\n")
 mean(jack)= 3.77 mean = 3.77
> cat("var  =",round(sqrt(sum((n-1)*(jmean-mean(jmean))^2)/n),3),
     "var =",round(sqrt(var(x0)/n),3),"\n")
 var = 0.88 var = 0.88.
```

The illustrative data show that the jackknife mean and variance estimates are identical to the usual estimates of the mean and variance from a normal distribution, which is true in general.

The jackknife and bootstrap estimators likely produce similar estimates when the estimator $s(\mathbf{x})$ is simple (simple is defined rigorously in [2]). For nonlinear or complicated estimates, however, the jackknife procedure becomes less efficient. Like the bootstrap estimation process, the jackknife estimate breaks down in attempts to estimate an "unsmooth" statistical summary, such as the median or range.

Jackknife estimates require an inflation factor to approximate the distribution of the estimator $\hat{\theta}$. The nature of the jackknife process yields jackknife replicates that are not much different from the original data. This "closeness" underestimates the distribution of the estimator $\hat{\theta}$ because $n - 1$ of the jackknife sampled observations are identical to $n - 1$ of the original observations. The quantities $(n - 1)[\hat{\theta}_{(i)} - \hat{\theta}_{(.)}]$ estimate the distribution of the sample estimator $\hat{\theta}$ in a way similar to the bootstrap estimates $[\hat{\theta}_{[i]} - \hat{\theta}_{[.]}]$.

BIAS ESTIMATION

Both the bootstrap and jackknife estimators provide an estimate of any bias associated with the estimator $\hat{\theta}$. The quantities

$$bias(bootstrap) = \hat{\theta}_{[.]} - \hat{\theta} \quad and \quad bias(jackknife) = (n-1)[\hat{\theta}_{(.)} - \hat{\theta}]$$

estimate the bias present in the estimator $\hat{\theta}$. If, for example, $\hat{\theta}_{(.)} - \hat{\theta} = 0$, then the estimator $\hat{\theta}$ is unbiased. The sample mean ($\hat{\theta} = \bar{x}$) and the jackknife estimated sample mean ($\hat{\theta}_{(.)} = \bar{x}$) are identical, verifying that the sample mean is an unbiased estimator of the population mean. The bootstrap and jackknife estimates of bias generally produce similar values since the jackknife bias estimator is approximately a special case of the bootstrap bias estimator.

The logic behind resampling estimators of bias is that the sample estimate $\hat{\theta}$ is in a sense the "population parameter." The resampling creates a series of estimates from a "population" with a known value of θ, namely $\hat{\theta}$. Therefore, the deviations from $\hat{\theta}$ of the resampling estimator ($\hat{\theta}_{[.]}$ or $\hat{\theta}_{(.)}$) measure bias. However, these bias estimates frequently have large standard errors. The potentially high variability suggests that interpretation of these estimates of bias should be tempered with the knowledge that they are possibly unstable. For example, using the estimated bias to correct an estimated value may not be worthwhile (even misleading) unless the precision of the estimated bias is high.

Estimation of the standard deviation based on values sampled from a standard normal distribution illustrates the estimation of bias. The following example S-code produces 2000 bootstrap replicate estimates of the standard deviation based on $n = 10$ sampled observations and computes the bias:

```
> sd<- function(x){sqrt(var(x))}
> n<- 10
> x<- rnorm(n)
> iter<- 2000
> temp<- matrix(sample(x,n*iter,replace=T),n,iter)
> sx<- apply(temp,2,sd)
> # bias estimate
> sd(x)-mean(sx)
[1] 0.0717223.
```

The estimate of the standard deviation is, as usual,

$$\hat{\theta} = \hat{s}d = \sqrt{\frac{\sum(x_i - \bar{x})^2}{n-1}} \quad i = 1, 2, 3, \cdots, n$$

and is computed with the S-function $sd(\ )$. Comparing the bootstrap estimate $\hat{s}d_{[.]}$ with the estimated standard deviation $\hat{s}d$ based on the original sample of $n = 10$ observations yields an estimated bias of 0.072. Rather complex theoretical considerations [9] produce a parametric estimated bias of

0.077. Clearly, bootstrap/jackknife estimates of bias are most useful when theoretical or model-based values are not available.

TWO-SAMPLE TEST—BOOTSTRAP APPROACH

As might be expected, the distribution of the bootstrap estimates also provides an opportunity to evaluate specific hypotheses concerning the sampled population. Bootstrap replicates produce an estimate of the distribution of $\hat{\theta}$, making it possible to evaluate the likelihood that various postulated values of θ are consistent with the collected data. If a hypothesis generated value θ_0 is much greater or much less than the estimate $\hat{\theta}_{[.]}$, then θ_0 becomes suspect as a candidate for "explaining" important aspects of the data. In other words, if the bootstrap distribution indicates that θ_0 is an unlikely value in light of the observed data, then it is not a plausible choice for a parameter associated with the population sampled. The difference between $\hat{\theta}_{[.]}$ and θ_0 measured in standard deviations is

$$z = \frac{\hat{\theta}_{[.]} - \theta_0}{\hat{se}_{[.]}}$$

leading to an estimate of a "significance level" since z usually has an approximate standard normal distribution for moderately large sample sizes (e.g., $n > 30$ or so).

A two-sample "test" based on a bootstrap approach is yet another way to utilize bootstrap replicate estimates. The previous data comparing cholesterol levels between type-A and type-B individuals illustrate. From the data in Table 1.5, the mean difference in cholesterol levels is $\bar{d} = \bar{x} - \bar{y} = 34.750$ (x = type-A and y = type-B) based on $n_1 = n_2 = 20$ sampled individuals. A bootstrap estimate provides a comparison of these two groups without assumptions about the population sampled. Bootstrap replicates are created by sampling $n_1 = 20$ "observations" from the type-A group (x) and $n_2 = 20$ "observations" from the type-B group (y), again with replacement. A distribution of bootstrap-estimated mean differences,

$$\bar{d}_{[i]} = \bar{x}_{[i]} - \bar{y}_{[i]},$$

provides the basis for investigating questions about the relationship between behavior type and cholesterol levels.

A "test" of significance and a 95% level confidence interval for the mean difference in cholesterol levels generated from 2000 bootstrap replicates is

```
> # atype contains n1=20 observations for type-A individuals
> # btype contains n2=20 observations for type-B individuals
> iter<- 2000
```

```
> d<- NULL
> for (i in 1:iter) {
  xtemp<- sample(atype,n1,replace=T)
  ytemp<- sample(btype,n2,replace=T)
  d[i]<- mean(xtemp)-mean(ytemp)
  }
> dbar<- mean(d)
> se<- sqrt(var(d))
> # distance from 0 in standard deviations
> z<- dbar/se
> pvalue<- 2*(1-pnorm(abs(z)))
> cbind(dbar,se,z,pvalue)
         dbar         se        z         pvalue
[1,] 34.66565   14.56030  2.380833   0.008641462
> # 95% limits of mean cholesterol levels
> quantile(d,c(0.025,0.975))
    2.5%       97.5%
 8.64625    59.90125.
```

The bootstrap estimated mean $\bar{d}_{[.]} = 34.666$ hardly differs from $\bar{d} = 34.750$. From a testing point of view, interest might focus on the difference between $\bar{d}_{[.]}$ and $d_0 = 0$ (no difference in cholesterol levels). Measuring this difference in terms of standard deviations gives $z = 2.381$, making it unlikely (p-value = 0.009) that a value of zero would be the underlying parameter generating the observed difference in mean levels of cholesterol. The 95% confidence interval (8.646, 59.901) indicates a range of plausible values of the mean difference and $d_0 = 0$ is not within this range, again implying that the observed difference between the mean levels of cholesterol is not likely to be a random deviation from zero.

Parallel to the t-test, eight values of $\bar{d}_{[i]}$ out of the 2000 generated are less than zero giving an estimated "significance level" = 8/2000 = 0.004, which is similar to the previously calculated value 0.007 (generated from a t-distribution—Chapter 1) or

```
> p<- sum(ifelse(d<0.0,1,0))/iter
> # previous parametric t-value = 2.562
> pvalue<- 1-pt(2.562,38)
> cbind(p,pvalue)
        p        pvalue
[1] 0.004   0.007247993.
```

TWO-SAMPLE TEST—RANDOMIZATION APPROACH

A bootstrap two-sample "t-test" consists of resampling each of two samples producing an estimate of the distribution of the mean difference. A randomization test similarly produces a distribution of the mean difference but under the hypothesis that no difference exists between the two sampled populations. Instead of resampling each of the two samples, the randomization procedure requires the original samples to be combined. Once the samples are com-

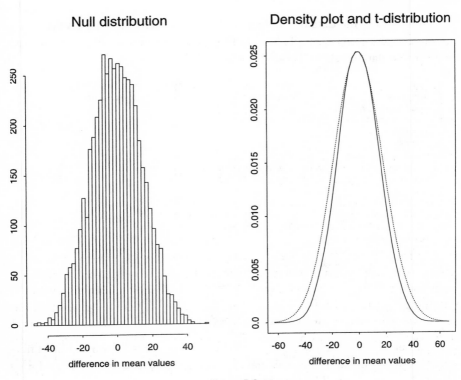

Figure 5.8

bined, a sample of n_1 observations is randomly selected, leaving n_2 observations (total sample size = $n = n_1 + n_2$), completely ignoring the binary classification variable. There are $\binom{n}{n_1}$ possible different resamples. When n is small, all possible selections are enumerated and when n is large, a sample of the possible selections is used. In both cases, the difference between the mean of the selected values (based on n_1 values) and the mean of the unselected values (based on n_2 values) is calculated. The difference between these two mean values is due strictly to random variation. Since each sample is selected at random, no reason exists for the mean of the selected values to differ from the mean of the unselected values, except chance variation. A series of these random differences produces a picture of the distribution of the mean differences when the hypothesis of "no difference" is true. Such a distribution is called the null distribution. Once sufficient numbers of random mean differences are calculated, it is possible to evaluate any particular difference in terms of this null distribution. Specifically, the likelihood associated with the original observed mean difference between the two samples is readily assessed.

To illustrate, the data on cholesterol levels and behavior type (A versus B) are once again used. Example S-code to produce a randomization test for the two-sample data given in Table 1.5 is

```
> # atype contains n1=20 observations for type-A individuals
> # btype contains n2=20 observations for type-B individuals
> d<- c(atype,btype)
> # randomization -- null distribution
> iter<- 5000
> difbar<- NULL
> for (i in 1:iter) {
   v<- sample(1:length(d),length(atype),replace=F)
   difbar[i]<- mean(d[v])-mean(d[-v])
   }
> quantile(difbar,seq(0,1,0.1))
     0%    10%    20%    30%    40%    50%  60%   70%
 -50.65 -19.05 -12.95  -8.05  -4.15  -0.25 3.55  7.45
    80%    90%   100%
  11.75  18.45  46.45
> dmean<- mean(atype)-mean(btype)
> p<- sum(ifelse(difbar>dmean,1,0))/iter
> cat("observed difference =",round(dmean,3),"\n",
    "p-value (randomization test) =",round(p,4),"\n")
 observed difference = 34.75
 p-value (randomization test) = 0.0068.
```

An estimated null distribution is created based on *iter* = 5000 random differences between mean values calculated from n_1 = 20 and n_2 = 20 randomly selected observations. The observed difference $\bar{d}_A - \bar{d}_B$ = 34.75 is not likely to have arisen by chance since only 34 null values among the 5000 random mean differences are greater than 34.75 yielding a "*p*-value" = 34/5000 = 0.0068. Once again a resampling approach produces a result similar to the formal *t*-test (*p*-value = 0.0072; one tail—Chapter 1). Figure 5.8 is a histogram of the 5000 generated mean differences and the corresponding smoothed estimated density function (solid line). Also included is the distribution of the *t*-statistic (dotted line) showing the close correspondence between a null distribution generated from a randomization procedure and a parametric null distribution generated by assuming that cholesterol levels among type A and type B individuals have the same mean and are normally distributed with equal variances.

Only a single example of a randomization test is presented as a contrast to the bootstrap approach. Alternative procedures based on randomization exist for most parametric-based statistical tests. Furthermore, it is usually relative simple to construct randomization tests for new situations not easily analyzed with available statistical tools. S-functions are particularly efficient in the context of resampling strategies. A complete description of other randomization strategies is found elsewhere [10].

Estimation : Least Squares

LEAST SQUARES PROPERTIES

Historically, one of the first rigorous methods used to estimate the parameters of an analytical model was the least squares approach. Least squares estimates are those parameter values that produce the smallest total squared distance between the observed data and model generated estimates. For n observations, the parameter estimates are chosen so that

$$Q = \sum (observation_i - model.value_i)^2 \qquad i = 1, 2, 3, \cdots, n$$

is minimum. Any other choice of the parameter estimates makes the least squares criterion Q larger. The resulting estimates, under certain conditions [1], are unbiased with minimum variance for all sample sizes. These conditions are generally fulfilled by a linear model making the least squares method the usual choice to estimate the model parameters.

A multivariable linear model, as before, is

$$y_i = a + b_1 x_{i1} + b_2 x_{i2} + b_3 x_{i3} + \cdots + b_k x_{ik} + e_i \qquad i = 1, 2, 3, \cdots, n$$

where n = the number of observations and k = the number of variables measured on each observation. In matrix notation, this model is expressed as

$$y = XB + e$$

where y represents a vector of n dependent observations, X represents an $n \times (k + 1)$ array of independent values, B represents a vector of $k + 1$ parameters (to be estimated), and e represents a vector of n error terms. The first column of the array X consists of ones and the next k columns consist of the observed values of the independent variables. The error terms are required to be uncorrelated with mean zero and constant variance (represented by σ^2). It is remarkable that least squares estimation places no restrictions on the x-values. The least squares criterion Q, in matrix notation, is expressed as

$$Q = (y - XB)'(y - XB)$$

for the linear model case. The Gauss–Markov theorem (named after the originators of the method) states that the least squares estimate of the vector of parameters B is given by

$$\hat{B} = (X'X)^{-1} X'y$$

as long as the inverse of $\mathbf{X'X}$ exists. The estimate $\hat{\mathbf{B}}$ makes Q as small as possible. In previously defined symbols, the estimate of the vector $\mathbf{B}$ is $\hat{\mathbf{B}} = \{\hat{a}, \hat{b}_1, \hat{b}_2, \cdots, \hat{b}_k\}$. Although the S-language contains several functions that directly execute a least squares analysis (e.g., *lsfit*( ), *glm*( ), and *lm*( ), primarily), the following explores in detail the underlying process that produces the estimates and the important analytic quantities.

Using the previous data on birth weight, maternal height, maternal weight, weight gained during pregnancy (Table 4.2), and the same linear model, the following S-code estimates the vector of parameters $\mathbf{B}$. In this case, $\mathbf{B} = \{a, b_1, b_2, b_3\}$ and

```
> # read array: bwt, height, weight and gain (columns)
> indata<- read.table("bwt.data",header=T)
> # changes data frame into a conventional n by k+1 matrix
> xtemp<- data.matrix(indata)
> n<- nrow(xtemp)
> k<- ncol(xtemp)-1
> x<- cbind(rep(1,n),xtemp[,-1])
> y<- xtemp[,1]
> # estimates the regression coefficients
> b<- solve(t(x)%*%x)%*%t(x)%*%y
> round(b,4)
>             [,1]
>           2.9155
>   ht     -0.0060
>   wt      0.0125
> gain      0.0428.
```

The data frame *indata* must be changed to a conventional S-array using the S-function *matrix.data<- data.matrix(frame.name)* so that matrix algebra methods can be applied.

An important part of the least squares estimation process is an estimate of the variability associated with y_i or, in other terms, an estimate of *variance*(e_i) $= \sigma^2$. An estimator of this variance is

$$S_{Y|\mathbf{x}}^2 = \frac{1}{n - (k + 1)} \sum (y_i - \hat{y}_i)^2$$

where $\hat{y}_i$ represents an estimated value of the dependent variable. Estimated values of the dependent variables $\hat{y}_i$ are, again in matrix notation, $\hat{\mathbf{Y}} = \hat{\mathbf{X}}\mathbf{B}$. The estimate of $S_{Y|\mathbf{x}}^2$ is then

```
> # calculation of the estimated values
> yhat<- x%*%b
> # calculation of the residual values
> res<- y-yhat
> quantile(res,c(0,0.25,0.5,0.75,1))
       0%         25%        50%        75%       100%
 -2.411053  -0.2569752  0.03002075  0.339125  1.479748
> ssr<- sum(res^2)
```

```
> s2<- ssr/(n-k-1)
> cat("\n","estimated variance of y =",round(s2,4),"\n")

estimated variance of y = 0.3339.
```

The estimate $S^2_{Y|x}$ is a key element in the estimation of the variability associated with each estimated regression coefficients $\hat{b}_j$. The Gauss–Markov theorem goes on state that the variances and covariances of the estimated parameters contained in $\hat{\mathbf{B}}$ are

$$variance\ of\ \hat{\mathbf{B}} = (\mathbf{X}'\mathbf{X})^{-1}\sigma^2$$

which are estimated by

$$variance(\hat{\mathbf{B}}) = (\mathbf{X}'\mathbf{X})^{-1}S^2_{Y|x}.$$

The estimated variance/covariance array associated with the regression coefficients from the birth weight data is

```
> # variance/covariance array associated with the estimates b
> v<- solve(t(x)%*%x)*s2
> round(v,8)
                   ht           wt         gain
      0.73527038 -0.00468563  0.00055134 -0.0000077
  ht -0.00468563  0.00003188 -0.00000782 -0.0000004
  wt  0.00055134 -0.00000782  0.00001227  0.0000001
gain -0.00007710 -0.00000392  0.00000056  0.0000044.
```

A summary of the fit of a linear model, as mentioned earlier, arises from comparing the observed values (y_i) with the model generated estimated values $(\hat{y}_i)$. The residual sum of squares (residual deviance) is a direct comparison of these two quantities where

$$residual\ sum\ of\ squares = \sum(y_i - \hat{y}_i)^2.$$

The total sum of squares (null deviance) is expressed as

$$total\ sum\ of\ squares = \sum(y_i - \bar{y})^2.$$

A fragment of S-code that produces these sums of squares is

```
> ssr<- sum(res^2)
> cat("residual sum of squares =",round(ssr,4),
    "degrees of freedom",n-k-1,"\n")
residual sum of squares = 76.1205 degrees of freedom 228

> ss0<- sum((y-mean(y))^2)
> cat("total sum of squares =",round(ss0,4),
    "degrees of freedom",n-1,"\n")
total sum of squares = 94.3886 degrees of freedom 231.
```

The difference is fundamental since, as noted, comparison of these two quantities measures the simultaneous influence of the k independent variables.

Up to this point no assumptions have been made nor are they required about the distributional form of the error terms. Least squares estimates are "best" (minimum Q) regardless of the distribution of the population sampled. However, to make inferences based on the estimated values it is usually assumed that the error terms are uncorrelated and sampled from normal distributions with the same variances. Based on these requirements, a formal test of the simultaneous influence of the three independent variables (expected $R^2 = 0$?) is

```
> df1<- n-k-1
> f<- ((ss0-ssr)/k)/(ssr/df1)
> pvalue<- 1-pf(f,k,df1)
> round(cbind(f,pvalue),k)
        f   pvalue
[1,] 18.239     0.
```

Another important summary of the effectiveness of the linear model is the squared multiple correlation coefficient and is calculated by

```
> # squared multiple correlations coefficient
> r2<- cor(yhat,y)^2
> cat("\n","squared multiple correlation coefficient =",
    round(r2,4),"\n")

 squared multiple correlation coefficient = 0.1935.
```

The individual "adjusted" impact of each independent variable can be assessed using the quantity

$$t\text{-}value = t_j = \frac{\hat{b}_j - b_j}{\sqrt{variance(\hat{b}_j)}}$$

since t_j has a Student's t-distribution distribution with $n - (k + 1)$ degrees of freedom when b_j represents the regression coefficient associated with the independent variable x_j. The estimate $variance(\hat{b}_j)$ comes from the diagonal elements of the estimated variance/covariance array. Results from the least squares estimation process can be summarized as a series of significance tests of the k regression coefficients under the hypothesis that $b_j = 0$ or

```
> sb<- sqrt(diag(v))
> tvalues<- b/sb
> pvalues<- 2*(1-pt(abs(tvalues),n-k-1))
> round(cbind(b,sb,tvalues,pvalues),4)
           b       sb   tvalues   pvalues
      2.9155   0.8575    3.4001    0.0008
ht   -0.0060   0.0056   -1.0698    0.2858
wt    0.0125   0.0035    3.5740    0.0004
gain  0.0428   0.0066    6.4760    0.0000.
```

Although least squares estimation is typically applied to estimate the elements of a linear model, least squares estimation and maximum likelihood estimation are related when the data are normally distributed. Inspection of the likelihood function associated with maximum likelihood estimation of the linear model parameters from normally distributed data shows that the least squares and maximum likelihood estimates of the regression coefficients are identical (maximizing the likelihood function L is the same as minimizing the least squares criterion Q).

NON-LINEAR LEAST SQUARES ESTIMATION

Models designed to reflect the influences of a series of independent variables on an observed outcome need not be restricted to linear relationships. Frequently non-linear expressions accurately summarize a relationship between dependent and independent variables. Least squares estimation is also useful in the non-linear case. The least squares estimates are again those parameter estimates that minimize the sum of the squared distances between the observed and model estimated values. Non-linear least squares estimates are achieved with the S-function *nls*( ) ("nls" for non-linear least squares). The process is implemented using an input formula, along much the same lines as the *glm*( ) function. The general form of the *nls*( )-function is

$$S.object <- nls(\sim formula, data.frame, start = list(<initial\ values>) \cdots) \ .$$

The option *data.frame* identifies the data to be used to calculate the least squares estimates of the parameters found in the expression given by the *~formula* option. Initial parameter values required to begin the iterative estimation process are communicated by a *list* option labeled *start*.

Table 5.3 contains the mean weight gained during pregnancy for the second and third trimesters by 13,202 women collected over the years 1980–1990.

To characterize the non-linear trend in maternal weight gain, the amount gained during pregnancy (y) for each week of pregnancy (x) is modeled by

$$weight\ gain = y_i = a \times b^{x_i} \qquad i = 1, 2, 3, \cdots, 28.$$

To estimate the parameters a and b, the S-function *nls*( ) is applied and

```
> # gdata = data frame with 28 pairs (x=weeks, y=gain)
> otemp<- nls(~y-a*b^x,gdata,start=list(a=3,b=1))
> summary(otemp)

Formula:  ~ y - a * b^x

Parameters:
     Value  Std. Error   t value
a 3.41719 0.029296100   116.643
b 1.03966 0.000278183  3737.340

Residual standard error: 0.107819 on 26 degrees of freedom

Correlation of Parameter Estimates:
         a
b -0.974.
```

Table 5.3. Mean weight gained (kilograms) during pregnancy (weeks) by 13,202 women, University of California Moffit Hospital, San Francisco (1980–1990)

week	gain	week	gain
13	5.67	27	9.89
14	5.80	28	10.32
15	6.18	29	10.84
16	6.20	30	10.93
17	6.61	31	11.32
18	6.80	32	11.62
19	7.25	33	12.28
20	7.51	34	12.75
21	7.74	35	13.33
22	7.97	36	13.86
23	8.37	37	14.48
24	8.80	38	14.89
25	9.05	39	15.64
26	9.32	40	16.23

The estimated model is then

$$weight\ gain = \hat{y}_i = 3.417 \times 1.040^{x_i}.$$

That is, the quantity $Q = \sum(y_i - \hat{y}_i)^2$ is minimized by the choices $\hat{a} = 3.417$ and $\hat{b} = 1.040$. A plot of the observed data (solid line) and the estimated curve (dotted line) is given in Figure 5.9.

Using a logarithmic transformation applied to this particular model yields alternative estimates of the parameters a and b. Taking the logarithm of the dependent variable linearizes the model so that

$$\log(weight\ gain) = \log(y_i) = \log(a) + \log(b)x_i = A + Bx_i.$$

Ordinary least squares estimation leads to estimates of the parameters A and B where

```
> b<- lsfit(x,log(y))$coef
> b
 Intercept          X
  1.225154 0.0390244
> exp(b)
 Intercept          X
    3.40469 1.039796.
```

An estimate of a is $\hat{a} = e^{\hat{A}} = e^{1.225} = 3.405$ and, similarly, an estimate of b is $\hat{b} = e^{\hat{B}} = e^{0.039} = 1.040$, which only slightly differ from the direct non-linear least squares estimates.

It is not always possible to transform a model to be a linear function of the dependent variable and use ordinary least squares estimation. Such a case arises when cancer mortality rates (dependent variable) are related to a work-

Maternal weight gain by weeks of gestation -- n = 13,202

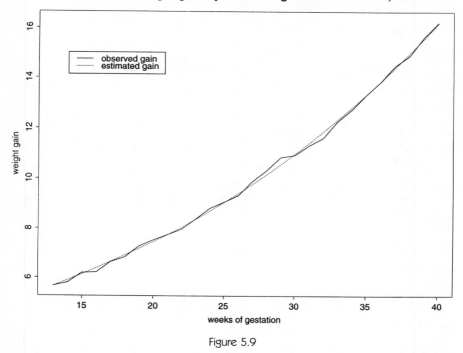

Figure 5.9

er's age and possibly related to cumulative exposure to ionizing radiation (independent variables) in a non-linear fashion. Data collected from workers at the Oak Ridge National Laboratory (1943–1972) allow exploration of the risk of radiation exposure (Table 5.4).

A nonlinear model relating age and exposure to the rate of cancer deaths is

$$rate_i = (1 + bx_i)e^{cy_i^2}$$

where x represents the level of lifetime radiation exposure measured in milliseiverts (mSv) and y represents the reported age at death. The cancer mortality rates among Oak Ridge workers in Table 5.4 are computed for each of the 56 exposure/age categories as

$$mortality\ rate = \frac{deaths}{person - years} \times 100,000.$$

To find the least squares estimates of the parameters b and c, the quantity

$$Q = \sum [rate_i - (1 + bx_i)e^{cy_i^2}]^2 \qquad i = 1, 2, 3, \cdots, 56$$

Table 5.4. Deaths, person-years and cancer mortality rates for workers at Oak Ridge National Laboratory (1943–1972) classified by exposure and age

mSv/age	<45	45–49	50–54	55–59	60–64	65–69	>69
mSv=0							
deaths	0	1	4	3	3	1	3
person-years	29901	6251	5251	4126	2778	1607	1358
rate/100,000	0.0	16.00	76.18	72.71	107.99	62.23	220.91
mSv=0–19							
deaths	1	5	4	10	11	16	11
person-years	71382	16705	13752	10439	7131	4133	3814
rate/100,000	1.40	29.93	20.09	95.79	154.26	387.13	288.41
mSv=20–39							
deaths	0	2	1	2	0	2	3
person-years	6523	2423	2281	1918	1322	723	538
rate/100,000	0.0	82.54	43.84	104.28	0.0	276.63	557.62
mSv=40–59							
deaths	0	0	1	1	0	2	3
person-years	2341	972	958	816	578	375	303
rate/100,000	0.0	0.0	104.28	122.25	0.0	533.33	990.10
mSv=60–79							
deaths	0	0	0	0	0	1	0
person-years	1363	478	476	387	225	164	150
rate/100,000	0.0	0.0	0.0	0.0	0.0	609.76	0.0
mSv=80–99							
deaths	0	0	0	1	0	0	0
person-years	779	296	282	251	193	125	69
rate/100,000	0.0	0.0	0.0	398.41	0.0	0.0	0.0
mSv=100–119							
deaths	0	0	0	0	1	0	1
person-years	520	188	217	184	109	60	23
rate/100,000	0.0	0.0	0.0	0.0	917.43	0.0	4347.83
mSv≥120							
deaths	0	0	1	3	1	2	2
person-years	2104	1027	1029	827	555	297	153
rate/100,000	0.0	0.0	97.18	362.76	180.18	673.40	1307.19

Note: mSv = milliseiverts (0.1 rem)—a measure of radiation exposure

is minimized. Analogous to the linear regression case, the values for b and c that make the sum of squares Q as small as possible are the least square estimates, denoted $\hat{b}$ and $\hat{c}$. The following reads a file containing the Oak Ridge data forming the data frame (*xdata*) necessary for the estimation process:

```
> # age, msv, deaths and pyears defined in the data file
> xdata<- read.table("ridge.data",header=T)
> rate<- deaths*100000/pyears
```

The data are now available to various S-functions where each of the 56 rows of the data frame *xdata* is a specific cell from Table 5.4 and the columns contain the variables age (years), exposure (mSv), deaths, and person-years. These data are identified in the exterior data file *ridge.data* by the first row which lists the variable names to be used in the S-analysis (*age, msv, deaths,* and *pyears*). The non-linear least squares estimates of the model parameters *b* and *c* from the cancer risk model using the Oak Ridge cancer data are:

```
> otemp<- nls(rate~(1+b*msv)*exp(c*age^2),xdata,
    start=list(b=0.01,c=0.005))
> summary(otemp)

Formula: rate ~ (1 + b * msv) * exp(c * age^2)

Parameters:
            Value        Std. Error       t value
b       0.03692890      0.040888700      0.903156
c       0.00113725      0.000178233      6.380680

Residual standard error: 504.272 on 54 degrees of freedom.
```

Alternatively, the "input" parametric model can be expressed as an S-function. Instead of describing the statistical model by means of the ~*formula* option in the *nls*( )-command, an S-function is called by *nls*( ) providing some flexibility in applying a nonlinear least squares analysis. For example,

```
> rvalues<- function(b,c,msv,age){rate-(1+b*msv)*exp(c*age^2)}
> otemp<- nls(~rvalues(b,c,msv,age),xdata,
    start=list(b=0.01,c=0.005))
```

gives the same results as putting the expression to be minimized directly into the *nls*( )-function.

The sum of squares Q is minimized but the minimum value may not be sufficiently small to produce satisfactory estimated values $\hat{y}_i$. It is prudent to assess the fit of the estimated model. The 56 estimated rates (*rate0*), based strictly on the model and the estimated parameters ($\hat{b}$ and $\hat{c}$) are given by

```
> f<- coef(otemp)
> rate0<- (1+f[1]*msv)*exp(f[2]*age^2)
> round(t(matrix(rate0,7,8)),2)
       [,1]   [,2]   [,3]    [,4]    [,5]    [,6]     [,7]
[1,]  10.00  13.01  22.98   42.95   84.98  177.96   263.09
[2,]  13.70  17.82  31.46   58.81  116.36  243.68   360.25
[3,]  21.09  27.43  48.43   90.53  179.12  375.13   554.57
[4,]  28.47  37.04  65.41  122.25  241.88  506.57   748.88
[5,]  35.86  46.65  82.38  153.97  304.64  638.01   943.20
[6,]  43.25  56.26  99.35  185.70  367.40  769.45  1137.52
[7,]  50.64  65.87 116.32  217.42  430.17  900.89  1331.83
[8,]  54.33  70.68 124.80  233.28  461.55  966.61  1428.99
> round(cor(rate0,rate),3)
[1] 0.608.
```

The correlation between the observed and estimated values begins to summarize the fit of the model. For the Oak Ridge data, the correlation between observed and estimated rates is 0.608.

A formal chi-square criterion reflects the agreement between the estimated and the observed numbers of deaths where

```
> ex<- pyears*rate0/100000
> x2<- sum((deaths-ex)^2/ex)
> pvalue<- 1-pchisq(x2,54)
> cbind(x2,pvalue)
           x2         pvalue
[1,] 53.16674    0.5065055
```

also shows a fair degree of correspondence between the model estimates and the observations.

The influences of the two independent variables on the rate of cancer mortality are graphically displayed by

```
> # a0 and m0 = xy-coordinates
> a0<- seq(min(age),max(age),1)
> m0<- seq(min(msv),max(msv),1)
> # surface height = z
> z<- outer(a0,m0,function(a0,m0){(1+f[1]*m0)*exp(f[2]*a0^2)})
> persp(a0,m0,z,xlab="age",ylab="mSv",zlab="rate",
    zlim=c(0,1500))
> title("Nonlinear fit -- Oak Ridge data")
```

Figure 5.10 displays the estimated relationship of age, exposure, and the rate of cancer. The cancer mortality rates are plotted on the vertical axis and the "floor" represents pairs of age and exposure values over their observed ranges. The plot indicates that the greatest impact of age and exposure, by far, is experienced by the older and highly exposed workers. Otherwise, the overall influence of radiation exposure appears minimal ($\hat{b} = 0.037$ and t-value = 0.903 yielding the p-value = 0.367 from the *summary(otemp)* S-function) after accounting for the influence of a worker's age.

Another S-function can be used to estimate the parameters of a nonlinear model. The function *ms( )* ("ms" for minimum sum) minimizes nonlinear functions in conjunction with a data frame. Applied to nonlinear least squares estimation, the results are essentially the same as those using *nls( )* but the S-function *ms( )* is useful in other contexts. The general form is

S.object<– ms(~formula, data.frame, start = list(<initial values>) ...).

The S-function *ms( )* produces parameter values that minimize the given *formula* starting with the initial values identified by the *list* option. Applied to the Oak Ridge data and the cancer risk model, the "minimum sum" approach yields

Nonlinear fit -- Oak Ridge data

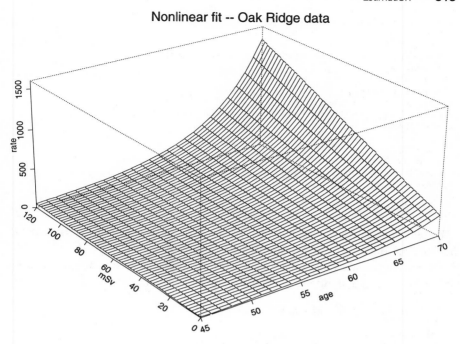

Figure 5.10

```
> otemp0<- ms(~(rate-(1+b*msv)*exp(c*age^2))^2,xdata,
    start=list(b=0.03,c=0.001))
> coef(otemp0)
        b            c
 0.0368943    0.001137397
```

which hardly differs from the nonlinear least squares estimates.

The *ms*( )-function calculates the values that minimize expressions other than the sums of squares associated with least squares estimation. For example, the *ms*( )-function can be used to find maximum likelihood estimates. Using the trivial fact that the values that maximize a function are also those values that minimize the negative of the function, parameters that maximize a likelihood function result from applying the *ms*( ) command.

For example, consider the exponential distribution. The following S-program produces 50 random exponential variables ($\lambda = 2$) and the maximum likelihood estimate of the parameter λ is $\hat{\lambda} = 1/\bar{x} = 1.948$. Using the S-function *ms*( ) also produces the maximum likelihood estimate. The log-likelihood expression is $log(L) = nlog(\lambda) - \lambda\sum x_i$ where $x_1, x_2, x_3, \cdots, x_n$ represent a sample of n independent observations from the same exponential distribution (parameter $= \lambda$). The "minimum sum" estimation of λ is

```
> # exponential distribution "data"
> n<- 50
> x<- rexp(n,2)
> # maximum likelihood estimate (closed-form)
> 1/mean(x)
[1] 1.947868
> # ms-estimation
> edata<- data.frame(x=x)
> temp<- ms(~(-n*log(u)+u*sum(x)),edata,start=list(u=2))
> coef(temp)
         u
 1.947868
> # equivalently, the sum is implicit
> temp<- ms((-log(u)+u*x),edata,start=list(u=2))
> coef(temp)
         u
 1.947868.
```

The simple data frame created with the command $data.frame(x = x)$ communicates the data vector x to the $ms( )$-function.

Consider another example where a random sample of $n = 50$ observations is selected from a standard normal distribution, then

```
> # standard normal distribution "data"
> n<- 50
> x<- rnorm(n)
> # maximum likelihood estimates closed-form
> mean(x)
[1] -0.3618082
> ((n-1)/n)*var(x)
[1] 0.8755047
> # ms-estimation
> ndata<- data.frame(x=x)
> temp<- ms(~(n*log(v)/2+sum(0.5*(x-m)^2/v)),ndata,
       start=list(m=0,v=1))
> coef(temp)
          m            v
 -0.3618082    0.8755046
> # equivalently, the sum is implicit
> temp<- ms(log(v)/2+0.5*(x-m)^2/v,ndata,
       start=list(m=0,v=1))
> coef(temp)
          m            v
 -0.3618082    0.8755046.
```

In certain situations sampled values fall below a limit of detection. The actual value of the observation cannot be determined because of limitations in the measurement method. All that is known is that the value is below a certain point (left censored). For example, when benzene exposure (ppm) samples collected from refinery workers are chemically analyzed, exposure levels below a certain point cannot be determined. Such a data set is contained in the S-vector x where

$$x = \{0.02, 0.18, 0.06, 0.09, 0.03, 0.04, 0.6, 0.04, 0.02, 0.04, 0.09, 0.10\}.$$

These 12 measured benzene values are above the limit of detection of $c = 0.015$ (ppm) and $k = 5$ observations were below this value (i.e., censored). The total sample consists of $n = 17$ observations of which $k = 5$ values are left censored (fall below 0.015). Furthermore, it is assumed that these data are a random sample from a normal distribution with mean μ and standard deviation σ. It is these parameters that are to be estimated. The likelihood function associated with a left censored (at point c_0) sample of n independent normally distributed observations is

$$likelihood = L = f(x_1|\mu, \sigma)f(x_2|\mu, \sigma)f(x_3|\mu, \sigma) \cdots f(x_{n-k}|\mu, \sigma) \times P^k$$

where

$$f(x_i|\mu, \sigma) = \frac{1}{\sigma\sqrt{2\pi}} e^{-\frac{1}{2}\left[\frac{x_i - \mu}{\sigma}\right]^2} \quad \text{and} \quad P = P(X \le c_0) = \frac{1}{\sqrt{2\pi}} \int_{-\infty}^{(c_0-\mu)/\sigma} e^{-\frac{1}{2}z^2} dz.$$

Observations are measured if they exceed c_0 and are simply counted if they fall below c_0. The value represented by P is the probability an observation falls below the limit of detection (i.e., less then c_0—censored). The log-likelihood function follows directly as

$$log\text{-}likelihood = \log(L) = -(n - k) \log(\sigma) - \frac{1}{2\sigma^2} \sum (x_i - \mu)^2 + k \log(P)$$
$$i = 1, 2, 3, \cdots, n - k.$$

Since the terms not involving the parameters μ and σ do not influence the estimation process, they are, as before, ignored in the likelihood function. S-code that calculates this log-likelihood value is

```
> clike<- function(x,n,k,c0,m,s){
    z<- (c0-m)/s
    -(n-k)*log(s)-0.5*sum(((x-m)/s)^2)+k*log(pnorm(z))
  }
```

where $x =$ vector of $n - k$ observations, $k =$ number of censored observations (below the point denoted c_0). The symbols $m =$ mean and $s =$ standard deviation represent the parameters describing the sampled normal population. The maximum likelihood estimates of the mean μ and the standard deviation σ (S-symbols m and s) can be found using the S-function $ms(\ )$. The S-function $clike(\ )$ is the log-likelihood function and since $ms(\ )$ finds the minimum of a function and not the maximum, $-clike(\ )$ is used. The estimated values that result from applying the $ms(\ )$-function are contained in the vector $S.object\$parameters$. Example S-code to find the maximum likelihood estimates of the mean and standard deviation from the left censored benzene data is

```
> # data
> x<- c(0.02,0.18,0.06,0.09,0.03,0.04,0.6,0.04,0.02,
    0.04,0.09,0.10)
> # number of censored values
> k<- 5
> n<- k+length(x)
> # limit of detection
> c0<- 0.015
> cat("xbar =",round(mean(x),4),"estimated variance =",
    round(var(x),4),"\n")
  xbar = 0.1092 estimated variance = 0.026
> #maximum likelihood estimation
> xin<- data.frame(x=x)
> est<- ms(-clike(x,n,k,c0,m,s),list(m=mean(x),
    s=sqrt(var(x))),data=xin)
> cat("estimated mean =",round(est$parameters[1],4),"\n",
    "estimated standard deviation =",
    round(est$parameters[2],4),"\n")

  estimated mean = 0.0438
  estimated standard deviation = 0.1731.
```

As in previous applications, the option *list* contains the initial values to start the iterative estimation process. The biased mean and standard deviation based on the $n - k$ measured observations serve as initial values and typically produce values sufficiently close to the mean and standard deviation of the sampled (uncensored) distribution ($k \ll n$) to allow the process to converge to the maximum likelihood estimates. The mean and standard deviation based on the 12 measured values are $\bar{x} = 0.109$ (biased; too large) and $S = 0.026$ (biased; too small). The maximum likelihood estimates $\hat{\mu} = 0.044$ and $\hat{\sigma} = 0.173$ are free of bias from the censoring.

The ms( )-function can be applied to estimate the parameters of multi-parameter models. To illustrate, the parameters from the logistic model describing the influence of gender and coffee consumption on case (pancreatic cancer) and control status are again estimated. The data are given in Table 4.7 (n_i = number of case/control observations with r_i cases in each of eight coffee consumption/gender categories) and the associated likelihood function is

$$L = \prod \binom{n_i}{r_i} p_i^{r_i} (1 - p_i)^{n_i - r_i}$$

and becomes

$$\log(L) = -\left\{\sum (n_i - r_i)(a + b_1 x_{i1} + b_2 x_{i2}) + \sum n_i \log[1 + e^{-(a+b_1 x_{i1}+b_2 x_{i2})}]\right\}$$

when

$$p_i = \frac{1}{1 + e^{-(a+b_1 x_{i1}+b_2 x_{i2})}} \qquad i = 1, 2, 3, \cdots, 8.$$

The value p_i represents the logistic probability of case status in the ith coffee consumption/gender category. The values which produce the minimum of the negative log-likelihood function are the maximum likelihood estimates of the three model parameters a, b_1, and b_2. The same estimates were produced by the *glm*-function (Chapter 4). Terms not involving the logistic model parameters are not included in log-likelihood expressions since, as before, they have no influence on the maximum likelihood estimates. Example S-code to implement the *ms*( )-function estimates is

```
> # coffee consumption data
> n<- c(41,213,127,142,67,211,133,76)
> r<- c(9,94,53,60,11,59,53,28)
> # S-likelihood function
> like<- function(n,r,a,b1,b2){
    x1<- c(0,2,4,5,0,2,4,5)
    x2<- c(1,1,1,1,0,0,0,0)
    q<- a+b1*x1+b2*x2
    -(sum((n-r)*q)+sum(n*log(1+exp(-q))))
  }
> datain<- data.frame(r=r,n=n)
> ms(~-like(n,r,a,b1,b2),list(a=-2.0,b1=0.5,b2=0.5),
    data=datain)
parameters:
         a         b1         b2
 -1.187791 0.1382988 0.3972517

> # repeat of the glm/logistic analysis
> p<- r/n
> x1<- c(0,2,4,5,0,2,4,5)
> x2<- c(1,1,1,1,0,0,0,0)
> otemp<- glm(p~x1+x2,family=binomial,weights=n)
> otemp$coefficients
 (Intercept)        x1         x2
    -1.18779 0.1382988 0.3972516.
```

As expected, both approaches produce the same maximum likelihood estimates $\hat{a} = -1.188$, $\hat{b}_1 = 0.138$, and $\hat{b}_2 = 0.397$.

Problem set V

1. The state fish and game service requires salmon catches to be reported from any boat catching one or more fish. The boats that do not catch fish, do not report. The data are, therefore, truncated since the number of boats failing to catch fish are not recorded. An example of such data is

number of fish	1	2	3	4	5	6
boats	34	25	12	5	1	0

Assume that the number of salmon caught per boat are described by a Poisson distribution where

$$f(x_i|\lambda) = \frac{e^{-\lambda}\lambda^{x_i}/x_i!}{1 - e^{-\lambda}} \qquad i = 1, 2, 3, \cdots.$$

The symbol x_i represents the number of fish caught per boat. Use the S-function $ms()$ to find the maximum likelihood estimate of λ.

Using the scoring technique to estimate parameters, find the maximum likelihood estimate of λ and an estimate of its variance.

Use the $uniroot()$ S-function to find the maximum likelihood estimate of λ.

2. Consider the situation where the number of observations below c_0 is known but the actual values of the observations are not known (i.e., the distribution is left censored at c_0). Also the number of observations above c_0' is known but the actual values of the observations are not known (i.e., the distribution is also right censored at c_0'). Further assume that the sampled distribution is normally distributed with mean μ and standard deviation σ. Write and test an S-code program to estimate μ and σ for this doubly censored normal distribution from n observations where n_0 are left censored, n_0' are right censored and $n - n_0 - n_0'$ are measured values.

3. Consider the following model constructed to estimate the proportion of dizygotic twins where

probability of a like-sex twin pair = P(like-sex twin) = $M + D/2$ and
probability of an unlike-sex twin pair = P(unlike-sex twin) = $D/2$

where $D = 1 - M$ is the proportion of dizygotic (fraternal twins). A specific number of pairs of like-sex twins = 67 and unlike-sex twins = 42 are observed.

Find* the maximum likelihood estimate of D and its variance in closed form.

Use an S-code program to estimate D and its variance using scoring techniques.

Use a bootstrap procedure to estimate D and its variance.

4. A measure of skewness is

$$\hat{M} = \frac{\sum (x_i - \bar{x})^3}{n}$$

where $M = 0$ identifies a symmetric distribution using a sample of n observations. For the data {2, 5, 8, 2, 5, 9, 1, 4, 30} estimate M and its standard error using a bootstrap procedure (i.e., find $\hat{M}_{[\cdot]}$ and $\hat{se}(M_{[\cdot]})$ estimates).

Find the same estimates using the jackknife procedure.

Estimate M and its standard error using $n = 100$ values sampled from a standard normal distribution using both estimation techniques.

5. Consider the following 15 observations:

0.28, −1.21, 0.60, 0.14, 0.51, 0.19, −0.27, 0.45, 0.29, 0.40, 0.04, 0.60, 1.11, 0.90.

Use a bootstrap strategy to assess the likelihood this sample arose from a population with a mean value of 0 ($\mu_0 = 0$?).

6. A sample of data yields the following 2 × 2 table:

	disease	no disease	total
exposed	$a = 200$	$b = 120$	320
unexposed	$c = 80$	$d = 120$	200
total	280	240	520

The odds ratio measure of association between disease and exposure is estimated by $\hat{or}$ $= ad/bc$. Construct and test an S-program to find the bootstrap estimate of the bias associated with this estimate. The logarithm of the estimated odds ratio ($\log[\hat{or}]$) is another measure of association. Use an S-program to estimate the bias associated with this measure of association.

7. For the data

$$x = 5, 10, 15, 20, 25, 30, 35, 40, 45 \text{ and}$$
$$y = 0.08, 0.12, 0.22, 0.21, 0.27, 0.56, 0.70, 0.71, 0.84$$

use the model $y_i = [1 + e^{-(a+bx_i)}]^{-1}$ and $nls(\ )$-function to estimate a and b. Hint: use initial values $a_0 = -3$ and $b_0 = 0.1$.

Apply a linearizing transformation to y and again estimate the parameters a and b using ordinary least squares estimation.

8. Use a bootstrap procedure to estimate θ, its standard error, and the bias for

$$\hat{\theta} = \frac{1}{n}\sum(x_i - \bar{x})^2$$

where $n = 15$ and $x = \{12, 13, 23, 31, 41, 22, 44, 37, 14, 18, 24, 36, 51, 11, 32\}$.

Use a bootstrap procedure to estimate θ, its standard error, and the bias from a sample of $n = 100$ random values selected from a standard normal distribution.

9. For the two sets of $n = 15$ observations

$$x = \{1, 3, 2, 6, 8, 3, 8, 3, 9, 10, 15, 12, 18, 5, 2\}$$

and

$$y = \{10, 14, 15, 22, 28, 21, 14, 15, 12, 18, 33, 37, 33, 11, 12\}$$

write and test an S-program to assess the conjecture that x and y are samples of unrelated variables (*correlation* = 0) using a randomization strategy.

10. A simple Mendelian genetic system is represented by the following model:

$$\text{AA-homozygote frequency: } p^2$$
$$\text{Aa-heterozygote frequency: } 2pq$$
$$\text{aa-homozygote frequency: } q^2$$

where p represents the frequency of the A-gene and $q = 1 - p$ represents the frequency of the a-gene.

Find* the maximum likelihood estimate of p and its variance when n_1, n_2, and n_3 represent the respective observed counts of AA, Aa, and aa genotypes where

$$\log(L) = n_1 \log(p^2) + n_2 \log(2pq) + n_3 \log(q^2).$$

If $n_1 = 250$, $n_2 = 441$, and $n_3 = 314$, find the maximum likelihood estimates of p using S-tools to verify the "closed-form" estimate and variance.

If the laboratory determination of the homozygotes is subject to misclassification, the log-likelihood function is then

$$\log(L) = n_1 \log(p^2 + e) + n_2 \log(2pq) + n_3 \log(q^2 - e)$$

where e represents the proportion misclassified homozygotic types.

If $n_1 = 250$, $n_2 = 441$, and $n_3 = 314$, find the maximum likelihood estimates of p and e using S-tools. Also estimate the variance/covariance array for the estimates of p and e.

11. Generate two sets of $n = 100$ random variables where x and y have independent standard normal distributions.

Use bootstrap tools to estimate the correlation between x and $2x + y$ (i.e., *correlation*$(x, 2x + y)$). Also estimate the variance and bias associated with this estimate. Plot the histogram and the estimated density function of the estimated correlation coefficient.

*Solve theoretically and not with a computer program.

REFERENCES

1. Kendall, M. G. and Stuart A., *The Advanced Theory of Statistics, Volume 1*. Charles Griffin and Company, London, 1963.
2. Efron, B. and Tibshirani, R. J., *An Introduction to the Bootstrap*. Chapman & Hall, New York, NY, 1993.
3. Mantel, N., (1967) The detection of disease clustering and a generalized regression approach. *Cancer Research*, 27:209–220.
4. Selvin, S., *Statistical Analysis of Epidemiologic Data*. Oxford University Press, New York, NY, 1996.
5. Rosenman, R. H., Brand R., J., Sholtz, R. I., and Friedman M., (1976) Multivariate prediction of coronary heart disease during 8.5 year follow-up in the Western Collaborative Group study. *American Journal of Cardiology*, 37:903–910.
6. Kahn, H. A., *An Introduction to Epidemiologic Methods*. Oxford University Press, New York, NY, 1983.
7. Snedecor, G. W. and Cochran W. G., *Statistical Methods*. The University of Iowa State Press, Ames, IA, 1974.
8. Selvin, S., *Practical Biostatistical Methods*. Duxbury Press, Belmont, CA, 1995.
9. Johnson, N. L. and Kotz, S., *Continuous Univariate Distributions—1*. John Wiley & Sons, New York, NY, 1970.
10. Manly, B. F. J., *Randomization and Monte Carlo Methods in Biology*. Chapman and Hall, New York, NY, 1991.

6

Analysis of Tabular Data

TWO BY TWO TABLES

A 2×2 table is a fundamental description of the relationship between two binary variables. The S-language contains more than a half dozen functions that allow different approaches to the description/analysis of data contained in a 2×2 table. The general notation for two binary variables A and B can be expressed as a table or a cell by cell representation. The notation for a table is

	$b_1 = 1$	$b_2 = 0$
$a_1 = 1$	f_{11}	f_{10}
$a_2 = 0$	f_{01}	f_{00}

and for a cell by cell the representation is

x_1	X_2	frequency
1	1	$f_{11} = F_1$
1	0	$f_{10} = F_2$
0	1	$f_{01} = F_3$
0	0	$f_{00} = F_4$

The symbol F_i represents a cell frequency and the subscript i indicates a specific cell in the table where $i = 1, 2, 3, 4 = $ total number of cells in a 2×2 table. The values x_i are design variables indicating the levels of the categorical variables A and B. An example of such data comes from a clinical trial to evaluate a diet thought to reduce the symptoms of benign breast disease. A group of $n = 229$ women with disease were divided randomly into two groups. One group received the usual care and the other was additionally assigned a special diet (variable $B = $ treatment). After a year individuals were evaluated and assigned to categories "improved" and "failed to improve" (variable $A = $ outcome). The results are summarized in the following table for the most severely affected women ($n_1 = 129$):

	diet	no diet	total
improved	26	21	47
failed to improve	38	44	82
total	64	65	129

The question of the effectiveness of the diet can be approached from several perspectives. A chi-square test addresses the question as to whether the diet had any effect. More technically, the hypothesis that diet status and benign breast disease status are statistically independent is tested using Pearson's chi-square statistic. The S-function *chisq.test*( ) produces this test and

```
> x1<- c(26,21)
> n1<- c(64,65)
> d1<- rbind(x1,n1-x1)
> d1
    [,1] [,2]
x1   26   21
     38   44
> chisq.test(d1)
        Pearson's chi-square test with Yates'
          continuity correction
data:  d1
X-squared = 0.6376, df = 1, p-value = 0.4246.
```

The identical test is performed by *prop.test*( ) but includes the estimated proportions of improved patients in each group and a confidence interval for the difference observed between these two proportions (i.e., $\hat{p}_1 - \hat{p}_2 = 26/64 - 21/65 = 0.406 - 0.323 = 0.083$) where

```
> prop.test(x1,n1)

        2-sample test for equality of proportions
          with continuity correction

data:  x1 out of n1
X-squared = 0.6376, df = 1, p-value = 0.4246
alternative hypothesis: two.sided
95 percent confidence interval:
 -0.09787049  0.26421664
sample estimates:
 prop'n in Group 1 prop'n in Group 2
        0.40625           0.3230769.
```

Fisher's exact test also addresses the same question and

```
> fisher.test(d1)
        Fisher's exact test
data:  d1
p-value = 0.3636
alternative hypothesis: two.sided.
```

All three approaches indicate no important differences in improvement are observed between patients on the diet and patients who received the usual care.

A Pearson chi-square test applies to tables of any size (any number of rows and any number of columns) to evaluate statistical independence (example in Chapter 1). The S-function *prop.test*( ) is designed to compare a series of sample estimated values to a series of postulated proportions (e.g., is $p_1 = p_2 = p_3 = \cdots = p_k = p$?). However, both tests give the identical results when the question concerns equality (homogeneity) of the k proportions in a $2 \times k$ table. Fisher's exact test requires the marginal values of the table to be fixed and is recommended for tables containing small numbers of observations. For a 2×2 table with large numbers of observations in all four cells, the results from an exact test and the chi-square approaches will likely be similar.

Fisher's exact test is an application of hypergeometric probabilities (Chapter 3) to data from a 2×2 table. Notation for such a table is given in Table 3.2 (i.e., N = total number in the population, m = number with a specific characteristic, and n = total number sampled). The probability of the occurrence of a particular 2×2 table when the row variable is unrelated to the column variable is given by a hypergeometric probability for fixed (not random) values of N, m, and n. The cell frequency X is the random quantity observed from the data where X is defined as the number of sampled observations with the characteristic. The two-tail significance probability associated with a specific observed outcome is defined several ways. It is common to define a significance probability as the probability associated with the occurrences of all outcomes with probability less than or equal to the probability of the observed outcome. That is, for observed cell frequencies x_0, the two-tail p-value is the sum of all hypergeometric probabilities less than or equal to p_0 where $P(X = x_0) = p_0$. The sum is then the probability of an equal or more extreme result when no relationship exists between the two binary classification variables. Say the following table was observed:

	B present	B absent	total
A present	$X = 2$	4	6
A absent	8	6	14
total	10	10	20

The values corresponding to the symbols in Table 3.2 are $N = 20$, $m = 10$, $n = 6$, and $X = x_0 = 2$. Example S-code that calculates a hypergeometric significance probability is

```
> N<- 20
> m<- 10
> n<- 6
```

```
> x0<- 2
> x<- max(0,n+m-N):min(m,n)
> p<- dhyper(x,m,N-m,n)
> round(p,4)
[1] 0.0054 0.0650 0.2438 0.3715 0.2438 0.0650 0.0054
> p0<- dhyper(x0,m,N-m,n)
> cat("x0 =",x0,"  p0 =",round(p0,4),"\n")
  x0 = 2   p0 = 0.2438
> pvalue<- sum(p[p<=p0])
> cat("p-value = ",round(pvalue,4),"\n")
  p-value =  0.6285.
```

The probability 0.629 indicates that the result observed ($X = 2$) is likely, producing no evidence of an association between the binary variables A and B. The S-function *fisher.test*( ) gives the same result:

```
> a<- cbind(c(x0,m-x0),c(n-x0,(N-m-n+x0)))
> a
     [,1] [,2]
[1,]   2    4
[2,]   8    6
> fisher.test(a)

        Fisher's exact test

data:  a
p-value = 0.6285
alternative hypothesis: two.sided.
```

A second sample of women is relevant to this clinical trial. Data from the women who were not severely affected ($n_2 = 100$) are shown in the following table:

	diet	no diet	total
improved	18	13	31
failed to improve	32	37	69
total	50	50	100

To assess the degree of association between diet and improvement in disease status taking into account information from both tables (severely and not severely affected individuals), the Mantel–Haenszel test is often appropriate. When the relationship between row and column variables in a series of 2×2 tables differs only because of random variation (no interaction), a summary test based on the data from all tables is achieved using the S-function *mantelhaen.test*( ). The essence of the Mantel–Haenszel test is the comparison of observed values to corresponding values estimated from each of a series of 2×2 tables under the hypothesis that the variables used to construct each table (row and column variables) have independent influences. For the benign breast disease data, this test yields

```
> x0<- c(18,13)
> n0<- c(50,50)
```

```
> dtest<- array(c(x1,n1-x1,x0,n0-x0),c(2,2,2))
> dtest

, , 1
      [,1] [,2]
[1,]    26   38
[2,]    21   44


, , 2
      [,1] [,2]
[1,]    18   32
[2,]    13   37
> mantelhaen.test(dtest)

    Mantel-Haenszel chi-square test with
       continuity correction

data:  dtest
Mantel-Haenszel chi-square = 1.6957, df = 1, p-value = 0.192.
```

The Mantel–Haenszel odds ratio summarizes the relationship between two binary variables based on data from a series of 2×2 tables. A single odds ratio expresses the association based on combining data for each table. Again, it is assumed that the relationship between classification variables is the same in all 2×2 tables summarized making the underlying odds ratio the same in all k tables. The estimated odds ratios then differ only because of the influence of random variation. The expression for the Mantel–Haenszel estimated summary odds ratio is

$$\hat{or}_{MH} = \frac{\sum \dfrac{f_{11l}f_{22l}}{n_l}}{\sum \dfrac{f_{12l}f_{21l}}{n_l}} \qquad l = 1, 2, 3, \cdots, k = \text{number of tables}$$

where f_{ijl} represents the ith, j^{th} cell frequency in a series of k tables (2×2) denoted by l and n_l represents the total number of observations in each table. To summarize, the two tables ($k = 2$) from the diet data,

```
> or.mh<- function(datatab) {
  a0<- datatab[1,1,]
  b0<- datatab[1,2,]
  c0<- datatab[2,1,]
  d0<- datatab[2,2,]
  n0<- a0+b0+c0+d0
  sum(a0*d0/n0)/sum(b0*c0/n0)
   }
> or.mh(dtest)
[1] 1.500884.
```

where *datatab* represents a $2 \times 2 \times k$ table ($k = 2$, for the example).

Summarizing information from a series of 2×2 tables is more generally done with a logistic regression model (Chapter 4) but the results will be similar to the Mantel–Haenszel approach in most cases, particularly when all cells of the k tables contain large numbers of observations. The test of the impact of the diet among severely affected women and the test of the same association between disease and treatment stratifying on both severely and less severely affected individuals ($n_1 + n_2 = 229$) show no evidence of an influence of the diet on the symptoms of benign breast disease.

MATCHED PAIRS—BINARY RESPONSE

Another type of 2×2 table arises in the context of matched pair data. Observations are collected in pairs where the members of each pair are identical or nearly identical for a particular variable that interferes with assessing a specific relationship. Frequently, this variable is called a "confounder." For example, pairs of infants collected to study maternal smoking (smokers (S) versus non-smokers ($\bar{S}$)) and low birth weight (less than 2500 grams versus greater than or equal to 2500 grams) matched for the amount of weight gained by the mother during pregnancy produce the following 2×2 table:

		≥ 2500 smoker	≥ 2500 non-smoker	total
< 2500	smoker	15	40	55
< 2500	non-smoker	22	90	112
total		37	130	167

The values in the table are the numbers of pairs that possess the factors listed on the margins of the table—the total number of infants is $2(167) = 334$. Two types of pairs are concordant with respect to the mother's smoking exposure (S, S or $\bar{S}, \bar{S}$) and two types of pairs are discordant with respect to smoking exposure ($\bar{S}, S$ or $S, \bar{S}$). For example, there are 90 pairs where the first member of the pair is an infant whose mother is a non-smoker and the second member of the pair is an infant whose mother also does not smoke (concordant). Additionally, the first member of each pair weighs less than 2500 grams and the second member weighs equal to or greater than 2500 grams. The within pair association between smoking and low birth weight (measured as binary variables) is unaffected by maternal weight gain since all pairs of infants consist of mothers with essentially the same weight gain during pregnancy. A matched pairs pattern of data collection removes the confounding influence of a third variable (maternal weight gain in the example).

The McNemar matched pair test is designed to evaluate the degree of association between two binary classification variables. The test necessarily focuses on the discordant pairs since the concordant pairs give no direct information on the relationship between a factor and outcome. That is, the impact of smoking on birth weight cannot be assessed in groups where the smoking status is the same within all pairs (e.g., pairs concordant for smoking status—the 15 and 90 pairs). The McNemar test compares the observed proportion of discordant pairs $\hat{p}$ with the one factor present and the other absent among all discordant pairs to 0.5. If no association exists between smoking exposure and low birth weight, then the numbers of discordant pairs of each type differ only because of the influence of chance variation (p = 0.5). In symbols, let b represent the number of discordant pairs of one type (e.g., $(S,\bar{S})$-pairs) and c represent the number of discordant pairs of the other type (e.g., $(\bar{S},S)$-pairs). The expected value of b is $np = n/2$ and the variance of b is $np(1 - p) = n/4$ under the hypothesis (null hypothesis) that p = 0.5 where n represents the total number of discordant pairs ($n = b + c$). A test-statistic based on a normal approximation to the binomial distribution (Chapter 3) is

$$z = \frac{|\,b - n/2\,| - \frac{1}{2}}{\sqrt{n/4}} \quad \text{and} \quad z^2 = \frac{(|\,b - c\,| - 1)^2}{b + c}.$$

The test-statistic z has an approximate standard normal distribution when the expected proportion of discordant pairs is p = 0.5 and z^2 has an approximate chi-square distribution with one degree of freedom, called McNemar's test. The "correction factor" of one-half is included to improve the correspondence between the binomial (exact) and normal (approximate) distributions. The S-function *mcnemar.test*( ) applied to the smoking/birth weight data gives

```
> m<- matrix(c(15,22,40,90),2,2)
> m
      [,1] [,2]
[1,]    15   40
[2,]    22   90
> mcnemar.test(m)


          McNemar's chi-square test with
                continuity correction

ata:   m
McNemar's chi-square = 4.6613, df = 1, p-value = 0.0308.
```

The same issue is addressed with the S-function *binom.test*( ). This S-function allows the comparison of any observed proportion $\hat{p}$ to any specified proportion p. For the matched pair data, comparing the estimate $\hat{p} = b/n = 40/62 = 0.645$ with the postulated value p = 0.5 yields

```
> binom.test(m[1,2],(m[1,2]+m[2,1]),p=0.5)

          Exact binomial test

data:   m[1, 2] out of (m[1, 2] + m[2, 1])
number of successes = 40, n = 62, p-value = 0.03
alternative hypothesis: true p is not equal to 0.5.
```

The McNemar and the binomial tests are identical when a normal approximation is used in *binom.test*( ) (large sample size procedure—*correct* = *T*). However, for small numbers of pairs a binomial test produces an exact *p*-value where the McNemar procedure is somewhat less precise.

TWO BY *k* TABLE

An important data structure occurs when a binary variable (*y*) is classified into a series of numeric categories (*x*). Such data are summarized in a 2 × *k* table and address the question of dose/response or trend associated with the *x*-variable. The Oxford Childhood Cancer Study [1] classified children with cancer (*y* = 1) and their controls (*y* = 0) by the number of x-rays received by their mothers during pregnancy (*x*: {0, 1, 2, 3, 4, 5 or more x-rays}). The data are contained in Table 6.1.

Table 6.1. Case/control infants classified by the number of prenatal maternal x-rays (X), Oxford Childhood Cancer Study, 1953

	X = 0	X = 1	X = 2	X = 3	X = 4	X ≥ 5	total
case	7 332	287	199	96	59	65	8 038
control	7 673	239	154	65	28	29	8 188
total	15 005	526	353	161	87	94	16 226
$\hat{p}_i$	0.489	0.546	0.564	0.596	0.678	0.691	0.495

The five x-rays or more category is treated as five x-rays.

A first question of concern is whether the binary variable (rows) is related in any way to the category variable (columns). A typical Pearson chi-square test of independence or test of homogeneity ($p_1 = p_2 = p_3 = \cdots = p_k = p$) is directly applied and

```
> r1<- c(7332,287,199,96,59,65)
> r2<- c(7673,239,154,65,28,29)
> d<- rbind(r1,r2)
> d
   [,1] [,2] [,3] [,4] [,5] [,6]
r1 7332  287  199   96   59   65
r2 7673  239  154   65   28   29
> chisq.test(d)

          Pearson's chi-square test without Yates'
               continuity correction

data:  d
X-squared = 47.2858, df = 5, p-value = 0
```

shows a strong relationship (*p*-value < 0.001) between prenatal x-rays and the proportion of children diagnosed with cancer relative to the controls.

A next question concerns a linear "dose–response" relationship between the x-variable and the binary variable. This relationship is frequently explored in terms of proportions. For the Oxford study data, the relationship between the proportion of cases in each category $\hat{p}_i$ and the number of maternal x-rays is clearly seen (Figure 6.1—increasing solid line).

It is convenient to remember that data displayed in a $2 \times k$ table are n pairs of observations (x_{ij}, y_{ij}) where the cell frequency in the $2 \times k$ table indicate the number of identical pairs. For example, there are 7332 pairs where the mother did not receive an x-ray among the cases or $(x,y) = (0, 1)$ and there are 28 pairs where the mother received four x-rays among the controls or $(x,y) = (4, 0)$. To estimate a straight line $(p_i = a + bx_i)$ summary of the relationship between a series of proportions and a series of numeric x-values, three quantities are necessary. The variability of x is measured among the n observations by

$$1.\ \textit{sum of squares for } x = S_{xx} = \sum \sum (x_{ij} - \bar{x})^2.$$

The mean value $\bar{x}$ is $\Sigma\Sigma x_{ij}/n$ where n is the total number of pairs in the data set. Similarly, the variability of y is measured by

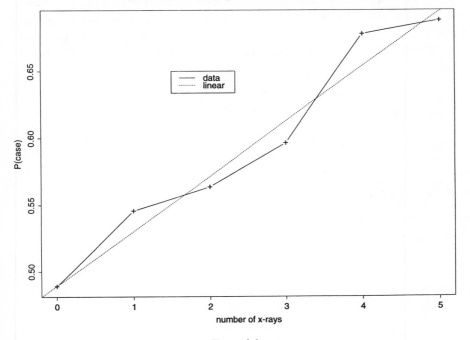

Case/control status by number of maternal x-rays

Figure 6.1

$$\text{2. } \textit{sum of squares for } y = S_{yy} = \sum\sum(y_{ij} - \bar{y})^2.$$

and joint relationship is summarized by

$$\text{3. } \textit{cross-product} = S_{xy} = \sum\sum(x_{ij} - \bar{x})(y_{ij} - \bar{y})$$

$$i = 1, 2 \text{ and } j = 1, 2, 3, \cdots, n_i.$$

The value $\bar{y}$ is the overall proportion of values where $y = 1$. For the childhood cancer data, $S_{xx} = 6733.58$, $S_{yy} = 4056.153$, $S_{xy} = 279.208$ and $\hat{p} = \bar{y} = 8038/16226 = 0.495$.

Short-cut formulas exist for these three sums of squares [2] but are not needed for a computer implementation. When the expected proportion of cases is represented by the line $p_i = a + bx_i$, an estimate of b and its variance are

$$\textit{estimated slope} = \hat{b} = \frac{S_{xy}}{S_{xx}} \quad \text{with} \quad \textit{variance}(\hat{b}) = \frac{S_{yy}}{(n-1)S_{xx}}.$$

The estimate $\hat{b}$ is the least squares estimate of the regression coefficient b (mentioned in Chapter 1 and discussed in detail in Chapters 4 and 5). To assess formally the estimate $\hat{b}$, the test-statistic $z^2 = \hat{b}^2/\textit{variance}(\hat{b})$ is calculated and has an approximate chi-square distribution with one degree of freedom when the proportion of responses within each category are not linearly related to the x-variable (that is, $b = 0$). The estimate $\hat{b}$ measures and summarizes the trend in the proportion across the values of the "dose" categories. For the childhood cancer data, example S-code to estimate b and evaluate its magnitude is

```
> # convert table into n paired observations
> x<- c(rep(0:(length(r1)-1),r1),rep(0:(length(r2)-1),r2))
> y<- c(rep(1,sum(r1)),rep(0,sum(r2)))
> table(y,x)
      0    1    2    3    4    5
0  7332  287  199   96   59   65
1  7673  239  154   65   28   29
> sxx<- sum((x-mean(x))^2)
> syy<- sum((y-mean(y))^2)
> sxy<- sum((y-mean(y))*(x-mean(x)))
> # chi-square test for trend
> b<- sxy/sxx
> b
[1] 0.04146503
> # or b<- lsfit(x,y)$coef[2]
> n<- sum(d)
> # linear chi-square
> v<- syy/((n-1)*sxx)
> linear<- b^2/v
> p.linear<- 1-pchisq(linear,1)
> round(cbind(linear,p.linear),3)
      linear p.linear
[1,] 46.311        0.
```

The chi-square statistic (46.311) clearly indicates that the slope estimated by $\hat{b} = 0.041$ is likely different from zero (p-value < 0.001).

For a $2 \times k$ table, the Pearson chi-square statistic can be partitioned into two meaningful pieces. The first piece reflects the linear relationship between the row binary variable and column "dose" variable and the second piece indicates the magnitude of the non-linearity in the relationship or

total chi–square value = *linear chi–square value* + *non–linear chi–square value*

For the childhood cancer data, the partition is calculated by

```
> # total chi-square
> total<- chisq.test(d)$statistic
> p.total<- chisq.test(d)$p.value
> # nonlinearity chi-square
> nonlinear<- total-linear
> p.nl<- 1-pchisq(nonlinear,length(r1)-2)
> round(cbind(linear,nonlinear,total),3)
          linear nonlinear   total
X-squared 46.311     0.975  47.286
> round(cbind(p.nl,p.linear,p.total),3)
            p.nl p.linear  p.total
> X-squared 0.914        0       0.
```

The relatively tiny nonlinear chi-square value (0.975) and, therefore, the extremely large linear component (46.311) verifies the astonishingly linear dose–response relationship between maternal x-ray exposure and the risk of childhood cancer in the Oxford study data (Figure 6.1—dotted line).

The Oxford data demonstrate a general property of case/control data. The risk of the disease cannot be estimated from the collected data. Obviously, the risk of childhood cancer is small ($\approx 1/100,000$) and is not estimated by the proportion of cases in a case/control study (i.e., proportion of cases = 0.495).

The linear relationship between X and Y in a $2 \times k$ table also can be evaluated by comparing the mean values of the x-variable for each level of the binary variable y and constructing a t-like statistic. The difference between the two means $\bar{x}_1$ (when $y = 1$) and $\bar{x}_0$ (when $y = 0$) is calculated and an estimate of the variance of the difference is given by

$$variance(\bar{x}_1 - \bar{x}_0) = \frac{S_{xx}}{n-1}\left(\frac{1}{n_1} + \frac{1}{n_0}\right)$$

for n_1 observations $y = 1$ and n_0 observations $y = 0$. Therefore, a two-sample "t-statistic" is

$$t\text{-like statistic} = z = \frac{\bar{x}_1 - \bar{x}_0}{\sqrt{variance(\bar{x}_1 - \bar{x}_0)}}$$

where the test-statistic z has an approximate standard normal distribution when the x-variable is unrelated to the binary y-variable (e.g., childhood cancer risk is unrelated to x-ray exposure). That is, the expected difference between the two mean values is zero. The mean number of x-rays among the cases is $\bar{x}_1 = 0.191$ and among the controls is $\bar{x}_0 = 0.122$. Applying this two-sample approach to Oxford study data gives

```
> # t-like test
> dd<- mean(x[y==1])-mean(x[y==0])
> vdd<- sxx*(1/sum(r1)+1/sum(r2))/(n-1)
> z<- dd/sqrt(vdd)
> pvalue<- 2*(1-pnorm(abs(z)))
> round(cbind(z,pvalue),3)
          z pvalue
[1,] 6.805      0
```

producing the identical result observed for the linear regression approach ($z^2 = (6.805)^2 = 46.311$). These two seemingly different perspectives on testing the linear association between X and Y are, in fact, identical in general.

The process of estimating and testing the linear relationship in a $2 \times k$ table is sometimes called a test of trend, measured by either $\hat{b}$ or $\bar{x}_1 - \bar{x}_2$.

MEASURES OF ASSOCIATION—2 × 2 TABLE

Four measures of association among the many possible indicate some of the ways the association between two binary variables in a 2×2 table can be summarized. Data on smoking illustrate. Smoking exposure histories on pairs of husbands (B) and wives (A) were collected and classified by their smoking status (Table 6.2).

Table 6.2. Smoking status (S = smokder and $\bar{S}$ = non-smoker) for pairs of husbands and wives

	S (husband)	$\bar{S}$ (husband)	total
S (wife)	42	22	64
$\bar{S}$ (wife)	32	81	113
total	74	103	177

Perhaps the most used measure of association applied to a 2×2 table is the odds ratio. The odds ratio, as the name indicates, is the ratio of two odds. For example, the odds of being a smoker among husbands is estimated by 42/22 when the wife smokes and 32/81 when the wife does not smoke, making the estimated odds ratio = (42/22)/(32/81) = 4.832. In general, the odds ratio is estimated by

$$\hat{o}r = \frac{(f_{11}/f_{12})}{(f_{21}/f_{22})} = \frac{(f_{11}/f_{21})}{(f_{12}/f_{22})} = \frac{f_{11}f_{22}}{f_{12}f_{21}}.$$

An odds ratio of 1.0 occurs when the odds are identical in each row (column) of a 2×2 table indicating no association exists between the categorical classification variables. The degree to which the odds ratio differs from 1.0 measures the association between the two binary variables.

The odds ratio has two important properties. If the number of observations in a row or column is multiplied by a constant, the odds ratio is unchanged. Also, the choice for coding of the binary variables does not affect the value of the odds ratio since $1/\hat{o}r$ reflects the same magnitude of association as $\hat{o}r$ itself. A disadvantage of using an odds ratio measure arises when f_{12} or f_{21} equals zero, making the value $\hat{o}r$ undefined. This problem is sometime corrected by adding one-half to the values in all four cells in the 2×2 table [3].

Three less popular measures of association are

1. *Yule's measure* $= Y = \dfrac{f_{11}f_{22} - f_{12}f_{21}}{f_{11}f_{22} + f_{12}f_{21}}$

2. *coefficient of contingency* $= C = \left[\dfrac{X^2}{X^2 + n}\right]^{\frac{1}{2}}$

3. *phi $-$ statistic* $= \Phi = \left[\dfrac{X^2}{n}\right]^{\frac{1}{2}}$

where X^2 is the Pearson chi-square statistic and n is the total number of observations in the table.

Applied to the husband/wife smoking data in Table 6.2,

```
> x<- rbind(c(42,22),c(32,81))
> x
>        [,1] [,2]
[1,]    42    22
[2,]    32    81
> or<- x[1,1]*x[2,2]/(x[1,2]*x[2,1])
> round(or,3)
[1] 4.832
> Y<- (x[1,1]*x[2,2]-x[1,2]*x[2,1])/
    (x[1,1]*x[2,2]+x[1,2]*x[2,1])
> round(Y,3)
[1] 0.657
> chi2<- chisq.test(x,correct=F)$statistic
> round(chi2,3)
X-squared
   23.374
> n<- sum(x)
> PHI<- sqrt(chi2/n)
> round(PHI,3)
[1] 0.363
> C<- sqrt(chi2/(chi2+n))
> round(C,3)
[1] 0.342.
```

MEASURES OF ASSOCIATION—$r \times c$ TABLE

Four parallel chi-square based measures of the association between categorical variables that apply to any two-way table with r = number of rows and c = the number of columns are:

1. $Cramer's\ V = V_0 = \left[\dfrac{X^2}{n \times min[(r-1),(c-1)]}\right]^{\frac{1}{2}}$

2. $Tschuprow's\ T = T_0 = \left[\dfrac{X^2}{n\sqrt{(r-1)(c-1)}}\right]^{\frac{1}{2}}$

3. $Cramer's\ C = C = \left[\dfrac{X^2}{X^2+n}\right]^{\frac{1}{2}}$ and

4. $phi\text{–}statistic = \Phi = \left[\dfrac{X^2}{n}\right]^{\frac{1}{2}}$.

Again, the chi-square statistic is represented by X^2 and the total number of observations in the table by n. These measures of association lack any interpretation in terms of probabilities and are only occasionally used. Note that $V_0 = T_0 = \Phi$ when $r = c = 2$.

Consider the smoking data (Table 6.2) expanded into four categories of smoking exposure given in Table 6.3.

Table 6.3. Smoker status (non-smoker, light, moderate, and heavy) by pairs of husbands (B) and wives (A)

	b_1 (non-smoker)	b_2 (light)	b_3 (moderate)	b_4 (heavy)	total
a_1 (non-smoker)	42	18	4	0	64
a_2 (light)	12	22	8	2	44
a_3 (moderate)	18	6	10	6	40
a_4 (heavy)	2	8	12	7	29
total	74	54	34	15	177

Note: light = 1–20 cigarettes per day, moderate = 21–30 cigarettes per day, heavy > 30 cigarettes per day

Applying these four chi-square measures of association gives

```
> xtemp<- c(42,18,4,0,12,22,8,2,18,6,10,6,2,8,12,7)
> x<-  matrix(xtemp,4,byrow=T)
> x
     [,1] [,2] [,3] [,4]
[1,]   42   18    4    0
[2,]   12   22    8    2
[3,]   18    6   10    6
[4,]    2    8   12    7
> n<- sum(x)
> chisq.test(x,correct=F)

 Pearson's chi-square test without Yates' continuity correction
```

```
data:  x
X-squared = 58.6607, df = 9, p-value = 0
> chi2<- chisq.test(x,correct=F)$statistic
> VO<- sqrt(chi2/(n*min((nrow(x)-1),(ncol(x)-1))))
> TO<- sqrt(chi2/(n*sqrt((nrow(x)-1)*(ncol(x)-1))))
> PHI<- sqrt(chi2/n)
> C<- sqrt(chi2/(chi2+n))
> round(cbind(VO,TO,C,PHI),3)
              VO    TO     C   PHI
X-squared 0.332 0.332 0.499 0.576.
```

Lambda measure of association

A lambda measure of association contrasts two estimated probabilities:

1. the maximum probability of predicting that an observation belongs to a specific row

with

2. the maximum probability of predicting that an observation belongs to a specific row given that the observation belongs to specific column.

The first probability is estimated by $f_{m.}/n$ where $f_{m.}$ is the largest row total and the second by $\Sigma f_{mj}/n$ where f_{mj} is the largest value in each column. The lambda measure contrasts these two probabilities in terms of the probabilities of not predicting an observation belongs to the right row or

$$\hat{\lambda}_c = \frac{probability\ of\ error\ (1) - probability\ of\ error\ (2)}{probability\ of\ error\ (1)}$$

$$= \frac{(1 - f_{m.}/n) - (1 - \Sigma f_{mj}/n)}{1 - f_{m.}/n}$$

$$= \frac{\Sigma f_{mj} - f_{m.}}{n - f_{m.}} \qquad j = 1, 2, 3, \cdots, c.$$

The "dot notation" is used to indicate sums. The symbol $x_{.j}$ means the sum is over the first subscript and the symbol $x_{i.}$ means the sum is taken over the second subscript. In a two-way table, for example, the first subscript indicates rows and $f_{i.}$ means the quantities represented by f are summed over the columns (i^{th} row total).

When categorical variables in a two-way table are exactly independent, the largest values within each column correspond to the row with the largest total, then Σf_{mj} equals $f_{m.}$ and $\hat{\lambda}_c = 0$. Therefore, values of $\hat{\lambda}_c$ near zero indicate that the row variable cannot be predicted from knowledge of the column variable and a value of $\hat{\lambda}_c$ different from zero reflects the degree of association.

A similar lambda measure of association is developed when interest is focused on the rows of a contingency table or

$$\hat{\lambda}_r = \frac{\Sigma f_{il} - f_{.l}}{n - f_{.l}} \qquad i = 1, 2, 3, \cdots, r.$$

where l indicates the column containing the largest value.

Often no reason exists to measure association in terms of rows or columns. A summary lambda measure is then created by a weighted average of $\hat{\lambda}_c$ and $\hat{\lambda}_r$ or

$$\hat{\lambda} = \frac{(n - f_{.l})\hat{\lambda}_r + (n - f_{m.})\hat{\lambda}_c}{(n - f_{.l}) + (n - f_{m.})}$$
$$= \frac{\Sigma f_{il} + \Sigma f_{mj} - f_{.l} - f_{m.}}{2n - f_{.l} - f_{m.}}.$$

The lambda correlations applied to the 4×4 table of smoking data (Table 6.3) give

```
> lam.cor<- function(x) {
  n<- sum(x)
  xmax<- apply(x,2,max)
  cmax<- max(apply(x,1,sum))
  rcol<- (sum(xmax)-cmax)/(n-cmax)
  xmax<- apply(x,1,max)
  rmax<- max(apply(x,2,sum))
  rrow<- (sum(xmax)-rmax)/(n-rmax)
  r<- ((n-rmax)*rrow+(n-cmax)*rcol)/(2*n-rmax-cmax)
  cbind(rcol,rrow,r)
  }
  round(lam.cor(x),3)
       rrow   rcol      r
[1,] 0.194 0.168 0.181.
```

The lambda measures of association can be applied to 2×2 tables but are most effective in larger tables.

MEASURES OF ASSOCIATION—TABLE WITH ORDINAL VARIABLES

Measures of association are important as a description of the strength of a relationship between classification variables A and B in a two-way table when the levels of the variables can be ordered. For example, the smoking exposure status of husbands and wives can be ordered (e.g., non-smoker < light < moderate < heavy). Several measures of association take advantage of the ordered nature of the categorical variables. These measures are based on a specialized way of counting pairs of observations. A typical pair of observations belongs to cell (i, j) and another belongs to cell (i', j'). Using other symbols, one observation belongs to categories a_i and b_j and the other to categories $a_{i'}$ and $b_{j'}$. Measures of association when the classification variables are ordinal are functions of the following four quantities:

P = total number of pairs of observations where either both $i > i'$ and $j > j'$ or both $i < i'$ and $j < j'$,

Q = total number of pairs of observations where either both $i < i'$ and $j > j'$ or both $i < i'$ and $j > j'$,

T_a = total number of observations where $i = i'$, and

T_b = total number of observations where $j = j'$.

If the variables A and B are associated, then both P and Q tend to be extreme and when no association exists P and Q tend to be equal. Functions of P and Q, therefore, serve to measure association with a value constructed to be between -1 and 1. Four examples are:

Goodman and Kruskal (cited in [4]) suggested a measure frequently called the gamma-measure of association where

$$\gamma = \frac{P - Q}{P + Q}.$$

Kendall's τ-statistic (cited in [4]) measures association and is defined by

$$\hat{\tau} = \frac{2(P - Q)}{\sqrt{(P + Q + T_a)(P + Q + T_b)}}.$$

Two related measures suggested by Somers [5] are

$$S_{b|a} = \frac{P - Q}{P + Q + T_b}$$

and

$$S_{a|b} = \frac{P - Q}{P + Q + T_a}.$$

Again apply these measures to the smoking data:

```
> #convert x (4 by 4) into n = 177 paired observations
> a0<- rep(1:nrow(x),apply(x,1,sum))
> b0<- rep(rep(1:ncol(x),nrow(x)),array(t(x)))
> table(a0,b0)
    1   2   3  4
 1 42  18   4  0
 2 12  22   8  2
 3 18   6  10  6
 4  2   8  12  7
> # count the pair types
> a<- outer(a0,a0,"-")
> b<- outer(b0,b0,"-")
> P<- sum(ifelse(a*b>0,1,0))/2
> Q<- sum(ifelse(a*b<0,1,0))/2
> Ta<- (sum(ifelse(a==0,1,0))-sum(x^2))/2
> Tb<- (sum(ifelse(b==0,1,0))-sum(x^2))/2
> cbind(P,Q,Ta,Tb)
          P    Q   Ta   Tb
[1,] 6404 1916 2458 3108
> #Goodman and Kruskal (gamma)
```

```
> (P-Q)/(P+Q)
[1] 0.5394231
> #Kendal's tau
> 2*(P-Q)/sqrt((P+Q+Ta)*(P+Q+Tb))
[1] 0.8087767
> #Sommer's r=b|a
> (P-Q)/(P+Q+Tb)
[1] 0.3927196
> #Sommer's r=a|b
> (P-Q)/(P+Q+Ta)
[1] 0.4164038.
```

A simple and often effective measure of association from tabular data is achieved by assigning numeric values to each category and calculating the Pearson correlation coefficient based on the n pairs of observations described by a two-way table. For example, the smoking data consists of 177 pairs and making the assignments non-smoker = $a_1 = b_1 = 1$, light smoker = $a_2 = b_2 = 2$, moderate smoker = $a_3 = b_3 = 3$, and heavy smoker = $a_4 = b_4 = 4$ yields

```
> # Pearson correlation
> cor(a0,b0)
[1] 0.4862099.
```

Kendall's τ-measure of association also applies to pairs of observations that are not contained in a table. Similar to the use in a two-way table, Kendall's τ is a function of the count of the similar pairs (same sign) and dissimilar pairs (opposite sign). The process starts with forming all possible pairs among each of the two variables. Then, counting the number of pairs where both the within pair differences have the same sign (P) and the number of pairs where the within pair differences have the opposite sign (Q), Kendall's measure of association is

$$\hat{\tau} = \frac{P - Q}{P + Q}$$

when no observations are identical making $P + Q = n(n - 1)$. For example, a sample of $n = 12$ birth weights (grams) measured on fraternal (dizygotic) unlike-sex twins are

males: 2850, 2530, 2590, 2130, 3180, 2730, 3040, 2270, 2360, 2440, 2820, 3130
females: 2140, 2531, 2580, 2370, 3220, 2970, 3080, 2820, 2690, 2470, 2280, 3000.

The measure of association $\hat{\tau}$ is found with the S-function *tau*( ) or

```
> tau<- function(x,y) {
    x0<- outer(x,x,"-")
    y0<- outer(y,y,"-")
    p<- sum(ifelse(x0*y0>0,1,0))
    q<- sum(ifelse(x0*y0<0,1,0))
    (p-q)/(p+q)
    }
> # S-vector m contains the 12 male twin birth weights
> m<- c(2850,2530,2590,2130,3180,2730,3040,2270,2360,
```

```
    2440,2820,3130)
> # S-vector f contains the 12 female twin birth weights
> f<- c(2140,2531,2580,2370,3220,2970,3080,2820,2690,
    2470,2280,3000)
> round(tau(m,f),3)
[1] 0.303.
```

Kendall's tau-correlation and the gamma measure of association are essentially the same process. However, a contingency table contains a large number of identical observations (i.e., the values in the same cell) that are accounted for in the calculation of the measure of association (e.g., symbols T_a and T_b).

No reason exists to use a single measure of association. Different measures of association can reflect various aspects of the data and using several measures of association possibly identifies these differences. Most of the measures of association described have expressions that allow estimates of their associated sampling variability. However, the intent of these measures is usually descriptive and alternative analytic procedures exist to evaluate formally the observed magnitude of an association. For example, chi-square and log-linear (next section) analyses are designed specifically to investigate rigorously statistical issues arising from tabular data.

LOGLINEAR MODEL

Loglinear models are designed for exploring the relationships within a contingency table. The dependent variable is the cell frequency transformed by taking the logarithm. The independent variables are the classification variables used to create the table. Transforming the cell frequencies and using a linear model allows estimation and analysis using Poisson regression techniques (Chapter 4).

As noted, the symbol F_i represents a cell count and the subscript i indicates a specific cell in the table where $i = 1, 2, 3, 4 = $ total number of cells in a 2×2 table. Infants classified by birth weight status (birth weight < 2500 grams —$x_1 = 1$ and $\geq$ 2500 grams—$x_1 = 0$ for rows) and maternal smoking status (smokers—$x_2 = 1$, non-smoker—$x_2 = 0$ for columns) yield the following data:

	x_1	x_2	F_i
< 2500g/smoker	1	1	191
< 2500g/non-smoker	1	0	1120
$\geq$2500g/smoker	0	1	422
$\geq$2500g/non-smoker	0	0	4443

A loglinear model describing such a 2×2 table is

$$\log(F_i) = a + b_1 x_{i1} + b_2 x_{i2} + b_3 x_{i1} x_{i2}.$$

where the x_i-values are binary design variables representing the two levels of each categorical variable.

For this elementary case, the loglinear model is explicitly

$$\log(F_4) = a \qquad\qquad (\geq 2500g/\text{non-smoker}),$$

$$\log(F_3) = a + b_2 \qquad\qquad (\geq 2500g/\text{smoker}),$$

$$\log(F_2) = a + b_1 \qquad\qquad (< 2500g/\text{non-smoker}), \text{ and}$$

$$\log(F_1) = a + b_1 + b_2 + b_3 \quad (< 2500g/\text{smoker}).$$

Like previous Poisson models, the cell counts F_i are known or assumed to have independent Poisson distributions. The same analytic results occur when the cell counts have simple multinomial or product multinomial distributions [6]. Although the estimates of the four coefficients describing a 2×2 table are easily calculated by hand, the *glm*( ) function gives

```
> # f = vector containing the cell frequencies
> f<- c(191,1120,422,4443)
> x1<- c(1,1,0,0)
> x2<- c(1,0,1,0)
> otemp1<- glm(f~x1+x2+x1*x2,family=poisson)
> summary(otemp1,correlation=F)
Call: glm(formula = f~x1+x2+x1*x2, family = poisson)

Coefficients:
                  Value Std. Error     t value
 (Intercept)  8.3990851 0.01500244   559.848009
          x1 -1.3780011 0.03343546   -41.213758
          x2 -2.3540798 0.05093860   -46.214062
       x1:x2  0.5852693 0.09339808     6.266395

(Dispersion Parameter for Poisson family taken to be 1)
Null Deviance: 6779.84 on 3 degrees of freedom
Residual Deviance:  0 on 0 degrees of freedom

Number of Fisher Scoring Iterations: 1.
```

The coefficient $\hat{b}_3$ is the key parameter and measures the association between the binary variables used to form the rows (birth weight) and columns (smoking exposure) of the 2×2 table. If $\hat{b}_3$ is 0, then the linear model is additive making the row and column variables unrelated. As before, an additive model implies that the independent variables have completely separate influences on the dependent variable—the row variable does not influence the column variable and vice versa. The degree to which $\hat{b}_3$ differs from zero measures the strength of association. For a 2×2 table, $\hat{b}_3$ is a function of the odds ratio where $\hat{b}_3 = \log(\hat{or})$. For the birth weight example, $\hat{or} = e^{\hat{b}_3} = e^{0.585} = 1.795$. The identical odds ratio can be estimated directly from the data where $\hat{or} = (191)(4443)/(422)(1120) = 1.795$. When values estimated from a model are identical to values calculated directly from the data, the model is said to be saturated. Another property of a saturated model is that the residual deviance is zero. This occurs when the number of observations is equal to the number of parameters in the model (four in a 2×2 table). To illustrate in concrete terms that a saturated model exactly reproduces the data, from the example,

```
> exp(predict(otemp1))
   1    2    3    4
 191 1120  422 4443.
```

When birth weight and smoking are unrelated ($b_3 = 0$), the appropriate additive loglinear model is

$$\log(F_i) = a + b_1 x_{i1} + b_2 x_{i2}$$

and the *glm*-analysis becomes

```
> otemp0<- glm(f~x1+x2,family=poisson)
> summary(otemp0,correlation=F)
Call: glm(formula = f ~ x1 + x2, family = poisson)
Deviance Residuals:
       1         2        3         4
 4.98543 -1.787082 -2.83183 0.9175002

Coefficients:
               Value Std. Error    t value
(Intercept) 8.385289 0.01494627  561.02875
        x1 -1.311277 0.03111694  -42.14028
        x2 -2.205528 0.04255025  -51.83349

    (Dispersion Parameter for Poisson family taken to be 1)
    Null Deviance: 6779.84 on 3 degrees of freedom
    Residual Deviance: 36.90924 on 1 degrees of freedom

    Number of Fisher Scoring Iterations: 1.
```

The expected cell frequencies calculated under this model are

```
> exp(predict(otemp0))
         1          2         3         4
  130.1236   1180.876  482.8765  4382.124.
```

The expected values can be calculated directly. For the birth weight/smoking data, the estimated probability of a low birth weight infant is $P(birth\ weight < 2500) = 1311/6176 = 0.212$ ($x_1 = 1$) and the estimated probability a mother smokes is $P(smoker) = 613/6176 = 0.099$ ($x_2 = 1$). Therefore, the expected number of low birth weight infants born to mothers who smoke is estimated to be $6176(0.212)(0.099) = 130.124$ when smoking and birth weight are unrelated (i.e., P(A and B) = P(A)P(B)—statistical independence). The estimates for the other three cell frequencies follow the same pattern.

As before, the residual deviance provides a measure of the goodness-of-fit. The residual deviance from the smoking and birth weight data is 36.909, or

```
> sum(residuals(otemp0,type="deviance")^2)
[1] 36.90924.
```

A slightly different goodness-of-fit statistics is

```
> sum(residuals(otemp0,type="pearson")^2)
[1] 40.12554.
```

Both test-statistics have approximate chi-square distributions with one degree of freedom. The large chi-square values indicate that smoking and birth weight are likely associated (p-value < 0.001) since the additive model is not a plausible description of the data ($b_3 \neq 0$). Essentially the same chi-square value emerges from a classic Pearson chi-square approach to a 2×2 table ([4] or [7]). The S-version of the Pearson chi-square test *chi.test*( ) produces

```
> chisq.test(matrix(c(191,422,1120,4443),2,2))
            Pearson's chi-square test
              with Yates' continuity correction
data:   matrix(c(191, 422, 1120, 4443), 2, 2)
X-squared = 39.4823, df = 1, p-value = 0.
```

The "t value" associated with $\hat{b}_3$ in the saturated model also gives approximately the same result (i.e., $(6.266)^2 = 39.263$ from *summary(otemp1)*—"t value"). The four statistical tests address the same question, use the same test-statistic (approximate chi-square values with one degree of freedom) and primarily differ because they employ different approaches to approximate the chi-square distribution with one degree of freedom.

The loglinear approach applied to a $2 \times 2 \times 2$ table created by three binary variables illustrates the use of nested loglinear models to analyze the issues that arise in the analysis of tabular data. The saturated loglinear model (eight observations = eight parameters) is

$$\log(F_i) = a + b_1 x_{i1} + b_2 x_{i2} + b_3 x_{i3} + b_4 x_{i1} x_{i2} + b_5 x_{i1} x_{i3} + b_6 x_{i2} x_{i3} + b_7 x_{i1} x_{i2} x_{i3}.$$

The subscript i again indicates a cell in the table where $i = 1, 2, 3, \cdots, n = 8 =$ total number of cells in the $2 \times 2 \times 2$ table. Again, the x_i-values are binary design variables representing two levels of three categorical variables. Consider the birth weight and smoking data further classified by race x_3 (white—$x_3 = 0$ and black—$x_3 = 1$), then

x_1	x_2	x_3	F_i	count
1	1	0	F_1	118
1	0	0	F_2	866
0	1	0	F_3	288
0	0	0	F_4	3672
1	1	1	F_5	73
1	0	1	F_6	254
0	1	1	F_7	134
0	0	1	F_8	771

The saturated loglinear model applied to the analysis of these data gives

```
> # f = vector containing the cell frequencies
> f<- c(118,866,288,3672,73,254,134,771)
> x1<- c(1,1,0,0,1,1,0,0)
> x2<- c(1,0,1,0,1,0,1,0)
> x3<- c(0,0,0,0,1,1,1,1)
> otemp1<- glm(f~x1+x2+x3+x1*x2+x1*x3+x2*x3+x1*x2*x3,
    family=poisson)
> summary(otemp1,correlation=F)

Call: glm(formula = f~x1+x2+x3+x1*x2+x1*x3+x2*x3+x1*x2*x3,
    family = poisson)

Coefficients:
                   Value    Std. Error        t value
(Intercept)   8.20849175    0.01650246     497.4102179
         x1  -1.44460684    0.03777652     -38.2408647
         x2  -2.54553127    0.06119276     -41.5985721
         x3  -1.56080338    0.03961500     -39.3993054
      x1:x2   0.55233099    0.11564542       4.7760730
      x1:x3   0.33425274    0.08161550       4.0954564
      x2:x3   0.79568270    0.11182243       7.1155909
   x1:x2:x3  -0.04935724    0.19942218      -0.2475013

(Dispersion Parameter for Poisson family taken to be 1)
Null Deviance: 9260.431 on 7 degrees of freedom
Residual Deviance: 0 on 0 degrees of freedom

Number of Fisher Scoring Iterations: 1.
```

The estimated coefficient $\hat{b}_7$ indicates whether the association between birth weight and smoking exposure is likely the same for both races as measured by two odds ratios. Specifically, $\hat{b}_7 = 0$ occurs when the odds ratio from one 2×2 table is identical to the odds ratio from the other 2×2 table. The degree to which $\hat{b}_7$ differs from zero measures the lack of equality between these two odds ratios; sometimes referred to as a measure of homogeneity (e.g., white observations—$\hat{or}_1 = 1.737$ versus black observations—$\hat{or}_2 = 1.654$). For the birth weight data, $\hat{b}_7 = -0.049$ and $e^{\hat{b}_7} = e^{-0.049} = 0.952$, which is the ratio $\hat{or}_1/\hat{or}_2 = 1.654/1.737 = 0.952$. The coefficient associated with the three-variable product term, in fact, measures the degree to which any pair of odds ratios differs between the two levels of the other variable.

Like the 2×2 table, the coefficient associated with each pairwise product term potentially reflects the degree of association between the two categorical variables. These summary measures of association are based on combining information from both 2×2 subtables. Therefore, accurate (unbiased) estimates of the pairwise associations are only possible when the underlying association is the same within each 2×2 subtable ($\hat{b}_7$ is at least small and inconsequential). That is, the odds ratios from each subtable differ only because of sampling variation. The "t value" calculated for the $x1 : x2 : x3$ term or a comparison of the saturated model with the model where the three-way product term is deleted ($b_7 = 0$) provides formal tests of homogeneity between subtables.

A loglinear model requiring each odds ratio to be the same for all levels of the third variable ($b_7 = 0$—$or_1/or_2 = 1$) is

$$\log(F_i) = a + b_1 x_{i1} + b_2 x_{i2} + b_3 x_{i3} + b_4 x_{i1} x_{i2} + b_5 x_{i1} x_{i3} + b_6 x_{i2} x_{i3}$$

and the estimates from the illustrative birth weight/smoking data are

```
> otemp0<- glm(f~x1+x2+x3+x1*x2+x1*x3+x2*x3, family=poisson)
> summary(otemp0,correlation=F)

Call: glm(formula = f~x1+x2+x3+x1*x2+x1*x3+x2*x3,
    family = poisson)
Deviance Residuals:
     1       2       3      4       5      6      7       8
 0.114 -0.042 -0.073 0.020 -0.145 0.078 0.108 -0.046

Coefficients:
                 Value Std. Error       t value
(Intercept)  8.2081534 0.01644852    499.020851
        x1  -1.4428351 0.03707177    -38.920052
        x2  -2.5408890 0.05813175    -43.709147
        x3  -1.5588552 0.03880041    -40.176256
     x1:x2   0.5356726 0.09429772      5.680652
     x1:x3   0.3259687 0.07452370      4.374027
     x2:x3   0.7801173 0.09265514      8.419580

(Dispersion Parameter for Poisson family taken to be 1)
Null Deviance: 9260.431 on 7 degrees of freedom
Residual Deviance: 0.0612935 on 1 degrees of freedom

Number of Fisher Scoring Iterations: 2.
```

Comparison of the residual deviances reflects, as usual, the difference between two nested models. The residual deviance associated with a saturated loglinear model ($b_7 \neq 0$) is as always zero (perfect fit; $D_1 = 0$ with $df_1 = 0$) and the residual deviance when $b_7 = 0$ is $D_0 = 0.061$ with $df_0 = 1$. Then, $D_0 - D_1 = 0.061$ has an approximate chi-square distribution with one degree of freedom when these two models differ only because of random variation. A more extreme difference than 0.061 arises by chance alone with probability 0.804 ($1 - pchisq(0.061, 1)$ returns 0.804) indicating that the term $x1 : x2 : x3$ does not make an important contribution to the model's fit. The result is similar to directly evaluating the coefficient from the saturated model, where $z = \hat{b}_7/S_{\hat{b}_7}$ = $-0.049/0.199 = -0.248$ yields a p-value of 0.804 (from $summary(otemp1)$) for $x1 : x2 : x3$). The Pearson chi-square goodness-of-fit statistic applied to the same data is

```
> sum(residuals(otemp0,type="pearson")^2)
[1] 0.0612554
```

and differs only slightly from the residual deviance measure of goodness-of-fit. These three test-statistics (difference in residual deviance, z-statistic, and

Pearson chi-square) measure the same issue (homogeneity) and are usually similar, particularly for tables with at least moderately large numbers of observations in all cells. For the birth weight example data, these tests indicate that no evidence exists that the odds ratio measuring association between any two variables differs between the levels of a third variable. More specifically, no evidence exists that the association between birth weight and smoking differs between the two races.

The absence of a substantial "three-way" effect means that summarizing the pairwise associations with the estimated coefficients $\hat{b}_4$, $\hat{b}_5$, and $\hat{b}_6$ from the homogeneous model accurately reflect the associations between birth weight and smoking exposure ($x1 : x2$), birth weight and race ($x1 : x3$), and smoking exposure and race ($x2 : x3$). In other words, the estimated relationships within the two 2×2 subtables are sufficiently homogeneous ($\hat{b}_7 \approx 0$) to be combined to summarize the pairwise associations.

The small chi-square statistic (i.e., a small and negligible $\hat{b}_7$-value) implies that the next step in an analysis of a $2 \times 2 \times 2$ table involves assessment of the estimated coefficients associated with the pairwise product terms from the homogeneous model. The test-statistic $z_j = \hat{b}_j / S_{\hat{b}_j}$ produces a formal assessment of the association between pairs of independent variables. For example, $z = 0.536/0.094 = 5.681$ (from *summary(otemp0)* for $x1 : x2$) is a test-statistic with an approximate standard normal distribution when birth weight and smoking status are unrelated ($b_4 = 0$). A value greater than 5.681 is extremely unlikely (p-value < 0.001) leading to the inference that the data provide strong evidence of an association between birth weight and smoking exposure adjusted for race. The two other pairwise relationships (birth weight and race, smoking exposure and race or $x1 : x3$ and $x2 : x3$) are similarly assessed. A series of nested models can also be compared to evaluate the pairwise associations. As before, the two approaches generally produce similar results.

The estimated cell frequencies based on homogeneity among the subtables ($b_7 = 0$) are, as usual, calculated with *predict( )* and from the birth weight model

```
> ex<- exp(predict(otemp0))
> # f = observed and ex = expected frequencies
> round(cbind(x1,x2,x3,f,ex),3)
  x1 x2 x3    f        ex
1  1  1  0  118   116.758
2  1  0  0  866   867.242
3  0  1  1  288   289.242
4  0  0  0 3672  3670.758
5  1  1  1   73    74.242
6  1  0  1  254   252.758
7  0  1  1  134   132.758
8  0  0  1  771   772.242.
```

The odds ratios, as required by the model, are identical for each subtable when calculated from these estimated values. For example, the smoking/birth weight association in whites is estimated by

$$or_1 = (116.758)(3670.758)/(867.242)(289.242) = 1.709$$

and in blacks

$$or_2 = (74.242)(772.242)/(252.758)(132.758) = 1.709.$$

More directly, $\hat{b}_4 = 0.536$ and $e^{\hat{b}_4} = e^{0.536} = 1.709$ summarizes the birth weight/smoking association accounting for race. The odds ratios measuring the birth weight/race association ($e^{\hat{b}_6} = e^{0.326} = 1.385$) and the smoking/race association ($e^{\hat{b}_5} = e^{0.780} = 2.181$) are also identical at both levels of the third variable. The estimated coefficients (estimated odds ratios) are fundamental summaries of the relationships among the categorical variables used to create the $2 \times 2 \times 2$ contingency table as long as $b_7 = 0$ or, at least, $\hat{b}_7$ is small and inconsequential. For the example birth weight data, the pairwise associations are summarized by $summary(otemp0)$ and, most importantly,

association	symbols	$\hat{b}_j$	$\hat{or}$	z_j	p-value
birth weight/smoking	$x1 : x2$	0.536	1.709	5.681	<0.001
birth weight/race	$x1 : x3$	0.326	1.385	4.374	<0.001
smoking/race	$x2 : x3$	0.780	2.181	8.420	<0.001

MULTIDIMENSIONAL—k-LEVEL VARIABLES

Loglinear models apply to any size table constructed from any number of categorical variables with any number of levels. Two not very important differences arise when a table is larger than a $2 \times 2 \times 2$ table. First, association between variables with more than two levels cannot be expressed in terms of odds ratios. Second, the unordered categorical variables with more than two levels need to be communicated to the S-analysis using specialized design variables. Nevertheless, coefficients associated with the pairwise terms in the linear model remain potential summary measures of pairwise associations and three-variable coefficients indicate the degree of homogeneity among these pairwise relationships.

To illustrate, data collected on ABO blood types of parents and the gender of their child are given in Table 6.4. The parental variables consist of four levels (A, B, AB, and O blood types—mother's and father's blood type are coded 1, 2, 3, and 4). The fact that these values indicate unordered categories and not a sequence of consecutive integers must be communicated to the *glm*( ) function. The S-function *factor*( ) converts the variable named between the parentheses into an unordered categorical variable. For example, if

```
> c1<- c(1,2,3,4,1,2,3,4,1,2,3,4,1,2,3,4)
> c1
 [1]  1 2 3 4 1 2 3 4 1 2 3 4 1 2 3 4
> c1+3
 [1]  4 5 6 7 4 5 6 7 4 5 6 7 4 5 6 7
> f1<- factor(c1)
> f1
 [1]  1 2 3 4 1 2 3 4 1 2 3 4 1 2 3 4
> f1+3
Error in Ops.factor(f1, 3): "+" not meaningful for factors.
```

The newly created variable $f1$ is interpreted by *glm*( ) and other S-functions as a four-level categorical variable where the categories have no specific ordering.

"Factoring" turns a variable identifying the k levels of a categorical variable into $k - 1$ dummy or design variables. There are a number of ways design variables represent categories but the end results of the analysis are unaffected. One approach consists of using 0's and 1's to indicate membership in a specific category. Continuing the four-level example, the value 1 (type-A) is replaced with the vector variable {1, 0, 0, 0}, the value 2 (type-B) is replaced with the vector variable {0, 1, 0, 0}, the value 3 (type-AB) is replaced with the vector variable {0, 0, 1, 0} and the value 4 (type-O) is replaced with the vector variable {0, 0, 0, 1}. Only three of these "factored" variables are necessary to identify four categories when a constant term is included in the model. "Factoring" a variable into a set of design variables automatically produces $k - 1$ new variables that are interpreted by S-functions as representing a k-level unordered categorical variable.

To further illustrate, if the first six fathers in the ABO data have blood types {A, O, O, A, AB, B} coded as {1, 4, 4, 1, 3, 2}, then "factoring" produces

father	ABO	code	factor (vector)
father 1	A	1	000
father 2	O	4	001
father 3	O	4	001
father 4	A	1	000
father 5	AB	3	010
father 6	B	2	100

Table 6.4. Number of children by mother ABO-blood type, father ABO-blood type, and the sex of the child

father/mother	A	B	AB	O
MALE				
A	114	218	24	267
B	231	685	63	843
AB	33	71	8	94
O	308	877	84	1014
FEMALE				
A	93	206	30	293
B	237	640	51	803
AB	37	72	9	101
O	279	800	79	989

or

	mother	father	sex	count
1	1	1	1	114
2	1	2	1	231
3	1	3	1	33
4	1	4	1	308
5	1	1	0	93
6	1	2	0	237
7	1	3	0	37
8	1	4	0	279
9	2	1	1	218
10	2	2	1	685
11	2	3	1	71
12	2	4	1	877
13	2	1	0	206
14	2	2	0	640
15	2	3	0	72
16	2	4	0	800
17	3	1	1	24
18	3	2	1	63
19	3	3	1	8
20	3	4	1	84
21	3	1	0	30
22	3	2	0	51
23	3	3	0	9
24	3	4	0	79
25	4	1	1	267
26	4	2	1	843
27	4	3	1	94
28	4	4	1	1014
29	4	1	0	293
30	4	2	0	803
31	4	3	0	101
32	4	4	0	989

Consider a model where the relationships among paternal blood type, maternal blood type, and the sex of their child are postulated as homogeneous. That is, the pairwise associations are assumed the same, except for random variation, at all levels of the other variable (i.e., the relationship between the child's gender and the father's blood type is the same regardless of the mother's blood type, the mother/father blood type association is the same for both male and female offspring, and the association between the child's gender and the mother's blood type is the same regardless of the father's blood type). Based on this assumption, the corresponding estimates and summaries using a homogeneous loglinear model (no $x1 * x2 * x3$ term—$b_7 = 0$) are

```
> # count = the 32 cell frequencies (vector)
> mother<- factor(mvalues)
> father<- factor(fvalues)
> otemp4<- glm(count~mother+father+sex+mother*father+
    mother*sex+father*sex,family=poisson)
> summary(otemp4,correlation=F)

Call: glm(formula = count ~mother +father+sex+mother*father
    +mother*sex+father*sex, family = poisson)

Deviance Residuals:
      Min        1Q        Median         3Q        Max
 -0.9519708 -0.1774194 -0.0005912162 0.1710533 0.9142597

Coefficients:
                        Value     Std. Error      t value
      (Intercept)   4.9828447320  0.030033017  165.91222915
          mother1   0.4374295500  0.028167674   15.52948808
          mother2  -0.5996342839  0.032518543  -18.43976450
          mother3   0.3281230122  0.011309967   29.01184556
          father1   0.4598822613  0.029988662   15.33520424
          father2  -0.5081671061  0.030658282  -16.57519848
          father3   0.3042732691  0.011293315   26.94277769
              sex   0.0212911041  0.038938787    0.54678396
   mother1father1   0.0808869798  0.025101667    3.22237482
   mother2father1  -0.0383780175  0.028776979   -1.33363608
   mother3father1   0.0222497693  0.010113951    2.19990877
   mother1father2  -0.0273780187  0.025712603   -1.06477041
   mother2father2   0.0049758644  0.029731671    0.16735905
   mother3father2  -0.0029802965  0.010430920   -0.28571751
   mother1father3   0.0281926469  0.009507670    2.96525289
   mother2father3  -0.0002970107  0.010913926   -0.02721392
   mother3father3   0.0015065947  0.003813792    0.39503852
       mother1sex   0.0054898733  0.032155906    0.17072675
       mother2sex  -0.0029250038  0.037329286   -0.07835681
       mother3sex  -0.0126489471  0.012863136   -0.98334859
       father1sex   0.0249467419  0.032964495    0.75677609
       father2sex  -0.0290977598  0.034170615   -0.85154335
       father3sex   0.0159122317  0.012337747    1.28971936

(Dispersion Parameter for Poisson family taken to be 1)
Null Deviance: 10201.46 on 31 degrees of freedom
Residual Deviance: 5.401238 on 9 degrees of freedom

Number of Fisher Scoring Iterations: 3.
```

Paternal (*father*) and maternal (*mother*) blood type codes are converted into unordered categorical variables where three coefficients measure the total influence of the $k = 4$ blood type categories for each parent. Specifically, *father*<– *factor*(*fvalue*) and *mother*<– *factor*(*mvalue*) produce S-design variables. The variable gender (*sex*) is binary {0,1} and is also an unordered categorical variable but does not requiring "factoring."

The residual deviance (5.401) indicates that this homogeneous model (no $x1 : x2 : x3$ term) is a good representation of the $4 \times 4 \times 2$ contingency table data (Table 6.4). The residual deviance has an approximate chi-square distribution with nine degrees of freedom yielding the probability of more extreme random differences between data and estimates by chance alone as 0.798 or

```
> 1-pchisq(otemp4$deviance,otemp4$df.residual)
[1] 0.7980234.
```

A classic chi-square approach also can be used to evaluate the goodness-of-fit of a loglinear model by directly comparing observed and estimated values. For the ABO example data:

```
> excount<- exp(predict(otemp4))
> x2<- sum((count-excount)^2/excount)
> df<- otemp4$df.residual
> pvalue<- 1-pchisq(x2,df)
> round(cbind(x2,df,pvalue),3)
        x2       df      pvalue
[1,] 5.395        9       0.799.
```

As noted, an approach based on the traditional chi-square statistic and one based on the residual deviance are usually similar (5.395 versus 5.401 for the ABO data).

Starting with the loglinear model requiring homogeneity among the variables (*otemp*4), a series of nested models is readily generated to evaluate the role of each of the three categorical (independent) variables or, for example,

model 1:

no relationships exist among the three variables (no pairwise associations).

model 2:

gender and parental blood type are unrelated (one pairwise association) and

model 3:

gender and paternal blood types are unrelated (two pairwise associations), and

model 4:

all three variables are pairwise related (three pairwise associations—homogeneous),

The evaluation of this sequence of nested models is achieved by

```
> otemp1<- glm(count~mother+father+sex,family=poisson)
> otemp2<- glm(count~mother+father+sex+mother*father,
      family=poisson)
> otemp3<- glm(count~mother+father+sex+mother*father+
      mother*sex,family=poisson)
> otemp4<- glm(count~mother+father+sex+mother*father+
      mother*sex+father*sex,family=poisson)
```

```
> anova(otemp1,otemp2,otemp3,otemp4)
```

```
Analysis of Deviance Table
Response: count
```

Terms	Res.Dev	Test	Df	Deviance
mother+father+sex	29.763			
mother+father+sex+mother*father	9.385	mother:father	9	20.378
mother+father+sex+mother*father+mother*sex	7.495	mother:sex	3	1.890
mother+father+sex+mother*father+mother*sex+father*sex	5.401	father:sex	3	2.094.

The sequence of test-statistics ("Deviance") shows no evidence of important associations between paternal or maternal blood types and the sex of the offspring. However, the analysis does indicate a likely systematic association between parental blood types (chi-square value = 20.378 with nine degrees of freedom yields a p-value of 0.016). A closer look at this analysis is generated by exploring observed and expected values for each of the 32 individual cells of the data table or, for example,

```
> ex<- exp(predict(otemp1))
> rvalues<- residuals(otemp1,type="pearson")
> round(cbind(mother,father,sex,count,ex,rvalues),3)
```

	mother	father	sex	count	ex	rvalues
1	1	1	1	114	87.811	2.795
2	1	2	1	231	250.596	-1.238
3	1	3	1	33	29.976	0.552
4	1	4	1	308	312.451	-0.252
5	1	1	0	93	83.984	0.984
6	1	2	0	237	239.676	-0.173
7	1	3	0	37	28.669	1.556
8	1	4	0	279	298.836	-1.147
9	2	1	1	218	235.283	-1.127
10	2	2	1	685	671.454	0.523
11	2	3	1	71	80.317	-1.040
12	2	4	1	877	837.191	1.376
13	2	1	0	206	225.030	-1.269
14	2	2	0	640	642.195	-0.087
15	2	3	0	72	76.818	-0.550
16	2	4	0	800	800.711	-0.025
17	3	1	1	24	22.942	0.221
18	3	2	1	63	65.471	-0.305
19	3	3	1	8	7.831	0.060
20	3	4	1	84	81.631	0.262
21	3	1	0	30	21.942	1.720
22	3	2	0	51	62.618	-1.468
23	3	3	0	9	7.490	0.552
24	3	4	0	79	78.074	0.105
25	4	1	1	267	290.330	-1.369
26	4	2	1	843	828.547	0.502
27	4	3	1	94	99.108	-0.513
28	4	4	1	1014	1033.060	-0.593
29	4	1	0	293	277.678	0.919
30	4	2	0	803	792.443	0.375
31	4	3	0	101	94.790	0.638
32	4	4	0	989	988.044	0.030.

The column labeled "rvalues" contains the Pearson residual values. These values measure individual standardized differences between the observed and expected counts by

$$r_i = \frac{count_i - estimate_i}{\sqrt{variance(estimate_i)}}$$

where *estimate*$_i$ is calculated under a specific model. The assumption that no associations exist (additivity) between any combination of the independent variables (*otemp*1—no product terms) produces the r_i-values (*rvalues* in the output) from the ABO data. The strictly additive model (Model 1) postulates purely separate effects from the three variables (independence). The Pearson residual values r_i identify where the estimated values are similar to the observed values and where they differ. Values greater than 1.6 in absolute value likely reflect important lack of fit. For the example data, the two largest deviations are associated with A-type fathers.

HIGH DIMENSIONAL TABLES

When four or more variables are used to create a table, evaluating all possible models becomes cumbersome and inefficient. There are $2^k - 1$ different models for a k-dimensional table. A primary analytic goal is to find a model that is as simple as possible but faithfully represents the relationships within a complex, high dimensional table. A starting point for selecting a simple but useful loglinear model to represent data from a high dimensional table is the saturated loglinear model. A saturated model has as many model parameters as there are cells in the table, offering little gain over that data itself. However, the estimates of the model coefficients and their standard errors begin to indicate the importance of each variable and combinations of variables in describing the tabular data. The simple fact that the coefficients associated with the inconsequential variables will likely be small and the coefficients associated with the important variables will likely be large relative to their standard errors provides a strategy for selecting a simpler model to represent the relationships within a table. The relative "importance" of each model coefficient $\hat{b}_j$ (model components) is evaluated by dividing by its standard error where $z_j = \hat{b}_j / S_{\hat{b}_j}$ ("t value" in *summary*( ) output).

Data on $n = 9,744$ births tabulated (Table 6.5) by race (white, black, Hispanic, and Asian), by birth weight (< 2500 grams and ≥ 2500 grams), by gestation (premature < 38 weeks and term ≥ 38 weeks), by parity (no previous pregnancies and one or more), and by gender (male and female) form a $4 \times 2 \times 2 \times 2 \times 2$ table with 64 cells.

Table 6.5. Numbers of infants classified by race (white, black, Hispanic, and Asian), birth weight (< 2500 grams versus ≥ 2500 grams), gestation (< 38 weeks versus ≥ 38 weeks), parity (0 versus 1 or more), and gender (male versus female)

	male			female	
race	≥ 2500 grams	< 2500 grams	race	≥ 2500 grams	< 2500 grams
PARITY = 0 AND GESTATION ≥ 38 WEEKS					
white	903	69	white	805	102
black	201	44	black	181	54
hispanic	258	23	hispanic	238	27
asian	368	71	asian	374	81
PARITY ≥ 1 AND GESTATION ≥ 38 WEEKS					
white	1089	129	white	1041	126
black	199	50	black	183	68
hispanic	216	29	hispanic	165	27
asian	453	103	asian	365	110
PARITY = 0 AND GESTATION < 38 WEEKS					
white	39	141	white	31	145
black	20	58	black	13	64
hispanic	20	68	hispanic	14	48
asian	29	36	asian	11	45
PARITY ≥ 1 AND GESTATION < 38 WEEKS					
white	57	163	white	37	135
black	6	50	black	11	44
hispanic	18	42	hispanic	5	41
asian	27	58	asian	17	60

One purpose of constructing this five-dimensional table is to assess the influence of previous pregnancies on the distribution of low birth weight infants. To understand the role of parity, a model is needed to accurately describe the relationships among race, birth weight, gestation, parity, and sex but as simply as possible. Once a model is established, the role of parity can be isolated from the other four variables. Table 6.6 displays the 64 estimates of the coefficients ($\hat{b}_j$) from the saturated model for these data (number of coefficients = 64 = number of cells in the table).

The key estimates from the saturated model are extracted with the S-commands

```
> b<- summary(otemp)$coefficients[,1]
> z<- summary(otemp)$coefficients[,3]
> zrank<- rank(-abs(z))
```

producing the corresponding columns $\hat{b}_j$, z_j, and "rank" in Table 6.6 where the S-object *otemp* is generated from the saturated model with all possible 64 terms (*Residual deviance* = 0).

The magnitude of the standardized coefficients (z_j) or their ranks identify those variables that play an important role in determining the cell frequencies (low ranks). Conversely, a number of the variables and combinations of vari-

Table 6.6. Coefficients from the saturated model ($\hat{b}_j$) and a reduced model ($\hat{b}_j'$); variables are race, birth weight, gestation, parity, and sex ($4 \times 2 \times 2 \times 2 \times 2$ table)

term	$\hat{b}_j$	z_z	rank	$\hat{b}_j'$	term	$\hat{b}_j$	z_j	rank	$\hat{b}_j'$
(Intercept)	4.263	207.797	1	4.278	race1gestsex	0.027	0.996	41	–
race1	−0.565	−21.159	4	−0.557	race2gestsex	−0.024	−1.269	36	–
race2	−0.236	−12.571	5	0.234	race3gestsex	−0.003	−0.262	58	–
race3	0.022	2.011	24	0.023	bwt:gest:sex	0.019	0.904	42	–
bwt	−0.123	−5.982	6	−0.133	race1bwtparity	0.040	1.515	31	–
gest	−0.717	−34.952	3	−0.703	race2bwtparity	0.015	0.791	46	–
sex	−0.056	−2.737	16	−0.051	race3bwtparity	0.002	0.140	61	–
parity	0.004	0.213	59	−0.006	race1gestparity	−0.050	−1.873	27	–
race1bwt	0.149	5.584	7	0.143	race2gestparity	0.000	−0.011	64	–
race2bwt	−0.035	−1.865	28	−0.038	race3gestparity	0.027	2.407	21	–
race3bwt	−0.005	−0.450	55	−0.005	bwt:gest:parity	−0.012	−0.578	51	–
race1gest	0.002	0.086	63	0.011	race1sexparity	0.053	1.986	25	–
race2gest	0.049	2.610	17	0.052	race2sexparity	−0.023	−1.225	38	–
race3gest	−0.061	−5.459	8	−0.060	race3sexparity	0.005	0.423	56	–
bwt:gest	0.760	37.055	2	0.749	bwt:sex:parity	−0.016	−0.765	47	–
race1sex	0.034	1.268	37	0.006	gest:sex:parity	0.016	0.799	45	–
race2sex	−0.046	−2.436	20	−0.021	race1bwtgestsex	−0.027	−1.029	40	–
race3sex	−0.006	−0.520	53	0.000	race2bwtgestsex	0.027	1.432	32	–
bwt:sex	0.083	4.049	10	0.067	race3bwtgestsex	0.021	1.854	29	–
gest:sex	−0.065	−3.145	14	−0.062	race1bwtgestparity	0.043	1.597	30	–
race1parity	−0.108	−4.030	11	−0.066	race2bwtgestparity	−0.002	−0.097	62	–
race2parity	−0.047	−2.521	18	−0.055	race3bwtgestparity	0.002	0.179	60	–
race3parity	0.040	0.577	12	0.022	race1bwtsexparity	−0.021	−0.799	44	–
bwt:parity	0.051	2.500	19	0.042	race2bwtsexparity	0.043	2.266	22	–
gest:parity	−0.064	−3.123	15	−0.057	race3bwtsexparity	−0.006	−0.520	54	–
sex:parity	−0.013	−0.633	49	−0.015	race1gestsexparity	0.024	0.890	43	–
race1bwtgest	−0.087	−3.263	13	−0.093	race2gestsexparity	−0.010	−0.538	52	–
race2bwtgest	0.024	1.284	35	0.022	race3gestsexparity	0.007	0.659	48	–
race3bwtgest	−0.055	−4.947	9	−0.054	bwt:gest:sex:parity	−0.007	−0.339	57	–
race1bwtsex	−0.017	−0.623	50	–	race1bwtgestsexparity	−0.057	−2.123	23	–
race2bwtsex	0.020	1.044	39	–	race2bwtgestsexparity	0.036	1.916	26	–
race3bwtsex	0.016	1.412	33	–	race3bwtgestsexparity	−0.016	−1.399	34	–

ables are seen to play only a small part in the model describing the relationships among the five variables used to create the table (high ranks). Eliminating these variables produces a simpler and potentially more useful model. For these data on newborn infants, the model selected includes the basic variables (*race, birthweight, gestation, sex, parity*), all pairwise combinations of these variables (*race * bwt, race * gest, bwt * gest, race * sex, bwt * sex, gest * sex, race * parity, bwt * parity, gest * parity, sex * parity*) and a single three-variable term (*race * bwt * gest*). The model has 29 parameters (listed as the first 29 lines in Table 6.6—$\hat{b}_j'$).

Using the S-function *glm( )* where

```
> otemp1<- glm(data~(race+bwt+gest+sex+parity)^2+gest*race*bwt,
    family=poisson
```

produces the estimated coefficients $\hat{b}_j'$ (Table 6.6). Comparing estimated and observed cell counts yields

```
> ex<- exp(predict(otemp1))
> xtemp<- (data-ex)/sqrt(ex)
> x2<- sum(xtemp^2)
> x2
[1] 44.01109
> 1-pchisq(x2,otemp1$df.residual)
[1] 0.141274
```

indicating that the simpler model (29 rather than 64 parameters) adequately represents the rather complex relationships among these five variables.

A specialized S-notation allows complex models to be communicated to the *glm*-function in a compact, short-cut form. For the example, the formula $(race + bwt + gest + sex + parity)\text{^}2$ is expanded to include all second order terms and all associated lower order terms, a model with 28 terms. The notation generalizes so that $(A + B + C + D + \cdots)\text{^}k$ produces all k-order terms and all associated lower order terms of the model involving the variables $A, B, C, D, \cdots$. The simplest case $(A + B)\text{^}2$ produces the model $A + B + A * B$. The expression $(A + B + C)\text{^}2$ expands to $A + B + C + A * B + A * C + B * C$. A similar S-convention also exists where naming only the highest k-order term in the *glm*-function produces an S-formula with the named term and all the hierarchical lower order terms. For example, $glm(data\text{~}A * B * C)$ expands to an eight-term model identical to $glm(data\text{~}A + B + C + A * B + A * C + B * C + A * B * C)$. For the birth weight data (Table 6.5),

```
> otemp<- glm(data~race*bwt*gest*sex*parity,family=poisson)
```

produces the 64-term saturated model where *data* is a vector containing the 64 cell counts and the saturated model produces 64 parameter estimates (Table 6.6).

To assess the role of parity, a model is postulated with the parity variable excluded from the previous 29-parameter model forming a 22-parameter model or

```
> otemp0<- glm(data~(race+bwt+gest+sex)^2+gest*race*bwt,
    family=poisson)
```

The fit of this model is dramatically changed by ignoring the parity variable. Specifically, the residual deviance including parity is 45.449 (*otemp1$deviance*) and excluding parity is 153.076 (*otemp0$deviance*). The difference of 107.627 has an approximate chi-square distribution with seven degrees of freedom when the two models differ by chance (p-value < 0.001). Despite the complicated relationships among the five variables in the table, the comparison of residual deviance values identifies a strong role of previous pregnancies in the distribution of the newborn data given in Table 6.5.

Searching a saturated model for important features to create a simpler model to describe and analyze tabular data is not a perfect solution to selecting an efficient model to represent high dimensional data. The values of the estimated coefficients and their estimated standard errors depend on the model used to make the estimates. The estimates derived from a saturated model differ, sometimes substantially, from those estimated from a model with fewer terms. The $\hat{b}_j'$-column in Table 6.6 shows the parallel estimates made from a simpler model ($\hat{b}_j$ versus $\hat{b}_j'$). The difference is caused by employing different models in the estimation process, producing different estimates as well as different estimated standard errors. It is not the least surprising that the estimates made from one model are not appropriate for another. Therefore, z-values reflecting the influences of the variables in the saturated model are only indications of the roles that variables might play in a more restricted model. Using a saturated model to choose an efficient subset of variables is a sensible but not a perfect model selection strategy due to the bias ("wrong model bias") in both the coefficients and their standard errors estimated from the saturated model.

Problem set VI

1. For the data in the following table, work out the estimated values of $\hat{a}$, $\hat{b}_1$, $\hat{b}_2$, and $\hat{b}_3$ for the saturated model algebraically:

a_i	b_i	f_{ij}	F_i	data
0	0	f_{00}	F_1	23
1	0	f_{10}	F_2	12
0	1	f_{01}	F_3	45
1	1	f_{11}	F_4	122

Verify the results using an S-program.

2. If n and p are parameters of a binomial distribution, then

$$z_0 = \frac{x - np}{\sqrt{np(1 - p)}} \quad \text{and} \quad z_1 \frac{x - np \pm 0.5}{\sqrt{np(1 - p)}}$$

provide approximate binomial probabilities (i.e., $pnorm \approx pbinom$). Compare the maximum difference between the exact binomial and normal approximated probabilities for $n = 10$, $p = 0.5$; $n = 20$, $p = 0.2$; $n = 50$, $p = 0.1$; and $n = 100$, $p = 0.05$.

3.   Consider the 2×4 table:

	$X = 0$	$X = 1$	$X = 2$	$X = 3$	total
$Y = 0$	1	7	15	40	63
$Y = 1$	4	19	34	42	99
total	5	26	49	82	162

Compute S_{xx}, S_{yy} and S_{xy}.

Calculate the chi-square statistics reflecting the total, linear, and non-linear influences. Demonstrate that the correlation between X and Y based on $n = 162$ pairs (X,Y), called the point biserial correlation coefficient, is directly related to the chi-square statistic reflecting the linear association or

$$r_{XY} = \sqrt{\frac{linear\ chi\ square\ statistic}{n - 1}}.$$

4. Show* algebraically that $or_1 / or_2 = e^{\hat{b}_7}$ when a saturated loglinear model is applied to a $2 \times 2 \times 2$ table where or_1 is the odds ratio calculated from one 2 by 2 subtable and or_2 is the odds ratio calculated from the other subtable.

5. An estimate of the variance of Yule's measure of association Y is

$$variance(Y) = \frac{1}{4}(1 - Y^2)^2 \left[\frac{1}{F_1} + \frac{1}{F_2} + \frac{1}{F_3} + \frac{1}{F_4} \right].$$

Create an S-function to calculate Y, the variance of Y and to construct an approximate 95% confidence interval for the expected value of Y. Show that Yule's Y is equivalent to the odds ratio measure $\hat{or}$ in a 2 by 2 table.

6. Demonstrate that the expected values calculated under the hypothesis of statistical independence (usual chi-square expected values—Chapter 1 example) are essentially the same as the estimates of the cell frequencies based on a loglinear additive model using the following data:

	b_1	b_2	b_3	b_4
a_1	12	8	22	4
a_2	5	3	11	2
a_3	26	17	44	10
a_4	53	38	82	18
a_5	108	75	167	44

7. Consider the following $2 \times 2 \times 2$ table:

x_1	x_2	x_3	F_i	count
1	1	0	F_1	$\hat{F}_1 = 11 + e$
1	0	0	F_2	$\hat{F}_2 = 8 - e$
0	1	0	F_3	$\hat{F}_3 = 12 - e$
0	0	0	F_4	$\hat{F}_4 = 37 + e$
1	1	1	F_5	$\hat{F}_5 = 22 - e$
1	0	1	F_6	$\hat{F}_6 = 5 + e$
0	1	1	F_7	$\hat{F}_7 = 3 + e$
0	0	1	F_8	$\hat{F}_8 = 7 - e$

Find the value e such that no interaction exists (i.e., $\hat{or}_1 = \hat{or}_2$). Display the "data" ($\hat{F}_i$) and show that the odds ratios measuring the association between any two variables at both levels of the third variable are the same. Use a loglinear model applied to the created "data" ($\hat{F}_i = F_i \pm e$ value) to show that the $x1 * x2 * x3$-term is zero (exact homogeneity).

* Solve theoretically and not with a computer program.

REFERENCES

1. Bithell, J. F. and Steward, M. A., (1975) Prenatal irradiation and childhood malignancy: A review of British data from the Oxford study. *British Journal of Cancer*, 31:271–287.
2. Selvin, S., *Statistical Analysis of Epidemiologic Data*. Oxford University Press, New York, NY, 1996.
3. Haldane, J. B. S., (1956) The estimation and significance of the logarithm of a ratio of frequencies. *Annals of Human Genetics*, 20:309–311.
4. Freeman, D. H., *Applied Categorical Data*. Marcel Dekker, New York, NY, 1987.
5. Upton, G. J. G., *The Analysis of Cross-tabulated Data*. John Wiley & Sons, New York, NY, 1978.
6. Bishop, Y. M. M., Fienberg, S. E., and Holland P. W., *Discrete Multivariate Analysis: Theory and Practice*. The MIT Press, Cambridge, MA, 1975.
7. Snedecor, G. W. and Cochran, W. G., *Statistical Methods*. The Iowa State University Press, Ames, IA, 1974.

7

Analysis of Variance and Some Other S-Functions

ANALYSIS OF VARIANCE

Analysis of variance is a special case of a general linear model where the dependent variable is continuous and the independent variables are categorical. This specialized statistical structure makes no real difference in principle. As before, the S-function *glm( )* can be used to evaluate differing analytic linear models by comparing specific residual deviances. However, differences exist in language and style so that separate S-functions are available particularly tailored to the analysis of variance approach. The following focuses on a few of the simplest but important data collection designs and the corresponding analysis of variance techniques.

ONE-WAY DESIGN

A one-way design involves a continuous dependent variable classified by a series of levels of a single categorical variable. The fundamental question is: does the response variable systematically differ among one or more of the categories? If the population mean values associated with each of k categories differ, these differences should be reflected in the sample mean values. Typically, a sample of size n_j observations is collected from each of the k categories and the sample mean values $\bar{y}_j$ calculated. Differences among these sample means are a basis to judge whether there is sufficient evidence to infer that differences exist among the k populations from which the data were sampled.

The symbol y_{ij} represents a measurement on the ith observation within the jth category. The notation for a sample of such data is displayed in Table 7.1. The symbol S_j^2, as before, represents the estimated variance based on n_j observations from within the jth category.

Table 7.1. Notation for a one-way table and corresponding analysis of variance

	category 1	category 2	category 3	$\cdots$	category k
observation 1	y_{11}	y_{12}	y_{13}	$\cdots$	y_{1k}
observation 2	y_{21}	y_{22}	y_{23}	$\cdots$	y_{2k}
observation 3	y_{31}	y_{32}	y_{33}	$\cdots$	y_{3k}
$\vdots$	$\vdots$	$\vdots$	$\vdots$	$\vdots$	$\vdots$
observation n_j	y_{n_11}	y_{n_22}	y_{n_33}	$\cdots$	y_{n_kk}
sample size	n_1	n_2	n_3	$\cdots$	n_k
sample mean	$\bar{y}_1$	$\bar{y}_2$	$\bar{y}_3$	$\cdots$	$\bar{y}_k$
sample variance	S_1^2	S_2^2	S_3^2	$\cdots$	S_k^2

Two sums of squares are the key elements for an analysis of data collected in a one-way design—the within sum of squares and the total sum of squares. The within sum of squares is calculated under the assumption that the data within each category are sampled from populations with different mean values but with the same variance. It is further assumed that these observations have at least an approximately normal distribution. The within sum of squares is defined as

$$SS_{within} = \sum\sum(y_{ij} - \bar{y}_j)^2 \quad \text{where } i = 1, 2, 3, \cdots, n_j \quad \text{and} \quad j = 1, 2, 3, \cdots, k.$$

The quantity represented by SS_{within} has a chi-square distribution with $n - k$ degrees of freedom when the normal populations sampled have different mean values. Alternatively, this sum of squares is expressed as a sum of the within category estimated variances each weighted by $n_j - 1$ or $SS_{within} = \sum(n_j - 1)S_j^2$. The within sum of squares, as the name implies, combines the variability within each of the k categories, producing a single summary reflecting the variation among the observed values unaffected by any differences among categories.

The total sum of squares is calculated to evaluate the conjecture that only random differences exist among the sampled observations. That is, the k populations of normally distributed data (with the same variance) differ only because of random variation. The total sum of squares reflects both the variability among the observations (random variation) and any influences from diffrences among the k categories where

$$SS_{total} = \sum\sum(y_{ij} - \bar{y}_{\cdot})^2 \quad \text{where } i = 1, 2, 3, \cdots, n_j \quad \text{and} \quad j = 1, 2, 3, \cdots, k.$$

The mean value $\bar{y}$ is estimated by combining all $n = \sum n_j$ observed values and computing a single mean value. When no differences exist among the k normal populations sampled, then the quantity represented by SS_{total} has a chi-square distribution with $n - 1$ degrees of freedom. The within sum of squares excludes the variation among groups and the total sum of squares includes any group to group variation. Comparison then reflects on the impact of the group classification on the measured outcome. Identical to the linear model approach (Chapter 4), a formal comparison of the within and the total sums of squares is accomplished by calculating

$$F = \frac{(SS_{total} - SS_{within})/k}{SS_{within}/(n-k)}.$$

The test-statistic F again has an F-distribution with k and $n-k$ degrees of freedom when differences among the $\bar{y}_j$ values are due strictly to random variation. The F-distribution, as always, allows a probability to be associated with the observed F-statistic leading to an assessment of the hypothesis that only random differences exist among the k sampled populations.

To illustrate, consider the data from the previous linear regression example (Table 4.1). Birth weight, maternal height, prepregnancy weight, and weight gained during pregnancy are formed into a data frame by

```
> dframe<- read.table("bwt.data",header=T)
> attach(dframe)
> summary(dframe)
         bwt             ht              wt             gain
Min.    :0.670   Min.   :144.7   Min.   :40.90   Min.   :1.20
1stQu.  :3.085   1stQu. :157.5   1stQu. :51.27   1stQu. :11.80
Median  :3.400   Median :162.6   Median :55.95   Median :15.85
Mean    :3.332   Mean   :163.2   Mean   :58.41   Mean   :15.72
3rdQu.  :3.719   3rdQu. :167.6   3rdQu. :61.85   3rdQu. :19.10
Max.    :4.780   Max.   :197.0   Max.   :122.20  Max.   :33.40.
```

The S-function that produces an analysis of variance object is *aov*( ), which has a general form much like the S-function *glm*( ) where

aov(*dependent variable~formula, data.frame,* $\cdots$).

The women participating in the birth weight study (Table 4.2) are classified into four ($k = 4$) categories based on their pregnancy weight gain (small, < 11 kilograms; normal, 11–16 kilograms; moderate, 16–22 kilograms; and extreme, > 22 kilograms) to create an analysis of variance illustration. These categories are formed with S-functions *cut*( ). Furthermore, the S-function *tapply*( ) produces summary values based on these categories and

```
> gcuts<- cut(gain,c(-99,11,16,22,99),
  label=c("small","normal","moderate","extreme"))
> cbind(tapply(bwt,gcuts,length),tapply(bwt,gcuts,mean),
  tapply(bwt,gcuts,var))
            [,1]      [,2]         [,3]
   small     48    2.885312   0.6906568
  normal     72    3.360389   0.2207134
moderate     85    3.475647   0.3131415
 extreme     27    3.601111   0.2541737.
```

The three summaries generated by *tapply*( ) are the sample sizes (n_j), the mean birth weights ($\bar{y}_j$), and the estimated variances (S_j^2) for the four weight gain categories. Mean birth weight appears to increase with increases in weight gained by the mother with moderate differences in estimated variability among the four categories. An analysis of variance formally evaluates the observed differences among the $k = 4$ mean values.

A one-way analysis of variance using the categorical variable *gcuts* and the S-function *aov*( ) produces an analysis of the observed differences among the sample birth weight means and

```
> # dframe = previously defined data frame
> gain0<- factor(gcuts)
> otemp<- aov(bwt~gain0,dframe)
> otemp
  Call:
  aov(formula = bwt ~ gain0, data = dframe)

Terms:
                          gain0    Residuals
    Sum of Squares     13.34472     81.04393
    Deg. of Freedom           3          228

  Residual standard error: 0.5962012
  Estimated effects may be unbalanced

> summary(otemp)
            Df   Sum of Sq   Mean  Sq   F Value           Pr(F)
  gain0      3    13.34472   4.448240   12.51418  1.323902e-07
Residuals 228    81.04393   0.355456.
```

The name of the S-object *otemp* (representing the S-object produced by the *aov*( ) function) executed as a command produces the first summary. The command *summary(otemp)* produces the second and more extensive summary. The "F Value" 12.514 is the *F*-statistic that results from comparing sums of squares SS_{total} (*total* = *gain0* + *Residual* = 94.388) and SS_{within} (*within* = *Residual* = 81.044) producing the associated significance probability, *p*-value < 0.001 ("Pr(F)" in the output).

The S-function *factor*( ) described in Chapter 6 in the context of a loglinear model plays the same role in the application of analysis of variance techniques. Say a series of categories are identified by letters such as *cats* = {"A","A","B","B","C","C","A","A","B", · · ·}, then the command *fcats*<– *factor(cats)* produces an unordered categorical variable that can be employed on the right-hand side of the *aov*( ) formula as an independent variable. As a general rule, independent variables identified in the *formula* option of the *aov*( ) command are categorical variables resulting from applying the S-function *factor*( ). In the weight gain example, the four integer values contained in the vector *gcuts* are transformed into design variables by the command *gain0*<–*factor(gcuts)* identifying four unordered categories.

Once the analysis of variance S-object is established (*otemp* in the example) several summary plots readily produce graphic displays of different aspects of the data and analysis. Plots showing the relative values of the mean ($\bar{y}_j$) and the median values (Figure 7.1), for the four weight gain categories, are produced by

```
> plot.design(otemp,main="Birth weigh data")
> plot.design(otemp,fun=median,main="Birth weigh data")
```

These two plots should be similar since the means and medians from each category should be close to the same value when the data are normally distributed. The two commands

```
> par(mfrow=c(1,2))
> plot(otemp,main="Birth weigh data")
```

produce Figure 7.2. The first plot (left side) shows the birth weight data again for the four weight gain categories and the second plot (right side) displays the distribution of the absolute values of the residual values by the same four categories. A basic diagnostic qqnorm plot (Figure 7.3) is produced by

```
> qqnorm(resid(otemp),main="Birth weigh data -- qqnorm")
> qqline(resid(otemp))
```

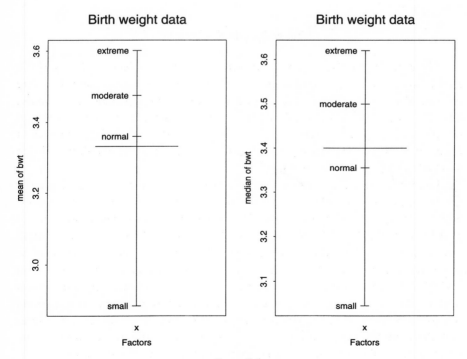

Figure 7.1

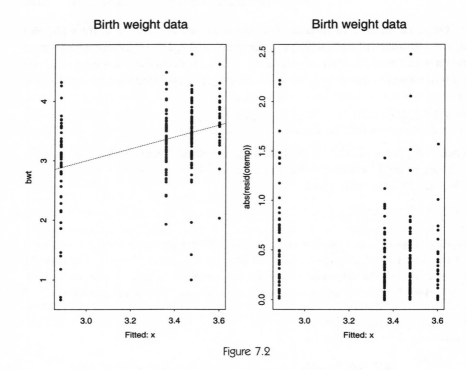

Figure 7.2

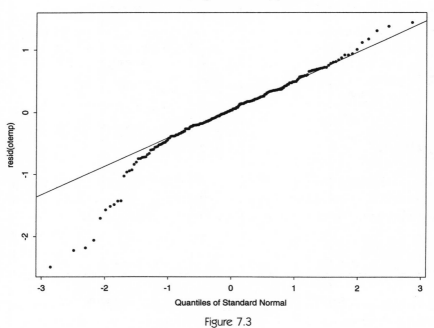

Figure 7.3

If the requirements underlying the analysis of variance are fulfilled, the qqnorm plot of the residual values should be close to the straight line plotted by *qqline*( ).

A nonparametric procedure parallel to a one-way analysis of variance is called the Kruskal–Wallis test. A nonparametric approach is most useful when the sampled data fail to fulfill the requirements of an analysis of variance. The procedure is distribution free since the observations are replaced with their ranks making the distribution that generated the data no longer relevant to the analysis. The basis of the Kruskal–Wallis test is the ranking of the observations (rank 1 = smallest value) without regard to the group membership. The ranks run from 1 to n ($n = \Sigma n_i$). The sum of the ranks from each of the k groups (R_i) is calculated producing k values $R_1, R_2, \cdots, R_k$. If no differences exist among the k populations sampled, then the expected value of each R_i-value is proportional to the number of observations in each category or

$$expected\ sum\ of\ the\ ranks\ within\ the\ i^{th}\ category = ER_i = n_i \frac{n+1}{2}.$$

The expected sum in the ith category is the overall average rank multiplied by the number of observations in that category (n_i). A test statistic to compare the k observed R_i-values to their expected values is

$$X^2 = \frac{12}{n(n+1)} \sum \frac{(R_i - ER_i)^2}{n_i} \qquad i = 1, 2, 3, \cdots, k$$

and X^2 has an approximate chi-square distribution with $k - 1$ degrees of freedom when the populations sampled have the same mean values [1]. A chi-square test to assess observed differences among k categories is easily implemented with the S-function *kruskal.test*(*dependent variable, categories*). For the birth weight data example,

```
> kruskal.test(bwt,gain0)
              Kruskal-Wallis rank sum test
data:  bwt and gain0
Kruskal-Wallis chi-square = 30.5005, df = 3, p-value = 0
alternative hypothesis: two.sided.
```

The Kruskal–Wallis test result is consistent with the parametric F-test (both p-values < 0.001) but, like most nonparametric approaches, is not based on a natural description of the relationships under investigation (R_i versus $\bar{y}_i$).

NESTED DESIGN

A special one-way data collection design is a nested or hierarchical pattern of classifying observations. The simplest nested design involves a single series of groups. Observations belong to a specific group and the data set consists of several different groups. For example, a number of orchards are selected for study, then a number of different types of trees are chosen from each orchard and measured for a particular property—trees are nested within orchards. When each type of tree appears only in one orchard, evaluating the joint of effects of orchard and tree type is not possible. Before an interaction, for example, can be evaluated, each type of tree must be sampled from each orchard.

The S-language allows the representation of a nested data structure by using either of two equivalent symbols, namely "/" or "%in%". When observations classified with respect to variable A (e.g., types of trees) are contained within a second group B (e.g., orchards), the nesting is communicated to the $aov()$ S-function by either B/A or $A\%in\%B$. The syntax B/A places the variable that is nested after the operator and the variable within which the variable is nested before the operator. The values represented by A and B are categorical classification variables.

To illustrate, consider $n = 12$ petroleum workers measured for exposure to o-xylene (parts per million). The data set consists of three refineries and samples were taken over six consecutive days of a week with measurements on two workers per day (no measurements on Sunday). The design is nested since the workers engage in different activities on different days of the week. The classification variables *refineries*, *days* (days of the week) and the dependent variable Y (the observed o-xylene levels) are:

refineries	1	1	1	1	2	2	2	2	3	3	3	3
days	1	1	2	2	3	3	4	4	5	5	6	6
Y	0.12	0.15	0.12	0.13	0.12	0.11	0.12	0.15	0.11	0.12	0.15	0.16

Days are nested within refineries or in S-notation *refineries/days*. To form a data frame

```
> y<- c(0.12,0.15,0.12,0.13,0.12,0.11,0.12,0.15,0.11,
       0.12,0.15,0.16)*100
> x1<- c(1,1,1,1,2,2,2,2,3,3,3,3)
> x2<- c(1,1,2,2,3,3,4,4,5,5,6,6)
> ydata<- data.frame(y=y,refineries=factor(x1),days=factor(x2))
> summary(ydata)
               y      refineries     days
Min.     :11            1:4          1:2
1st Qu.  :12            2:4          2:2
Median   :12            3:4          3:2
Mean     :13                         4:2
3rd Qu.  :15                         5:2
Max.     :16                         6:2.
```

The analysis of variance follows the prescribed pattern and

```
> otemp<- aov(y~refineries+refineries/days,ydata)
> summary(otemp)
                    Df Sum of Sq  Mean Sq  F Value      Pr(F)
  refineries         2         2 1.000000 0.545455 0.6058261
  days %in% refineries 3       21 7.000000 3.818182 0.0764733
  Residuals          6        11 1.833333.
```

The S-commands

```
> aov(y~refineries+days%in%refineries,ydata)
> aov(y~refineries/days,ydata
```

produce identical results. Analysis of the 12 petroleum workers indicates little difference in exposure levels among the refineries and marginal evidence of a difference among days within refineries.

TWO-WAY CLASSIFICATION WITH ONE OBSERVATION PER CELL

After a one-way design, a common data collection pattern is a two-way classification. Frequently, two characteristics (independent variables) serve to classify each observation (dependent variable) forming a two-way table. For example, cholesterol levels might be classified by gender (male or female) and, at the same time, by the individual's socio-economic status (low, medium, or high). Again, the dependent variable is a measured outcome value and the independent variables are categorical. Two-way data where one observation is sampled for each pair of categorical levels are typically displayed in the following table:

	column 1	column 2	column 3	$\cdots$	column c
row 1	y_{11}	y_{12}	y_{13}	$\cdots$	y_{1c}
row 2	y_{21}	y_{22}	y_{23}	$\cdots$	y_{2c}
row 3	y_{31}	y_{32}	y_{33}	$\cdots$	y_{3c}
	$\vdots$	$\vdots$	$\vdots$	$\vdots$	$\vdots$
row r	y_{r1}	y_{r2}	y_{r3}	$\cdots$	y_{rc}

where r = number of rows and c = number of columns forming an $r \times c$ table. The symbol y_{ij} represents one of the $n = rc$ measured outcomes but, in this case, i indicates the level of the row categorical variable and j indicates the level of the column categorical variable.

Specifically, three experimental methods ($c = 3$) of determining serum lead levels in an individual's blood are compared where measurements were made on blood drawn from six sampled individuals ($r = 6$). The total $n = 3 \times 6 = 18$ observations are given in Table 7.2.

Table 7.2. Three methods of determining serum lead levels from blood sampled from six individuals

	method 1	method 2	method 3
individual 1	20	26	28
individual 2	34	32	38
individual 3	54	61	68
individual 4	38	40	46
individual 5	19	25	31
individual 6	40	38	54

The analysis of variance of a two-way classification addresses the questions: do non-random differences exist among the row mean values and do non-random differences exist among the column mean values? In terms of the serum lead example, this question focuses on the mean differences among individuals (rows) and among methods (columns). In this particular case, difference among individuals is not much of an issue, since it is expected that the six individuals will differ in lead exposure.

Analogous to the one-way analysis, the key analytic summaries are sums of squares. For a two-way pattern of data collection three sums of squares are at the core of the analysis—row, column, and residual sums of squares. The row sum of squares is defined by

$$1.\ SS_{rows} = c \sum (\bar{y}_{i.} - \bar{y})^2 \qquad i = 1, 2, 3, \cdots, r$$

where $\bar{y}_{i.}$ represents the mean of the ith row. The column sum of squares is analogously defined by

$$2.\ SS_{columns} = r \sum (\bar{y}_{.j} - \bar{y})^2 \qquad j = 1, 2, 3, \cdots, c$$

where $\bar{y}_{.j}$ represents the mean of the jth column. The dot in the subscript indicates sums of row or sums of column observations. For the serum lead data, the mean levels of the three methods of lead determination (columns) are: $\bar{y}_{.1} = 34.167$, $\bar{y}_{.2} = 37.000$, and $\bar{y}_{.3} = 44.167$ $(\Sigma y_{ij}/r = \bar{y}_{.j})$. The residual sum of squares is defined by

$$3.\ SS_{residual} = \sum \sum (y_{ij} - \bar{y}_{i.} - \bar{y}_{.j} + \bar{y})^2$$

where $\bar{y}$ is the mean of all n observations. The first two sums of squares measure the variability (lack of equality) among the row and the column means. Under specific conditions, the residual sum of squares measures the "background" variability of the dependent variable.

A fundamental requirement for a two-way analysis of variance with one observation per cell is that the structure underlying the sampled data can be described by an additive model (introduced in Chapter 2). More specifically, each value y_{ij} is a random sample from a normal distribution with mean $a + r_i$

+ c_j. As before, a represents a constant term, r_i represents the row variable influence and c_j represents the column variable influence. These mean values are estimated from sampled data by

$$estimated\ mean(y) = overall\ influence + row\ influence + column\ influence$$
$$= \hat{a} + \hat{r}_i + \hat{c}_j = \bar{y} + (\bar{y}_{i.} - \bar{y}) + (\bar{y}_j - \bar{y}).$$

The residual value associated with each observation is then

$$y_{ij} - estimated\ mean(y) = y_{ij} - [\bar{y} + (\bar{y}_{i.} - \bar{y}) + (\bar{y}_j - \bar{y})] = y_{ij} - \bar{y}_{i.} - \bar{y}_j + \bar{y}.$$

The residual sum of squares $SS_{residual}$ is the sum of the n squared residual values (one for each cell in the data table). If the data do not conform to an additive model, the residual values measure both the random variation associated with the dependent variable and the deviation from the additive model (interaction effects). However, the residual sum of squares reflects strictly random variation when the classification variables have additive effects.

If an S-vector $x1$ contains the column classification indicators, $x2$ contains the row classification indicators, and y is an S-vector of serum lead levels, then

```
> # data
> y<- c(20,26,28,34,32,38,54,61,68,38,40,46,19,25,31,40,38,54)
> # x1 = columns -- methods
> x1<- rep(c(1,2,3),6)
> # x2 = rows -- individuals
> x2<- rep(1:6,rep(3,6))
> methods<- factor(x1)
> methods
[1] 1 2 3 1 2 3 1 2 3 1 2 3 1 2 3 1 2 3
> persons<- factor(x2)
> persons
[1] 1 1 1 2 2 2 3 3 3 4 4 4 5 5 5 6 6 6
> ldata<- data.frame(y=y,methods=methods,persons=persons)
> summary(ldata)
        y          methods persons
 Min.   :19.00     1:6     1:3
 1st Qu.:28.75     2:6     2:3
 Median :38.00     3:6     3:3
 Mean   :38.44             4:3
 3rd Qu.:44.50             5:3
 Max.   :68.00             6:3
```

forms a data frame that becomes the basic input to the analysis of variance S-function. Assuming an additive relationship between methods and individuals as well as normally distributed data with the same variance regardless of the categorical classification, the analysis of variance S-function $aov()$ yields

```
> otemp1<- aov(y~methods+persons,ldata)
> summary(otemp1)
            Df   Sum of Sq   Mean Sq    F Value         Pr(F)
methods      2     318.778   159.3889   17.47259   0.0005452353
persons      5    2798.444   559.6889   61.35445   0.0000003534
Residuals   10      91.222     9.1222.
```

The output row labeled "methods" displays the contribution to the total variation from the differences among the three methods (columns). The output row labeled "persons" displays the contribution to the total variation from the differences among the six measured individuals (rows). The residual sum of squares reflects the variability in serum lead levels after accounting for the differences in methods of determination and the differences among individuals. The respective degrees of freedom are: $c - 1$ (columns), $r - 1$ (rows), and $(r - 1)(c - 1)$ (residual). The F-statistics ("F Value") show, as expected, large differences among individuals in serum lead levels and, additionally, significant differences in the three methods for determining the lead levels.

A more general approach to assessing the "row effects" and the "column effects" is once again based on comparing changes in the sums of squares from nested models. This approach was described in connection with the S-function $glm(\ )$ and the analysis of linear models (Chapter 4). The application to analysis of variance is not different in principle. For the serum lead example, primary interest concerns possible differences among methods; so the model ignoring any possible influences from the three methods is postulated yielding the one-way analysis of variance

```
> otemp0<- aov(y~persons,ldata)
> summary(otemp0)
            Df   Sum of Sq   Mean Sq    F Value        Pr(F)
persons      5    2798.444  559.6889   16.38114  5.365865e-05
Residuals   12     410.000   34.1667.
```

Comparison of the residual sum of squares from this restricted model (410.0) to the model including the influence of the methods (91.222) produces a measure of the impact associated with using different methods (columns) of serum lead determinations while accounting for the person to person variation (rows). The S-function $anov(\ )$ comparing these two models gives

```
    > anova(otemp0,otemp1)
    Analysis of Variance Table

    Response: y

      Terms Resid.  Df  RSS   Test   Df Sum of Sq F Value    Pr(F)
1    persons        12 410.00
2 methods+persons   10  91.22 +methods 2  318.7778 17.4726 0.000545.
```

These results are identical to the first analysis since both approaches are fundamentally the same.

Once the analysis of variance S-object is created (*otemp*1 in the example), there are a number of plots that supplement the analysis. Two versions of a plot addressing the assumption of additivity are created by

```
> par(mfrow=c(2,1))
> interaction.plot(persons,methods,y,
    main="Lead determination data")
> interaction.plot(methods,persons,y)
```

Figure 7.4 shows the results for the serum level data. If the row and column influences are additive, the lines in both versions of the plot will be parallel except for the influence of random variation. The example shows some deviation from parallel but it is hard to assess rigorously the magnitude of the influence of random variation on the observed pattern. A statistical test exists for non-additivity. Lack of additivity (interaction) can be investigated formally with a sophisticated analysis of variance model called "Tukey's one degree of freedom for non-additivity" [2].

Boxplots graphically display (Figure 7.5) the row and column distributions and are produced by the S-command

```
> plot.factor(ldata,main="Lead determination data")
```

where the input argument is the analysis of variance data frame. These plots are frequently based on extremely small numbers of observations (e.g., the individual mean levels of serum lead are based on three observations).

Much like the one-way analysis of variance, a plot of the residual values reflects on the conformity of the data to the basic underlying requirements of the analysis of variance. A qqnorm plot (Figure 7.6) and a residual plot (Figure 7.7) for the serum lead analysis are created by

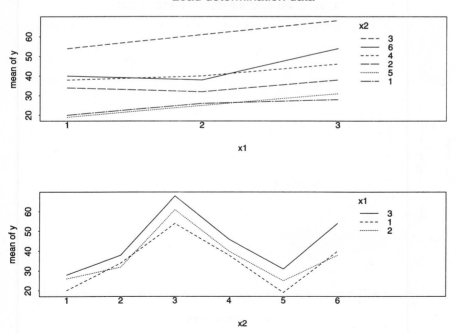

Figure 7.4

Lead determination data

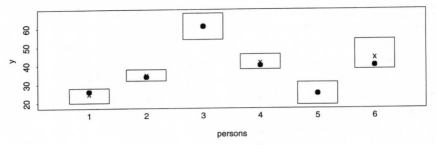

persons

Lead determination data

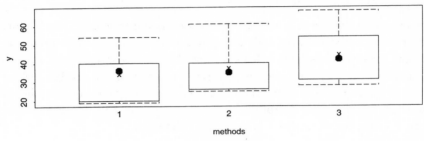

methods

Figure 7.5

Lead determination data -- qqnorm plot

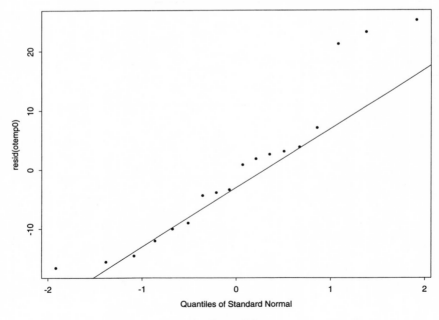

Quantiles of Standard Normal

Figure 7.6

```
> qqnorm(resid(otemp1),
    main="Lead determination data -- qqnorm plot")
> qqline(resid(otemp1))
> plot(resid(otemp1),fitted(otemp1),
    main="Lead determination -- residual plot)
```

It is a simple matter to evaluate differences among pairs of row or column means. For the serum lead data, the column means are

```
> ymean<- tapply(y,methods,mean)
> cat("column means",round(ymean,3),"\n")
   column means 34.167    37    44.167.
```

An estimate of the "background" variance assuming an additive model is the mean squared error (mse = 9.1222—labeled by $summary(\,)$ as "Mean Sq"). The mean squared error is an estimate of the common variance associated with the normally distributed data contained in each of the rc-cells of the two-way table. The mean squared error (mse) is estimated by dividing the residual sum of squares ($SS_{residual}$) by the associated degrees of freedom $(r - 1)(c - 1)$ and

```
> # calculation of the mean squared error
> df<- otemp1$df.residual
> mse<- sum(otemp1$residuals^2)/df
```

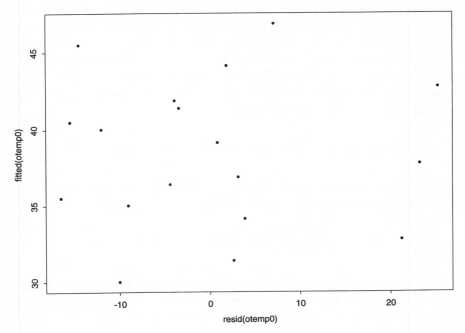

Lead determination data-- residual plot

Figure 7.7

The resulting value *mse* is an unbiased estimate of the "background" variability only when the row and column variables have additive effects. A series of *t*-tests comparing the three methods of determining serum lead is

```
> T.stat<- function(xbar,ybar,mse,df) {
  tstat<- (xbar-ybar)/sqrt(mse)
  pvalue<- 2*(1-pt(abs(tstat),df))
  cat("tstat = ",round(tstat,3),"   pvalue = ",
  round(pvalue,3),"\n")
  }
> # method 1 versus method 2
> T.stat(ymean[1],ymean[2],mse,df)
   tstat =  -0.938     pvalue =  0.37
> # method 1 versus method 3
> T.stat(ymean[1],ymean[3],mse,df)
   tstat =  -3.311     pvalue =  0.008
> # method 2 versus method 3
> T.stat(ymean[2],ymean[3],mse,df
   tstat =  -2.373     pvalue =  0.039.
```

The three tests, although not independent, indicate informally (no exact overall error rate) that methods 1 and 2 do not appear very different. However, differences between methods 2 and 3 as well as between methods 1 and 3 are unlikely to be due to random influences.

A parallel nonparametric test to assess influences of the row or column variables estimated from a two-way classification is called the Friedman test. The Friedman rank test is similar to the Kruskal–Wallis test. To assess the influences of the column variable ("treatment") the data are ranked from 1 to *c* within each row of a two-way table (e.g., treatment = methods = ranks = 1, 2, or 3). The sum of the ranks from the jth column (R_j) is calculated producing *c* values R_1, R_2, $\cdots$, R_c. If no differences exist among the *c* columns (treatments), then the expected value of each R_j-value is the average rank within rows multiplied by the number of rows or

$$\text{expected sum of the ranks within the } j^{th} \text{ column} = ER_j = r\frac{c+1}{2}.$$

For the serum lead data, $ER_j = 6(3 + 1)/2 = 12$. A test statistic to compare the *c* observed R_j-values to their corresponding expected values is

$$X^2 = \frac{12}{rc(c+1)} \sum (R_j - ER_j)^2 \qquad j = 1, 2, 3, \cdots, c$$

and X^2 has an approximate chi-square distribution with $c - 1$ degrees of freedom when only random variability causes differences within the rows of an $r \times c$ table [1]. This rank-based test applied to the serum lead data (Table 7.2) to compare the three methods of determination is

```
> friedman.test(y,methods,persons)
                    Friedman rank sum test
data:  y and methods and x2
Friedman chi-square = 9.3333, df = 2, p-value = 0.0094
alternative hypothesis: two.sided.
```

The result from the nonparametric approach is consistent with the parametric F-test. In both cases, the differences among methods appear due to non-random influences—p-value $= 0.001$ (parametric F-statistic) and p-value $= 0.009$ (nonparametric chi-square statistic).

   A fundamental purpose of a two-way classification is to account for the variability associated with one variable so that the analysis of the other variable has increased power (more likely to identify differences among row or column means when differences exist). Accounting for the variability among individuals, for example, produces a more powerful investigation of differences among the methods for determining lead levels. When the impact of either categorical variable on the dependent variable is assessed, the denominator of the F-statistic is based on the residual sum of squares ($SS_{residual}$). When a data collection design takes into account a specific variable, that source of variation can be removed from the residual sum of squares. The serum lead level from each individual was determined by all three methods (rows of Table 7.2) making it possible to remove the individual to individual variation from the residual sum of squares. This reduction usually increases the F-statistic, producing a more powerful approach.

   If the individual to individual variation is ignored and a one-way analysis performed, then the analysis of variance addressing differences among the three methods of serum lead determination is

```
> otemp<- aov(y~methods,ldata)
> summary(otemp)
              Df   Sum of Sq     Mean Sq     F Value       Pr(F)
methods        2     318.778    159.3889   0.8273734   0.4561936
Residuals     15    2889.667    192.6444.
```

The considerable increase in the residual sum of squares (denominator of the F-statistic) is due to the failure to account for the individual to individual variation causing an expected increase in the residual sum of squares over the two-way design. The residual sum of squares from the serum lead two-way analysis is 91.222 compared to 2889.667 from the one-way analysis, demonstrating the substantial increased power of the two-way design. Situations occasionally arise where classifying data into a two-way table produces a less efficient analysis of variance when compared to a one-way classification. Of course, the efficiency of a two-way analysis can be directly evaluated by contrasting it to a one-way analysis of variance using the same data ($aov(y~x1 + x2, \cdots)$ versus $aov(y~x1, \cdots)$, for example).

MATCHED PAIRS—MEASURED RESPONSE

As discussed in Chapter 6, an important data collection pattern is a matched pair design. McNemar's chi-square analysis applies to matched pair data when the response variable is binary but when the response studied (dependent variable) is a measured quantity, analysis of variance techniques are used.

Matched pair data can be viewed as a $r \times 2$ table with one observation per cell (a special case of the $r \times c$ table just discussed). The rows of the table are a series of r paired observations. The columns consist of observations classified by a binary independent variable ($c = 2$) and the cells of the table contain a measured response. For example, a sample of 24 pairs of infants (rows) are classified by birth weight status (low: < 2500 grams and normal: ≥ 2500 grams — columns) and the net weight gained during pregnancy by their mothers is recorded in each cell. Such data are given in Table 7.3 for small women (weight less than 50 kilograms).

Table 7.3. Matched pairs—maternal weight gain in small women (women < 50 kilograms) classified by their newborn's birth weight (< 2500 grams, bwt = 1 versus ≥ 2500 grams, bwt = 0) and matched for maternal prepregnancy weight

id	bwt	gain	ppwt*	id	bwt	gain	ppwt*	id	bwt	gain	ppwt*
1	1	6.1	40.9	9	1	6.9	46.8	17	1	7.2	47.7
1	0	21.0	40.9	9	0	7.7	46.8	17	0	13.2	47.7
2	1	9.2	43.0	10	1	8.4	46.8	18	1	7.2	47.7
2	0	10.0	43.0	10	0	9.3	46.8	18	0	9.0	47.7
3	1	3.4	44.5	11	1	12.1	46.8	19	1	8.4	48.2
3	0	15.4	44.5	11	0	9.3	46.8	19	0	7.2	48.2
4	1	4.4	44.5	12	1	11.2	46.8	20	1	10.6	48.2
4	0	18.1	44.5	12	0	11.4	46.8	20	0	11.7	48.2
5	1	6.1	44.5	13	1	6.4	47.3	21	1	11.0	48.2
5	0	19.3	44.5	13	0	7.3	47.3	21	0	11.7	48.2
6	1	1.0	45.5	14	1	5.0	47.7	22	1	15.0	48.2
6	0	1.5	45.5	14	0	5.3	47.7	22	0	14.7	48.2
7	1	8.4	45.5	15	1	17.6	47.7	23	1	11.2	48.6
7	0	8.9	45.5	15	0	21.1	47.7	23	0	12.0	48.6
8	1	6.5	45.5	16	1	0.0	47.7	24	1	6.5	49.1
8	0	8.8	45.5	16	0	22.3	47.7	24	0	15.1	49.1

*ppwt = prepregnancy weight

The $n = 24$ pairs are matched for mother's prepregnancy weight (Table 7.3). Therefore, the within pair differences observed in maternal weight gain are not influenced by prepregnancy weight. It is the same for both low and normal birth weight infants within each pair. A principal feature of a matched pair design, as before, is that the variable used to match the observations has little or no influence on comparisons within each pair. The data collection design eliminates the effects of a possibly confounding influence. The "match-

ing variable" is shown in Table 7.3 (prepregnancy weight = *ppwt*) to empha-
size the matched character of the data but the numerical values play no role in
the statistical analysis. An analysis of matched pairs, like the analysis of any
two-way classification, accounts for the among pair (rows) variation typically
increasing the probability of identifying (power) within pair differences.

The analysis of matched pair data takes several equivalent forms. A
matched *t*-test contrasts differences in mean values. For example, the mean
weight gained by mothers of low birth weight infants ($\bar{x}_{low}$ = 7.098) is compared to the mean weight gained by mothers of normal birth weight infants
($\bar{x}_{normal}$ = 12.138). Using the S-function *t.test*( ) gives

```
> # low = vector of 24 birth weights <2500 (bwt=1)
> # normal = vector of 24 birth weights >= 2500 (bwt=0)
> t.test(low,normal,paired=T)

        Paired t-Test

data:  low and normal
t = -3.2375, df = 23, p-value = 0.0036
alternative hypothesis: true mean of differences
    is not equal to 0
95 percent confidence interval:
 -6.931463 -1.526871
sample estimates:
 mean of x - y
   -4.229167
```

The same result is achieved by directly calculating the within pair differences and applying a *t*-test to evaluate the hypothesis that the observed mean
differs from zero by chance ($\bar{x}_{difference}$ = −4.229) or again using the S-function
t.test( ) gives

```
> t.test(low-normal,mu=0)

One-sample t-Test

data:  low - normal
t = -3.2375, df = 23, p-value = 0.0036
alternative hypothesis: true mean is not equal to 0
95 percent confidence interval:
 -6.931463 -1.526871
sample estimates:
 mean of x
 -4.229167
```

For matched pair data considered as a two-way classification, an analysis
of variance of the $r \times 2$ table (rows = pairs and columns = birth weights)
produces identical results where

```
> # id = pairs and bwt = birth weight classifications (0,1)
> otemp<- aov(gain~factor(id)+bwt)
> summary(otemp)
            Df Sum of Sq  Mean Sq  F Value      Pr(F)
bwt          1   214.6302 214.6302 10.48144 0.0036372
factor(id)  23   554.4198  24.1052  1.17718 0.3494880
Residuals   23   470.9748  20.4772.
```

The p-value ("Pr(F)" in summary) comparing columns is identical to the t-test generated p-values since the significance probability for an F-statistic with 1 and k degrees of freedom is same as that associated with a two-tail t-statistic with k degrees of freedom (e.g., $F = 10.481 = t^2 = (-3.238)^2$). All three analyses, as before, require the dependent variable (maternal weight gain) to be normally distributed with the same variance within all cells of the $r \times 2$ table.

A parallel nonparametric matched pair procedure is the Wilcoxon signed rank test designed to be free of assumptions about the structure of the sampled population. The distribution of the response variable is again not an issue because observed differences are replaced by ranks. The Wilcoxon signed rank test starts with ranking the absolute values of n observed within pair differences. A test statistic W is then calculated where W is the sum of the ranks associated with the observed positive (or negative) differences. An extreme value of W indicates the likely presence of non-random within pair influence. The expected value of W is $EW = n(n + 1)/4$ and the variance of W is $variance(W) = n(n + 1)(2n + 1)/24$ when only random differences exist within pairs [1]. When the number of pairs compared is moderately large (n greater than 20 or so), then

$$z = \frac{W + 0.5 - EW}{\sqrt{variance(W)}}$$

has an approximate standard normal distribution when the observed differences within pairs arise by chance alone. An analysis of these ranks reflects the within pair differences and the S-function $wilcox.test(\ )$ executes the test. For the birth weight data,

```
> wilcox.test(low,normal,exact=F,paired=T)
          Wilcoxon signed-rank test
data:   low and normal
signed-rank normal statistic with correction Z = -3.3575,
   p-value = 8e-04
alternative hypothesis: true mu is not equal to 0.
```

The option $exact = T$ is used for small samples of data because an approximation based on the normal distribution fails to give an accurate p-value. The nonparametric signed rank test produces results similar to the parametric analysis of variance of the birth weight data. Both approaches show that maternal weight gained during pregnancy is strongly associated with an infant's birth weight classified as below and above 2500 grams while eliminating any influences from prepregnancy maternal weight.

A matched pair design can be expanded to include one case and several controls (C). A 1 : C set of matched observations is designed, for example, so that all $1 + C$ members have the same or close to the same levels of a potentially confounding variable. The birth weight matched pairs could be expanded so that three additional "normal" weight infants ($C = 4 = $ controls) are compared to a low birth weight infant (case) where all five mothers belong to a set with essentially the same prepregnancy weight. Again, any within set differences cannot be attributed to prepregnancy weight. The analysis of a $1 : C$ set of matched data offers nothing new. The t-test approach is no longer possible but an analysis of variance ($aov(\ )$ S-function) applied to the two-way table serves to identify differences among the columns (within set differences). The data are treated as an $r \times (1 + C)$ table (r sets = rows and $1 + C$ controls = columns). Analogous to matched pair data, any observed within set differences cannot be attributed to the "matching variable" but only to random or systematic differences associated with the column classification.

TWO-WAY CLASSIFICATION WITH MORE THAN ONE OBSERVATION PER CELL

A natural extension of the two-way data collection design with one observation per cell is the situation where more than one observation per cell is available. The analysis follows the same pattern used for a two-way table based on a single observation per cell with one major difference. It is possible to measure separately the deviation from an additive model and the random variation associated with the dependent variable. If the number of observations in each cell of a two-way table is denoted as n_{ij} (again, i^{th} row and j^{th} column), then the residual sum of squares is

$$residual\ sum\ of\ squares = \sum\sum(n_{ij} - 1)s_{ij}^2$$

where s_{ij}^2 is the usual estimated variance calculated from the n_{ij} observations within each of the rc cells in the table. The residual sum of squares directly measures the variation of the dependent variable and does not depend on the data conforming to an additive model as required by the one observation per cell case. However, like the previous analysis of variance models, the data are required to be sampled from normally distributed populations with the same variances.

The first step in a two-way analysis is to compare the sum of squares measuring the magnitude of any non-additivity (interaction) to the residual sum of squares. When more than one observation per cell is available, calculating a sum of squares measuring non-additivity (interaction sum of squares) is somewhat complicated except when all cells have the same number of observations ($n_{ij} = n$). However, the S-function $aov(\ )$ produces this sum of squares, which is a critical part of the assessing of the row and column influences. When the row and column variables have additive influences, both interaction and residual sums of squares reflect only random variation. Furthermore, if no appreciable interaction exists, then the row means directly measure the influences of the row categorical variable separately from any influences of the column variable and, conversely, the column mean values directly measure the influences of the column categorical variable separately from any influences of the row variable. This same property of additivity is discussed in Chapter 2 and is an explicit assumption for a two-way analysis of variance when only one observation per cell is available.

Again using the data from Table 4.1 and classifying birth weights by maternal prepregnancy weight (four categories—light, < 50 kilograms; normal, 50–55 kilograms; heavy, 55–72 kilograms; obese, >72 kilograms) and maternal net weight gain (four categories—small, < 11 kilograms; normal, 11–16 kilograms; moderate, 16–22 kilograms; extreme, > 22 kilograms) produces the following summary two-way tables (n_{ij} = count of observations/cell, $\bar{y}_{ij}$ = mean, values and $s_{ij}/\sqrt{n_{ij}}$ = standard error of the mean):

```
> wcut<- c(-99,50,55,72,99)
> gcut<- c(-99,11,16,22,99)
> gain0<- cut(gain,gcut,label=c("small","normal",
    "moderate","extreme"))
> wt0<- cut(wt,wcut,label=c("light","normal","heavy","obese "))
> tapply(bwt,list(wt0,gain0),length)
>           small  normal  moderate     extreme
light        13     15       17          7
normal       12     20       23          8
heavy        19     30       35          9
obese         4      7       10          3
> round(tapply(bwt,list(wt0,gain0),mean),3)
           small     normal     moderate     extreme
light      2.406     3.083      3.244        3.487
normal     3.238     3.425      3.495        3.619
heavy      2.888     3.387      3.568        3.619
obese      3.370     3.657      3.504        3.767
se<- function(x){sqrt(var(x)/length(x))}
> round(tapply(bwt,list(wt0,gain0),se),3)
           small     normal     moderate     extreme
light      0.304     0.060      0.177        0.144
normal     0.159     0.093      0.107        0.157
heavy      0.162     0.078      0.067        0.238
obese      0.174     0.325      0.245        0.126.
```

A complete two-way analysis of variance for data with more than one observation per cell requires the comparison of four models. They are:

model 0: $y\sim$ variable 1 + variable 2 + interaction between variables 1 and 2 (non-additive model)
model 1: $y\sim$ variable 1 + variable 2 (additive model)
model 2: $y\sim$ variable 2 (variable 1 removed)
model 3: $y\sim$ variable 1 (variable 2 removed).

These four models applied to the birth weight data give

```
> otemp0<- aov(bwt~wt0+gain0+wt0*gain0)
> summary(otemp0)
             Df    Sum of Sq   Mean Sq   F Value        Pr(F)
wt0           3      7.17939   2.393130   7.14572    0.0001346
gain0         3     12.34236   4.114121  12.28447    0.0000002
wt0,gain0     9      2.52761   0.280845   0.83858    0.5813141
Residuals   216     72.33929   0.334904

> otemp1<- aov(bwt~wt0+gain0)
> summary(otemp1)
            Df   Sum of Sq   Mean Sq   F Value         Pr(F)
wt0          3     7.17939   2.393130   7.19215   0.0001245086
gain0        3    12.34236   4.114121  12.36431   0.0000001623
Residual 225      74.86689   0.332742

> otemp2<- aov(bwt~gain0)
> summary(otemp2)
             Df   Sum of Sq   Mean Sq   F Value          Pr(F)
gain0         3    13.34472   4.448240  12.51418   1.323902e-07
Residuals   228    81.04393   0.355456

> otemp3<- aov(bwt~wt0)
> summary(otemp3)
            Df   Sum of Sq   Mean Sq    F Value         Pr(F)
wt0          3     7.17939   2.393130   6.256602   0.0004241809
Residuals  228    87.20926   0.382497.
```

For the additive model, any non-additivity is assumed to be due to random variation and, therefore, is reflected as part of the residual sum of squares. The residual sum of squares in the additive model (*otemp*1—74.867) is the sum of the interaction and residual sum of squares from the non-additive model (*otemp*0—2.528 + 72.339 = 74.867). The S-function *anov*() succinctly compares the results from these models.

To assess the impact of maternal weight gain on infant birth weight, then

```
> anova(otemp3,otemp1,otemp0)
Analysis of Variance Table

Response: bwt

  Terms Resid. Df      RSS    Test   Df Sum of Sq F Value     Pr(F)
1          wt0   228 87.20926
2  wt0 + gain0   225 74.86689  +gain0  3  12.34236 12.28447 0.0000002
3  wt0 * gain0   216 72.33929 wt0:gain0 9  2.52761  0.83858 0.5813141.
```

To assess the impact of prepregnancy weight on birth weight, then

```
> anova(otemp2,otemp1,otemp0)
Analysis of Variance Table

Response: bwt

 Terms Resid. Df      RSS      Test Df  Sum of Sq  F Value     Pr(F)
1       gain0 228 81.04393
2 wt0 + gain0 225 74.86689      +wt0  3   6.177035 6.148063 0.000498
3 wt0 * gain0 216 72.33929 +wt0:gain0 9  2.527606 0.838584 0.581314.
```

If the analysis shows substantial non-additivity, the row and column means do not directly reflect the influences of the two categorical variables, as noted.

A strong interaction implies that comparisons among the row values depend on the specific columns being considered and, vice versa, comparisons among the column values depend on the specific rows being considered. Therefore, the row and column sums of squares do not meaningfully summarize the separate influences from the row and column categorical variables unless their effects are at least approximately additive (negligible interaction).

The birth weight data show no important evidence of non-additivity. The interaction between maternal weight gain and prepregnancy weight (in S-terms; $wt0 * gain0$) is not significantly large where $SS_0 = 72.339$ (interaction present) and $SS_1 = 74.867$ (interaction ignored) produces a p-value = 0.581. The test of significance derives from comparing the residual sum of squares from the model $bwt\tilde{\ }wt0 + gain0 + wt0 * gain0$ to the residual sum of squares from the additive model $bwt\tilde{\ }wt0 + gain0$ (last line in the $anova(\ )$ summaries). The lack of interaction makes the assessment of the influence of maternal weight gain on an infant's birth weight relatively straightforward. The pattern of comparing differences in residual sums of squares calculated from nested models yields, as before, an F-statistic ("F Value") and a significance probability ("Pr(F)"). Comparison of the additive model $bwt\tilde{\ }wt0 + gain0$ with the model $bwt\tilde{\ }wt0$ measures the impact of the $gain0$ (maternal weight gain) accounting for prepregnancy weight. The resulting difference in the sums of squares 12.342 (differences between models 1 and 3; labeled "Sum of Sq") yields a p-value less than 0.001. Similarly, comparison of the additive model $bwt\tilde{\ }wt0 + gain0$ with the model $bwt\tilde{\ }gain0$ measures the impact of the $wt0$ (prepregnancy weight). The resulting difference in sums of squares is 6.177 (differences between models 1 and 2) and also yields a p-value less than 0.001.

If additivity is not a plausible data structure, then the row and column sums of squares potentially produce misleading summary results. A significant interaction requires the row comparisons to be considered separately for some or all columns (a series of one-way comparisons). Similarly, the column comparisons must be made within some or all rows. In the face of a strong interaction, a two-way classification/analysis is no longer useful in the investigation of the separate influences of the independent variables and is frequently replaced by a series of one-way comparisons.

LEAPS—A MODEL SELECTION TECHNIQUE

Data sets occasionally contain a large number of independent variables; sometimes more than are necessary to adequately describe the relationship between a dependent variable and a series of independent variables. It is frequently desirable to choose from among such variables a subset that parsimoniously predicts the dependent variable. In fact, the main purpose of some studies is to find a subset of independent variables that provides good prediction of an outcome. A typical approach to evaluating the influence of a series of independent variables on a dependent variable is a multivariable regression equation (Chapter 4).

The selection of the "best" predictors, one way or another, involves the fit of the predicted values to the observed data. A number of criteria measure the correspondence between predicted and observed values in a statistical analysis. However, many of these criteria are monotonic functions. Monotonic in the sense that they continue to increase (or decrease) as variables are added to the analysis. No clearly "best" set of predictors emerges. Two examples of such criteria are the squared multiple correlation coefficient and the residual sum of squares. Other criteria exist, however, that do not have this monotonic property. These criteria reach a maximum or minimum value as differnent combinations of independent variables are included in the regression equation, making it possible to select a subset of "best" variables for a regression model. Three examples of such criteria are the adjusted R-squared, the *PRESS* (predicted sum of squares), and Mallow's *Cp* criteria [3].

Regression analysis data almost always produce an important question: what variables should be included in the regression model? A simple answer is to include all possible relevant variables. However, this solution potentially leads to a large unmanageable equation, which is frequently not useful in identifying the important contributors to predicting values of the outcome variable. Furthermore, a large and complex regression model, on occasions, is plagued by unstable estimates that can become less of a problem in models with fewer variables. But, most importantly, a simple representation of the relationships within a data set is usually better than a complex one.

The process of choosing a "best" subset of explanatory variables to produce a parsimonious regression model takes several directions. The most direct approach to variable selection involves a series of regression analyses based on all possible combinations of the collected independent variables. Using a summary criterion such as the residual sum of squares, the relative worth of each combination of independent variables is judged. For example, five maternal variables relevant to predicting birth weight are: height, prepregnancy weight, height squared, prepregnancy weight squared, and prepregnancy weight multiplied by height. In symbols, the five-variable regression model for the ith observation is

$$bwt_i = a + b_1 ht_i + b_2 wt_i + b_3 ht_i^2 + b_4 wt_i^2 + b_5 (wt_i \times ht_i)$$

where bwt_i represents the birth weight of the ith infant. Using this expression as a starting point, the selection of a "best" expression for the prediction of birth weight involves $2^5 - 1 = 31$ regression analyses using all possible combinations of these five independent variables. The model including all five measured variables produces the smallest residual sum of squares (i.e., "fits the best"). This is a mathematical fact of the least squares estimation. A full regression equation (all variables), however, is often unnecessary. Regression models made up of a subset of variables are often useful descriptions of the data since they frequently produce negligible changes in the goodness-of-fit, as measured by only small increases in the residual sum of squares over the minimum value. This is the case for the birth weight model. The full model (five variables) produces a residual sum of squares = 87.378. The model (four variables)

$$\textit{birth weight of the } i^{th} \textit{ infant} = bwt_i = a + b_1 ht_i + b_2 wt_i + b_3 ht_i^2 + b_4 wt_i^2$$

barely increases the sum of squares (87.378 to 87.387).

Another approach to selecting a "best" regression model uses a stepwise selection process. A forward stepwise procedure starts with a constant term and consists of adding variables to a regression equation until a stopping criterion is reached. At that point, the included variables are said to "best" describe the dependent variable. A backwards stepwise procedure starts with all measured independent variables in the model and consists of deleting variables until again a stopping criterion is reached. The popularity of stepwise approaches is largely due to the fact that they are easily implemented using widely available standard statistical computer packages.

A stepwise procedure is implemented with the S-command *step( )*. An S-object is created in the usual fashion by *S.object<– glm(dependent variable~formula, · · ·)*; then the command *step(S.object)* finds the "best" model using the variables specified by the S-formula in the *glm*-function. A stepwise criterion known as AIC (Akaike Information Criterion [4]) provides one of many available criteria to eliminate the variables that contribute little to the model. Each step of the stepwise process is displayed unless the option *trace = F* is used. The AIC criterion is not the only possibility and a complete discussion of the extensive number of model selection strategies is found elsewhere [4].

Using the S-function *step( )* and the birth weight data yields

```
> otemp<- glm(bwt~ht+wt+ht^2+wt^2+wt*ht)
> step(otemp,trace=F)
Call:
glm(formula = bwt ~ ht + wt + I(ht^2))

Coefficients:
  (Intercept)         ht          wt       I(ht^2)
    -25.04458  0.3375191  0.01224954  -0.001027481

Degrees of Freedom: 232 Total; 228 Residual
Residual Deviance: 87.8674.
```

The AIC criterion selects the "best" model as

$$\text{birth weight of the } i^{th} \text{ infant} = bwt_i = -25.045 + 0.338ht_i + 0.012wt_i - 0.001ht_i^2.$$

Although stepwise procedures produce a subset of "best" variables, they are not without problems. Forward analysis and backward analysis applied to the same set of independent variables does not always produce the same "best" equation. Neither procedure guarantees a regression model with the smallest sum of squares for a fixed subset size. For a fixed number of variables there exists a regression equation with the smallest residual sum of squares ("best-fit for a specific size"). Only exhaustively calculating the residual sum of squares for all possible regression equations with a fixed number of variables always produces the combination of variables that most accurately predicts the dependent variable. Furthermore, stepwise procedures require the user to choose rather complicated and usually arbitrary stopping criteria (e.g., AIC).

An approach to model selection is available that does not involve a stepwise process but rather evaluates all possible models. The S-function *leaps( )* implements such a process and produces the "best" subset of independent variables based on the choice of a non-monotonic criterion. The general form of the *leaps( )* command is

$$leaps(x, \ y, \ method = `` < criterion > ", \ nbest = k)$$

where x is an array of independent variables (rows = observations and columns = variables), y is a S-vector of dependent variables, the option *method* identifies the model selection criterion, and *nbest* indicates the number of "best" models to be selected (output). The application of *leaps( )* is illustrated with a model selection criterion called Mellow's Cp but applications using other choices (e.g., R-squared adjusted) are, in principle, the same. The *leaps( )* S-function uses the chosen criterion to select the "best" model or models and by means of a subtle and efficient algorithm ([5] or [6]) considers all possible models (up to $k = 30$ variables; $2^{30} - 1$ models!).

Mallow's Cp criterion is a function of the mean squared error. The mean squared error consists of a component measuring bias and a component measuring lack of fit. The details of this measure are given elsewhere [4]. The important feature is that the Cp-value is a function of fit of the model and the bias incurred from employing less than all possible k independent variables. Cp-values are extreme when the fit is poor or the bias is large. Therefore, the S-function *leaps( )* determines the subset of variables with the minimum value of Cp-value producing the "best" or a series of "best" regression models. The minimum Cp-value, in a concrete but somewhat arbitrary sense, produces a potentially simpler model that is both relatively unbiased and a relatively good representation of the data.

Table 7.4. *All possible models for predicting infant birth weight from maternal height and weight (size = number of model parameters)*

model	size	Mallow's Cp
wt	2	5.229
ht*wt	2	6.334
wt^2	2	6.357
ht	2	15.188
ht^2	2	15.359
wt + wt^2	3	6.477
wt + ht*wt	3	6.889
wt + ht^2	3	7.012
ht + wt	3	7.098
ht^2 + ht*wt	3	7.220
ht + ht*wt	3	7.454
wt^2 + ht*wt	3	8.184
ht^2 + wt^2	3	8.281
ht + wt^2	3	8.327
ht + ht^2	3	11.821
ht + wt + ht^2	4	3.265
ht + ht^2 + ht*wt	4	3.284
ht + ht^2 + wt^2	4	4.479
ht + wt + ht*wt	4	7.981
wt + wt^2 + ht*wt	4	8.055
wt + ht^2 + wt^2	4	8.061
ht + wt + wt^2	4	8.184
ht^2 + wt^2 + ht*wt	4	8.280
wt + ht^2 + ht*wt	4	8.618
ht + wt^2 + ht*wt	4	8.859
ht + ht^2 + wt^2 + ht*wt	5	4.082
ht + wt + ht^2 + wt^2	5	4.448
ht + wt + ht^2 + ht*wt	5	5.265
ht + wt + wt^2 + ht*wt	5	9.769
wt + ht^2 + wt^2 + ht*wt	5	10.054
ht + wt + ht^2 + wt^2 + ht*wt	6	6.000

Continuing the example of predicting birth weight from maternal height and weight, Table 7.4 shows all 31 possible models constructed from the five independent variables along with the Cp-values calculated for each model. The data for these calculations come from Table 4.2. The minimum Cp-value is 3.265 and corresponds to the model

$$\textit{birth weight of the } i^{th} \textit{ infant} = bwt_i = a + b_1 ht_i + b_2 wt_i + b_3 ht_i^2.$$

This is the same model selected by the AIC criteria using *step( )* but in general these two approaches are not guaranteed to pick the same "best" model. The Cp-values and variable selection are produced by the following S-code:

```
> # variable labels
> vnames<- c("ht","wt","ht^2","wt^2","ht*wt")
> d<- matrix(scan("bwt.dat"),4)
> y<- d[1,] # birth weight
> x1<- d[2,] # maternal height
> x2<- d[3,] # maternal weight
> x<- cbind(x1,x2,x1^2,x2^2,x1*x2)
> # produces "leaps" object
> otemp<- leaps(x,y,method="Cp",nbest=31,names=vnames)
> summary(otemp)
        Length Class        Mode
    Cp     31              numeric
  size     31              numeric
 label     31            character
 which    155              logical
   int      1              logical
> cbind(otemp$label,otemp$size,round(otemp$Cp,3))
                [,1]                    [,2]      [,3]
  [1,] "wt"                            "2"    "5.229"
  [2,] "ht*wt"                         "2"    "6.334"
  [3,] "wt^2"                          "2"    "6.357"
  [4,] "ht"                            "2"    "15.188"
  [5,] "ht^2"                          "2"    "15.359"

        ------                          --    -----
        ------                          --    -----
        ------                          --    -----
        ------                          --    -----

 [27,] "ht,wt,ht^2,wt^2"               "5"    "4.448"
 [28,] "ht,wt,ht^2,ht*wt"              "5"    "5.265"
 [29,] "ht,wt,wt^2,ht*wt"              "5"    "9.769"
 [30,] "wt,ht^2,wt^2,ht*wt"            "5"    "10.054"
 [31,] "ht,wt,ht^2,wt^2,ht*wt"         "6"    "6,000".
```

The values of the model selection criteria (i.e., Mallow's Cp in the example) plotted against the number of variables in the model ($size$) is a useful description of the variable selection possibilities. An S-plot follows from

```
> plot(otemp$size,otemp$Cp,pch=".",type="b",
    main="Birth weight data -- model selection")
```

and produces a plot of the Cp-values showing the relative magnitudes of the criteria for each of the 31 possible models (Figure 7.8).

For five independent variables, it is, perhaps, unnecessary to use an approach based on a statistical criterion to choose a "best" model. All possible 31 models can be readily estimated and compared. However, if the number of independent variables is much more than five, direct estimation of all possible cases becomes computationally formidable and frequently impractical to interpret. Continuing the birth weight example, including a third variable (maternal weight gain) produces $2^{10} - 1 = 1023$ possible regression equations. Using *leaps( )* with selection criterion *methods = "Cp"*, the five "best" models are found by

Birth weight data -- model selection

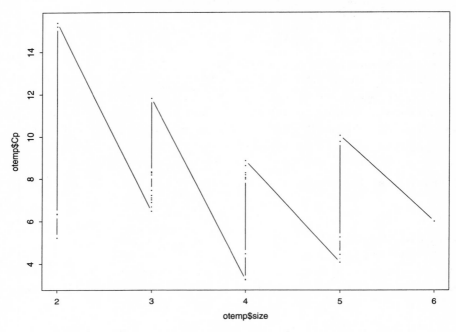

Figure 7.8

```
> y<- d[1,] # birth weight
> x1<- d[2,] # maternal height
> x2<- d[3,] # maternal weight
> x3<- d[4,] # maternal weight gain
> x<- cbind(x1,x2,x3,x1^2,x2^2,x3^2,x1*x2,
    x1*x3,x2*x3,x1*x2*x3)
> vnames<- c("ht","wt","gain","ht^2","wt^2","gain^2",
    "ht*wt","ht*gain","wt*gain","wt*ht*gain")
> otemp<- leaps(x,y,method="Cp",names=vnames)
> cp<- otemp$Cp
> ordcp<- order(cp)
> lmin<- otemp$label[ordcp]
> smin<- otemp$size[ordcp]
> cp<- sort(cp)
> cbind(lmin[1:5],smin[1:5],round(cp[1:5],3))
                                                   [,1]         [,2]    [,3]
[1,] "ht,wt,gain,ht^2,gain^2,ht*gain"              "7"    "4.844"
[2,] "ht,wt,ht^2,gain^2,wt*gain,wt*ht*gain"        "7"    "4.855"
[3,] "ht,wt,gain,ht^2,wt^2,gain^2,ht*gain"         "8"    "5.214"
[4,] "wt,gain,gain^2,wt*ht*gain"                   "5"    "5.241"
[5,] "wt,gain^2,wt*gain,ht*gain,wt*ht*gain"        "6"    "5.502".
```

A plot of the *Cp*-values against model *size* is given on the left side of Figure 7.9 for $k = size = 2$ to 11 (produced with the S-plot command used in the two-variable example). The second plot (right side) is the same plot focused on a more relevant range of *Cp*-values. Both the plot and the S-function show the "best" selected model to be

$$bwt_i = a + b_1 ht_i + b_2 wt_i + b_3 gain_i + b_4 ht_i^2 + b_5 gain_i^2 + b_6 ht_i \times gain_i$$

with the minimum *Cp*-value = 4.844.

The same variable selection process applied to linear regression can be used in conjunction with a logistic analysis. Two changes are necessary—the dependent variable must be transformed and a set of weights derived [7]. Once these two changes are made, the S-function *leaps*( ) can be used to select a "best" set of variables when the option *wt* =< *vector of weights* > is included. The option *method* =< *criterion* > again defines a model selection criterion.

PRINCIPAL COMPONENTS

An often effective approach to dealing with a complex multivariate measurement is to form a simpler summary value by combining the variables making

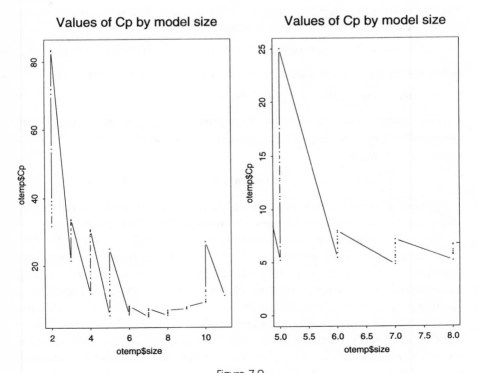

Figure 7.9

up the observation, sometimes called a canonical variable. Discriminant scores (Chapter 4) are an example of a canonical variable. For a k-dimensional observation represented by $\{x_{i1}, x_{i2}, x_{i3}, \cdots, x_{ik}\}$, a possibly effective canonical summary is a linear combination of these variables. That is, the ith observation is summarized as a sum of k measurements or

$$P_{i1} = a_{11}x_{i1} + a_{21}x_{i2} + a_{31}x_{i3} + \cdots + a_{k1}x_{ik}$$

A principal component (originated by Karl Pearson) is such a sum of the observed variables weighted by coefficients selected to give the summary specific properties. A second principal component summary can be calculated, also as a linear combination of the k variables, where

$$P_{i2} = a_{12}x_{i1} + a_{22}x_{i2} + a_{32}x_{i3} + \cdots + a_{k2}x_{ik}$$

and the weights are a second set of selected coefficients. In fact, up to k such principal component summaries can be formed where, in general,

$$P_{im} = a_{1m}x_{i1} + a_{2m}x_{i2} + a_{3m}x_{i3} + \cdots + a_{km}x_{ik}$$

is the mth principal component summary of the ith observation constructed from the set of k coefficients a_{jm}. The basic question is: how should the coefficients be chosen to give these canonical variables effective properties? The coefficients are chosen so that the principal component summaries have the following two statistically useful properties:

1. $variance(P_1) > variance(P_2) > variance(P_3) > \cdots > variance(P_k)$

and these k principal components are uncorrelated with each other or

2. $correlation(P_i, P_j) = 0$ for all pairs $i \neq j$.

The choice of the coefficients that produce the principal components canonical summaries does not change the overall variance but rather redistributes it. In symbols,

$$\sum variance(P_j) = \sum variance(x_j) \qquad j = 1, 2, 3, \cdots, k.$$

A principal component not only summarizes the multivariate measurement with a single value but does so with a simplified "data" structure.

Variability of a canonical summary statistic is a desirable property. The more variable an index or summary, the more likely it reflects important properties of the observation summarized. The converse is obviously true. If a summary index has little or no variability, then it is relatively useless as a summary since it takes on essentially the same value under all conditions. Additionally, when a series of summary values are uncorrelated, they potentially reflect different aspects of the data. The mathematical machinery of a principal component summary produces coefficients to construct canonical summary values with maximum variability that are uncorrelated. Data made up of high dimensional observations (k large) sometimes reduce to a few principal component summaries with a small loss of information. It is certainly ideal to reduce a large complex multivariate observation to a few effective canonical values. This reduction in "dimensionality" is most effective when there is a great deal of redundancy in the k measurements made on each observation. Using principal component values to represent a complex multivariate measurement is not always effective. An extreme case occurs when the original variables are all pairwise uncorrelated; then the principal component values make absolutely no change to the basic data structure.

To illustrate principal component analysis, data consisting of four variables measured on a mother (age, smoking exposure, height, and weight) and four variables measured on a father (age, smoking exposure, height, and educational level) are used ($k = 8$ measurements per observation). These measurements were made on each of the parents of $n = 38$ extremely small infants (birth weight less than the 5th percentile; Table 7.5).

Principal component values depend on the measurement units of the variables that make up the multivariate observations. If a variable is measured in feet rather than inches, the relationships among the resulting principal components will differ. When the k variables are measured in a variety of units (e.g., years, cigarettes smoked per day, inches, and pounds), the data are typically transformed so that all variables have mean value zero and unit variance. The standardization forces all variables to participate in the principal component analysis on an equal footing. Also, the standardized variables are commensurate making interpretation easier. Otherwise, unequal variances and differing measurement units can disrupt the interpretation of the principal component values, making these summaries less useful.

The S-function *scale*( ) is designed to perform this transformation. The input argument is an $n \times k$ array of data and the output is again an $n \times k$ array where the column values have means equal to zero (S-option *center* $= T$) and variances equal to one. For example, the S-function *scale*( ) applied to an array labeled x produces k sets of commensurate variables. Specifically,

```
> new.x<- scale(x,center=T)
```

produces the array *new.x* where the column means $= 0$ and the column variances $= 1$.

The first question addressed from the calculation of k principal components is: how much of the total variability is associated with the first several principal components? Unless most of the variation is concentrated in the first few principal components, this approach to simplifying a multivariate measurement is not very effective. The percent of variation associated with each principal component summary is

Table 7.5. *Birth weights and eight maternal/paternal variables *from parents of infants whose birth weight is less than the 5th percentile*

	bwt	maternal				paternal			
		age	cigs/day	height	weight	age	education	cigs/day	height
1	5.3	32	17	67	112	28	10	17	71
2	3.3	32	9	64	142	32	14	0	66
3	5.6	22	25	66	122	23	12	25	68
4	5.4	18	25	60	101	21	14	12	67
5	5.5	21	0	67	125	21	14	2	68
6	5.3	41	7	65	125	37	14	25	68
7	5.6	21	7	64	123	24	12	0	71
8	5.3	20	7	63	109	20	10	35	71
9	5.6	20	7	62	123	27	12	7	71
10	5.8	20	35	67	125	23	12	50	73
11	4.4	20	25	65	167	21	12	25	72
12	5.8	29	12	65	115	33	14	0	69
13	5.2	31	0	65	125	31	16	0	72
14	5.5	22	7	62	115	23	14	25	78
15	5.5	35	17	65	119	44	16	2	66
16	5.0	25	0	62	125	28	14	0	71
17	5.8	37	0	65	130	41	14	0	72
18	5.5	30	0	66	130	31	12	0	69
19	5.3	41	0	67	137	36	12	0	70
20	5.5	21	12	60	115	24	14	7	68
21	5.6	19	0	61	125	29	16	7	70
22	5.6	32	7	63	105	40	16	7	66
23	5.4	31	2	62	120	33	16	25	69
24	5.3	23	25	65	125	24	14	25	72
25	5.8	36	7	61	130	38	10	25	71
26	3.9	24	0	58	99	26	16	0	66
27	4.5	25	25	66	200	29	12	25	72
28	5.2	20	7	64	104	20	10	35	73
29	5.2	37	0	66	140	41	16	0	74
30	5.7	26	25	65	112	29	14	25	69
31	5.3	24	0	60	114	25	12	25	69
32	4.6	21	25	65	103	29	10	25	67
33	4.4	20	25	65	124	30	10	25	67
34	5.7	22	0	64	117	23	12	0	71
35	5.4	38	17	63	144	36	12	0	69
36	5.8	19	12	61	132	20	10	25	75
37	5.8	21	0	64	112	23	16	25	70
38	5.5	28	25	67	127	31	16	35	71

*bwt and maternal weight in pounts, age in years, cigarettes in reported number smoked per day, height in inches, and education in last grade completed.

$$\% \; variance \; associated \; with \; P_j = \frac{variance(P_j)}{\sum variance(P_j)} \times 100$$

yielding a measure of the relative effectiveness of principal component P_j as a summary.

The S-command *prcomp( )* produces a principal component S-object, which contains the elements of principal component analysis. When *lbwt.data* is an S-array (38×8) containing the 38 observations (rows) consisting of the eight parental variables (columns) from the low birth weight data (Table 7.5), then

```
> # standardization of the variables contained in lbwt.data
> bdata<- scale(lbwt.data,center=T)
> # p.object = principal component S-object
> p.object<- prcomp(bdata)
> summary(p.object)
> Length      Class           Mode
      sdev          8        numeric
rotation         64        numeric
        x        304        numeric

> # extract variances of the principal components
> v<- p.object$sdev^2
> round(v,2)
 [1] 2.68 1.82 1.12 0.73 0.68 0.57 0.28 0.10
> round(100*v/sum(v),1)
[1] 33.6 22.7 14.0 9.2 8.6 7.2 3.5 1.3
> round(100*cumsum(v)/sum(v),1)
[1] 33.6 56.3 70.3 79.5 88.1 95.2 98.7 100.0.
```

The S-vector *S.object$sdev* contains the standard deviations associated with each of the eight canonical principal components calculated from the standardized maternal/paternal data. Since the variability of each parental variable (x_j) is standardized; creating a variable (z_j) with unit variance, then $\sum variance(P_j) = \sum variance(z_j) = k = 8$. The first principal component "explains" 33.6% of the variability, the second principal component "explains" 22.7% and both variables "explain" 56.3% of the variability of the original observations. The first two principal components reduce an eight-dimensional observation to a bivariate observation with an average 44.7% "loss of information." The first three principal components summarize 70.3% of the total variance. These and the remaining variances (percentages) describe the effectiveness of a reduced set of principal component summaries to reflect all eight variables.

The influence of each variable in a principal component summary is proportional to the magnitude of the associated coefficients when the data are standardized. The relative sizes of the coefficients can indicate an overall interpretation of a principal component summary. The coefficients from the example data are

```
> round(p.object$rotation,2)
      [,1]   [,2]   [,3]   [,4]   [,5]   [,6]   [,7]   [,8]
[1,] -0.49 -0.32  0.02 -0.16 -0.36  0.17  0.06 -0.69
[2,]  0.34 -0.33  0.52  0.18  0.16  0.23 -0.59 -0.19
[3,] -0.02 -0.58  0.14  0.10 -0.03 -0.78  0.13  0.10
[4,] -0.03 -0.52 -0.35  0.01  0.64  0.35  0.27  0.02
[5,] -0.51 -0.26  0.16 -0.03 -0.24  0.30 -0.19  0.68
[6,] -0.35  0.18  0.04  0.90  0.12 -0.01  0.07 -0.10
[7,]  0.45 -0.19  0.19  0.23 -0.46  0.32  0.59  0.09
[8,]  0.23 -0.21 -0.72  0.25 -0.38  0.01 -0.42  0.02.
```

The columns of the $k \times k$ array *S.object$rotation* contain the coefficients for each of the k principal components. The first column contains the coefficients of the first principal component, the second column the coefficients of the second principal component and so forth, up to the kth column.

For the low birth weight data,

$$P_{i1} = -0.49x_{i1} + 0.34x_{i2} - 0.02x_{i3} - 0.03x_{i4}$$
$$- 0.51x_{i5} - 0.35x_{i6} + 0.45x_{i7} + 0.23x_{i8}$$

is the ith value of the first principal component. The largest coefficients are associated with parental age and smoking exposure ($-0.49, 0.34, -0.51$, and 0.45) as well as father's educational level (-0.35). In this sense, the first principal component P_1 combines the simultaneous influences of age and smoking exposure of both parents. Similarly, the largest coefficients in the second principal component summary are associated with maternal height and weight (-0.58 and -0.52) indicating that "size" of the mother dominates this summary.

Specific principal component summary values for each infant can be extracted from the S-object generated by *prcomp()* where they are contained in an array labeled x or, for the example data, *p.object$x*. The k columns are the n values of the principal component summaries. The 38 values from each of the first two principal components from the scaled low birth weight data are

```
> p<- sweep(p.object$x,2,apply(p.object$x,2,mean))
> round(p[,1],3)
 [1]   0.534 -1.987  1.548  1.224 -0.126 -1.774  0.419  2.301
 [9]   0.505  3.246  2.123 -1.173 -1.635  1.542 -2.807 -0.712
[17]  -2.503 -1.177 -2.272  0.265 -0.543 -2.408 -1.132  1.417
[25]  -0.554 -1.175  1.097  2.473 -2.685  0.586  0.597  1.443
[33]   1.404  0.209 -1.580  2.528  0.360  0.420
> round(p[,2],3)
 [1]  -1.242  0.014 -0.567  2.219  0.489 -1.080  0.575  0.770
 [9]   0.909 -1.861 -1.738  0.012  0.026  0.571 -0.573  1.073
[17]  -0.953 -0.430 -1.655  1.963  1.717  0.859  0.675 -0.630
[25]  -0.619  3.503 -3.460  0.502 -1.470 -0.356  1.690 -0.063
[33]  -0.649  0.956 -1.166  0.328  1.231 -1.570
> # verify a few properties of principal components
> ptemp<- cbind(p[,1],p[,2])
> round(apply(ptemp,2,mean),3)
> [1]  0  0
```

```
> round(apply(ptemp,2,var),3)
[1] 2.685 1.818
> round(cor(ptemp),3)
     [,1] [,2]
[1,]   1    0
[2,]   0    1.
```

The *sweep*( )-command produces principal components with mean values equal to zero, for convenience.

Another view of the role each variable plays in determining the value of a principal component is achieved by correlating the principal component summary P_i with a specific variable x_j. A high correlation between the values P_i and the values x_j indicates that the principal component reflects the impact of variable x_j and, conversely, a low correlation indicates that a principal component score is not influenced by the variable x_j. Like the coefficients themselves, these correlations provide a measure of the role of each observed variable in determining the principal component values. The 8×8 correlation array containing all pairwise correlations between the eight parental variables and the eight principal components is (rows = variables and columns = principal components)

```
> round(cor(x,p),3)
        [,1]    [,2]    [,3]    [,4]    [,5]    [,6]    [,7]    [,8]
[1,] -0.803 -0.427  0.024 -0.134 -0.299  0.131  0.033 -0.218
[2,]  0.562 -0.450  0.555  0.156  0.133  0.177 -0.310 -0.062
[3,] -0.030 -0.785  0.148  0.090 -0.028 -0.589  0.067  0.031
[4,] -0.048 -0.698 -0.372  0.009  0.532  0.262  0.145  0.006
[5,] -0.836 -0.350  0.175 -0.026 -0.199  0.225 -0.099  0.216
[6,] -0.571  0.248  0.043  0.774  0.097 -0.005  0.036 -0.031
[7,]  0.744 -0.255  0.202  0.199 -0.379  0.245  0.310  0.029
[8,]  0.376 -0.287 -0.762  0.212 -0.318  0.007 -0.221  0.007.
```

Some examples are: the correlation between the 38 maternal ages (x_1) and the 38 values of the first principal component (P_1) is -0.803; the similar correlation between maternal age and the second principal component is -0.427. The correlation between maternal smoking (x_2) and the first principal component is 0.562. The correlation coefficients $(\mid cor(P_1, x_j) \mid > 0.5$—column 1) suggest that the first principal component reflects age and smoking exposure of the mother and age, education, and smoking exposure of the father (correlations > 0.5). The second principal component is associated with maternal size $(\mid cor(P_2, x_j) \mid > 0.6$—column 2). Similar results are observed by directly comparing the principal component coefficients derived from commensurate data.

Pairwise plots of the first several principal component summaries occasionally show clustering within a multivariate data set. Such a plot is (Figure 7.10) created by

```
> plot(p[,1],p[,2],pch="+",
  main="First and second principal components")
```

First and second principal components

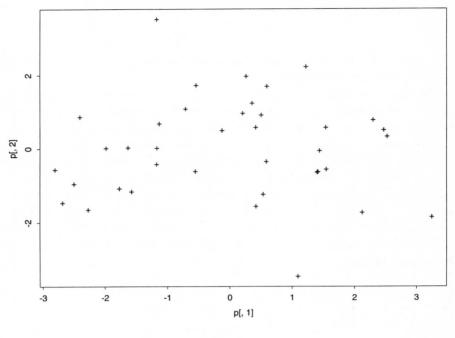

Figure 7.10

The parental variables summarized by the first two principal components do not seem to show any obvious clustering. A comprehensive plot of the patterns described by all pairs of principal component summaries is given by *pairs(S.object$x)* and specifically, for the example data *pairs(p.object$x)*.

Principal component values can serve to further describe the relationships within a data set. For example, the relationships between the birth weight in small infants and the "age/smoking" and "size" principal components can be explored. A bivariate linear regression analysis using birth weight (contained in an S-vector labeled *bwt* from Table 7.5) as the dependent variable and the first two uncorrelated principal component summaries as independent variables gives

```
> otemp<- lm(bwt~p[,1]+p[,2])
> summary(otemp)
Call: lm(formula = y ~ p[, 1] + p[, 2])
Residuals:
     Min        1Q Median       3Q      Max
  -1.956 -0.03362 0.1653 0.309 0.5583
```

```
Coefficients:
              Value Std. Error    t value   Pr(>|t|)
(Intercept)  5.2868    0.0923     57.2644     0.0000
    p[, 1]   0.0157    0.0571      0.2746     0.7853
    p[, 2]   0.0062    0.0694      0.0899     0.9289

Residual standard error: 0.5691 on 35 degrees of freedom
Multiple R-Squared: 0.002379
F-statistic: 0.04173 on 2 and 35 degrees of freedom,
  the p-value is 0.9592

Correlation of Coefficients:
        (Intercept) p[, 1]
p[, 1]      0
p[, 2]      0              0.
```

The regression analysis produces absolutely no indication that the "age/smoking" or "size" principal components are associated with the birth weights of these exceptionally small infants ($R^2 = 0.002$ with p-value $= 0.959$).

Another illustration of principal component analysis comes from the cereal contents data given previously (Table 2.10). The S-array *cereal* contains 30 observations made up of 11 measured variables (30 × 11 array) and

```
> # array = cereal (30 by 11) contains the data
> v<- prcomp(cereal)$sd^2
> round(v,2)
[1] 12231.37 5580.55 162.13   24.17   9.18   5.07   1.02   0.70
[9]     0.34       0.11    0.02
> round(100*v/sum(v),1)
[1] 67.9 31.0   0.9   0.1   0.1   0.0   0.0   0.0   0.0   0.0   0.0
> round(cumsum(100*v/sum(v)),1)
[1]  67.9  98.9  99.8  99.9 100.0 100.0 100.0 100.0 100.0.
```

The first two principal components "explain" essentially all the variation associated with the 11 measured variables (98.9%). A multidimensional measurement is, therefore, unnecessary since almost all the variation captured by the 11 cereal measurements is summarized by two variables. The principal component coefficients associated with each of the 11 variables are (columns):

```
> round(prcomp(cereal)$rotation,2)
       [,1]  [,2]  [,3]  [,4]  [,5]  [,6]  [,7]  [,8]  [,9] [,10] [,11]
[1,]   0.00  0.00  0.01  0.00 -0.01  0.04  0.05  0.00  0.01  0.08 -0.99
[2,]   0.02  0.00 -0.76  0.57 -0.24 -0.18  0.00  0.08 -0.02  0.01 -0.01
[3,]  -0.01  0.00 -0.63 -0.73  0.09  0.23 -0.02 -0.02  0.02  0.10  0.01
[4,]   0.00  0.00 -0.06 -0.08 -0.01 -0.02  0.19 -0.05 -0.08 -0.97 -0.07
[5,]   0.99  0.14  0.00 -0.02  0.01  0.00  0.00  0.00  0.00  0.00  0.00
[6,]  -0.14  0.99  0.00 -0.01 -0.01 -0.02 -0.02 -0.02  0.01  0.00  0.00
[7,]   0.01  0.02 -0.02  0.32  0.08  0.91 -0.06 -0.23  0.00 -0.04  0.03
[8,]   0.00  0.03  0.03  0.02  0.07  0.23  0.36  0.87 -0.22  0.03  0.02
[9,]  -0.01  0.01 -0.13  0.18  0.95 -0.16  0.00 -0.07 -0.14  0.00 -0.02
[10,]  0.00  0.01  0.01 -0.02 -0.12 -0.04  0.62 -0.40 -0.63  0.20  0.04
[11,]  0.00  0.00 -0.02  0.04  0.08  0.00  0.67 -0.10  0.72  0.07  0.05.
```

The first two principal components almost exclusively reflect two separate variables, namely the sodium and potassium measurements, which essentially are determined by the type of grain used to manufacture the cereal. In other words, once the cereal grain is identified, the other nine measurements add almost no new information.

A plot of the first two principal components created by

```
> p<- prcomp(cereal)$x
> plot(p[,1],p[,2],pch="*",
    main="Cereal classification by principal components")
> text(p[,1],p[,2],1:nrow(dtemp),adj=2,cex=0.5)
```

is shown in Figure 7.11. Almost the same plot occurs if the sodium and potassium measurements are plotted (x = sodium and y = potassium; n = 30) ignoring the other nine variables, which is another indication of the dominance of the sodium/potassium measurements. Some of the same patterns of clustering appear in the principal component plot (Figure 7.11) that are evident in the dendrogram of the same cereal data (Figure 2.34).

The S-function $text(x, y, labels)$ places labels on the current plot at the locations of specified points. The first two arguments are vectors of the xy-coordinates for the points and the third argument is a vector of labels to be assigned to the points (e.g., an integer labeling each cereal brand—Table

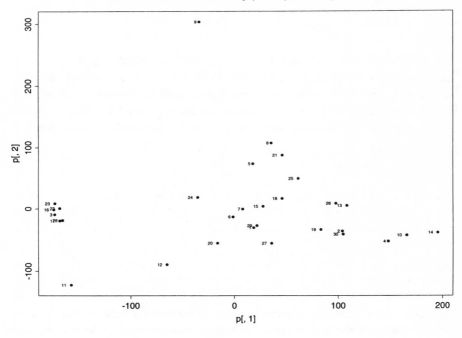

Figure 7.11

2.10). An option *adj* shifts the position of the label to the right or left of the plotted points (see *?text*) and the option *cex*, again, determines the size of the plotted label.

CANONICAL CORRELATIONS

Canonical correlations can be viewed as a generalization of a multivariable regression analysis with elements of a principal component summary. In a broad sense, a canonical correlation coefficient measures the association between two sets of multivariate observations. The technique, originally described by Hotelling [8], was first applied to investigate the association between reading and arithmetic abilities in school children. Two measurements of reading ability and two measurements of arithmetic skills were made. Interest focused on the association between these two bivariate observations. Simple correlation coefficients could be calculated describing the pairwise associations between the reading and arithmetic measures. However, these pairwise correlations do not take into account the undoubtedly high correlation between the two measures of reading skills and between the two measures of arithmetic skills.

A canonical correlations approach addresses the question of the relationship between pairs of multivariate observations by finding two linear combinations of the multivariate measurements that have the highest possible correlation. These linear combinations are yet another type of canonical summary. Specifically, if x_1 and x_2 represent values measuring reading ability and y_1 and y_2 represent values measuring arithmetic skills, then two canonical variables are formed

$$X = a_1x_1 + a_2x_2$$

and

$$Y = b_1y_1 + b_2y_2$$

where the coefficients a_j and b_j are chosen so that the correlation between X and Y is as large as possible. The correlation between X and Y then reflects the association between two bivariate measurements, math versus reading scores. A canonical correlation analysis is analogous to a regression analysis but instead of a single dependent variable, the "dependent variable" is a canonical variable based on a multivariate response such as the bivariate measure from a math or reading exam. Instead of k independent variables and one dependent variable, canonical correlations symmetrically summarize the association between a p-dimensional x-variable from one group and q-dimensional y-variable from another group.

The process of creating a canonical summary generalizes to any number of measurements per observation where

$$X_{i1} = a_{11}x_{i1} + a_{21}x_{i2} + a_{31}x_{i3} + \cdots + a_{p1}x_{ip}$$
$$X_{i2} = a_{12}x_{i1} + a_{22}x_{i2} + a_{32}x_{i3} + \cdots + a_{p2}x_{ip}$$

$$\vdots$$

$$X_{ip} = a_{1p}x_{i1} + a_{2p}x_{i2} + a_{3p}x_{i3} + \cdots + a_{pp}x_{ip} \qquad i = 1, 2, 3, \cdots, n.$$

The value X_{ij} represents the jth canonical variable for the ith observation constructed from p-dimensional data in one group. Also,

$$Y_{i1} = b_{11}y_{i1} + b_{21}y_{i2} + b_{31}y_{i3} + \cdots + b_{q1}y_{iq}$$
$$Y_{i2} = b_{12}y_{i1} + b_{22}y_{i2} + b_{32}y_{i3} + \cdots + b_{q2}y_{iq}$$

$$\vdots$$

$$Y_{iq} = b_{1q}y_{i1} + b_{2q}y_{i2} + b_{3q}y_{i3} + \cdots + b_{qq}y_{iq} \qquad i = 1, 2, 3, \cdots, n.$$

where the value Y_{ij} represents the jth canonical variable for the ith observation constructed from q-dimensional data in another group. The numbers of measured variables per observation are represented by p and q, respectively. The transformation produces n pairs of canonical measurements (X, Y) for each canonical summary.

Each set of coefficients is chosen, like the coefficients that generate principal components, to give the canonical summaries specific properties. The first set of coefficients (a_1 and b_1) are chosen so that X_1 and Y_1 have the largest possible correlation. The second set of coefficients (a_2 and b_2) are chosen so that X_2 and Y_2 have the next largest correlation and X_2 and Y_2 are uncorrelated with X_1 and Y_1. Similarly, the third set of coefficients (a_3 and b_3) are chosen so that X_3 and Y_3 have the next largest correlation and X_3 and Y_3 are uncorrelated with the other canonical variables. In symbols,

$$correlation(X_1, Y_1) > correlation(X_2, Y_2) > correlation(X_3, Y_3) > \cdots$$

and

$$correlation(X_i, X_j) = 0 \text{ and } correlation(Y_i, Y_j) = 0 \text{ when } i \neq j.$$

The property that the canonical variables are uncorrelated allows each canonical variable to possibly reflect different aspects of the multivariate measurements. Like principal component analysis, the first few canonical correlations are the most descriptive.

A special case arises when $q = 1$ ($Y_{i1} = y_{i1}$). The canonical correlation is then identical to the multiple correlation coefficient from a linear model based on the p independent variables and the single dependent variable y ($q = 1$).

To illustrate, a data set with two components, vital statistics variables and "demographic" variables, is investigated (Table 7.6). Four vital statistics for the 50 states and the District of Columbia are recorded—life expectancy of males in years (x_1), life expectancy of females in years (x_2), birth rate per 100,000 (x_3), and death rate per 100,000 (x_4). Also recorded are 51 values reflecting demographic characteristics—percent urban areas (y_1), percent of population earning more than 25,000 dollars (y_2), taxes in millions of dollars (y_3), and population density (y_4). The "health" observations are contained in the 51 × 4 S-array labeled y and the "demographic" variables are contained in the 51 × 4 S-array labeled x. The S-code that forms a correlation array displaying the 28 pairwise product-moment correlations is

```
> y<- cbind(exm,exf,births,deaths)
> y<- scale(y,center=T)
> x<- cbind(urban,income,taxes,density)
> x<- scale(x,center=T)
> data<- cbind(y,x)
> round(cor(data),3)
           exm     exf births deaths  urban income   taxes density
    exm  1.000   0.802 -0.237 -0.318  0.239 -0.570   0.141  -0.264
    exf  0.802   1.000 -0.043 -0.314 -0.105 -0.394  -0.153  -0.340
 births -0.237  -0.043  1.000 -0.628 -0.079  0.193  -0.242   0.043
 deaths -0.318  -0.314 -0.628  1.000 -0.134  0.282   0.078   0.266
  urban  0.239  -0.105 -0.079 -0.134  1.000  0.151   0.480   0.375
 income -0.570  -0.394  0.193  0.282  0.151  1.000   0.014   0.689
  taxes  0.141  -0.153 -0.242  0.078  0.480  0.014   1.000  -0.010
density -0.264  -0.340  0.043  0.266  0.375  0.689  -0.010   1.000.
```

These correlations show the pairwise relationships among the eight variables, particularly the correlation within the two components. The data are standardized to have mean zero and unit variance using the S-function *scale( )*. Standardizing the data does not affect the correlation array or the canonical correlations but is helpful when examining the relationships of each individual variable to the canonical summary variables. Like the principal component analysis, scaling the original data aids in the interpretation of the roles of the individual components that make up the canonical variables.

Canonical correlation analysis generated by the S-function *cancor( )* produces the relevant S-object and for the United States data

```
> c.object<- cancor(x,y)
> summary(c.object)
        Length Class   Mode
    cor    4           numeric
  xcoef 16           numeric
  ycoef 16           numeric
xcenter   4           numeric
ycenter   4           numeric.
```

The canonical correlations are

```
> c.object$cor
[1]    0.8262540    0.5220645    0.2331807    0.1662209.
```

Table 7.6. Data on 50 states plus the District of Columbia for health and demographic characteristics

state	vital records variables				demographic variables			
	exm	exf	births	deaths	urban	income	taxes	density
AL	66.17	74.35	19.4	9.8	58.4	26.2	297.7	68
AK	66.86	74.31	24.9	4.8	48.8	2.9	53.8	1
AZ	66.97	74.19	21.2	8.4	79.5	3.0	406.9	16
AR	66.98	74.74	18.5	10.7	50.0	18.3	162.2	37
CA	67.97	74.27	18.2	8.3	90.9	7.0	7365.3	128
CO	67.95	74.53	18.8	7.9	78.7	3.0	589.7	21
CT	68.93	74.88	16.7	8.6	77.3	6.0	981.5	624
DE	67.35	74.04	19.2	9.0	72.1	14.3	67.1	277
DC	65.16	72.77	20.1	11.7	100.0	71.1	457.8	12402
FL	67.49	74.85	16.9	11.0	80.5	15.3	1203.9	126
GA	65.88	74.08	21.1	9.1	60.3	25.8	629.0	79
HI	70.39	75.68	21.3	5.2	83.0	1.0	125.9	120
ID	67.72	74.82	20.3	8.6	54.3	0.3	112.2	9
IL	67.20	73.70	18.5	10.0	83.0	12.8	3130.0	199
IN	67.25	73.81	19.1	9.3	64.9	6.9	1247.2	144
IA	68.40	74.98	17.1	10.4	57.2	1.2	676.6	51
KS	68.53	75.24	17.0	9.7	66.1	4.7	522.1	28
KY	66.24	73.60	18.7	10.3	52.4	7.2	305.2	81
LA	66.16	73.93	20.4	9.2	66.1	29.8	500.1	81
ME	66.75	73.42	17.9	11.1	50.9	0.3	224.7	32
MD	67.48	74.16	17.5	8.4	76.6	17.8	996.8	397
MA	67.80	74.20	16.6	10.1	84.6	3.1	1929.5	727
MI	67.57	73.94	19.4	8.6	73.9	11.2	2184.7	156
MN	68.87	75.26	18.0	8.9	66.4	0.9	924.3	48
MS	65.74	74.06	22.1	10.5	44.5	36.8	189.8	47
MO	67.32	74.17	17.3	11.1	70.1	10.3	958.5	68
MT	66.74	74.08	18.2	9.5	53.6	9.3	191.1	5
NE	68.53	75.23	17.3	10.1	61.6	2.7	384.9	19
NV	65.69	72.83	19.6	7.9	80.9	5.7	136.3	4
NH	67.06	73.84	17.9	10.0	56.5	0.4	210.4	82
NJ	68.16	73.98	16.8	9.5	88.9	10.7	2475.6	953
NM	66.70	73.73	21.7	7.3	70.0	1.9	85.3	8
NY	67.60	73.70	17.4	10.3	85.6	11.9	7453.4	381
NC	66.35	74.33	19.3	8.8	45.0	22.2	526.3	104
ND	69.07	75.59	17.6	9.1	44.3	0.4	110.5	9
OH	67.42	73.82	18.7	9.4	75.3	9.1	2372.9	260
OK	67.38	74.59	17.5	10.5	68.0	6.7	334.7	37
OR	68.03	74.75	16.8	9.3	67.1	1.3	540.5	22
PA	67.24	73.47	16.3	10.8	71.5	8.6	2362.9	262
RI	68.02	74.16	16.5	10.0	87.0	2.7	200.3	905
SC	65.70	73.67	20.1	8.8	47.6	30.4	230.4	86
SD	68.71	75.27	17.5	9.9	44.6	0.3	174.1	9
TN	66.68	74.31	18.4	9.7	58.8	15.8	546.9	95
TX	67.72	74.36	20.6	8.4	79.8	12.5	1971.8	43
UT	68.96	75.18	25.5	6.7	80.6	0.6	167.6	13
VT	67.32	74.27	18.8	10.0	32.2	0.2	122.5	48
VA	67.27	74.38	18.6	8.4	63.1	18.5	819.5	117
WA	67.93	74.56	17.8	8.8	72.6	2.1	653.4	51
WV	65.35	72.82	17.8	11.5	39.0	3.8	167.7	72
WI	68.71	74.75	17.6	9.2	65.9	2.9	1181.7	81
WY	66.19	74.08	19.6	8.8	60.4	0.7	70.4	3

In symbols, the canonical correlations found in *S.object$cor* are *correlation*($X_1, Y_1$), *correlation*($X_2, Y_2$), *correlation*($X_3, Y_3$), $\cdots$, in descending order.

Each canonical variable is a linear combination created by multiplying each variable in a multivariate observation by its corresponding coefficient and summing the terms, forming a single variable. These coefficients are extracted from the S-object by *S.object$xcoef* and *S.object$ycoef* (columns) and for the United States data

```
> ya<- otemp$ycoef
> round(ya,3)
        [,1]    [,2]    [,3]    [,4]
[1,] -0.074  0.050  0.159 -0.016
[2,]  0.134  0.009  0.116  0.091
[3,] -0.034 -0.091 -0.079  0.111
[4,] -0.047 -0.144 -0.101 -0.120
> xa<- c.object$xcoef
> round(xa,3)
        [,1]    [,2]    [,3]    [,4]
[1,] -0.206 -0.139  0.012 -0.150
[2,]  0.149  0.166 -0.106  0.002
[3,]  0.027 -0.089  0.042 -0.210
[4,]  0.038 -0.143 -0.096 -0.153.
```

For example, the first X and Y canonical variables are

$$Y_{i1} = -0.074y_{i1} + 0.134y_{i2} - 0.034y_{i3} - 0.047y_{i4}$$

and

$$X_{i1} = -0.206x_{i1} + 0.149x_{i2} + 0.027x_{i3} + 0.038x_{i4} \qquad i = 1, 2, 3, \cdots, 51.$$

The *correlation*(X_1, Y_1) is 0.826 based on two sets of 51 "observations." No other linear combination of the x-values and y-values has a higher correlation.

Again, the magnitude of the coefficients that make up the linear combination do not directly indicate the relative roles of the variables in determining the variation of the canonical variables unless the data are standardized. A summary of the relationship between a measured value and a canonical value is again a product–moment pairwise correlation coefficient. Specifically, *correlation*(X_i, x_j) or *correlation*(Y_i, y_j) indicates the role of variables x_j or y_j in the make-up of the canonical variables X_i or Y_i. For the example United States data, the two correlation arrays are

```
> # cy = four canonical summaries -- vital statistics variables
> cy<- y%*%yb
> round(cor(cbind(cy,y)),3)
        cy[,1] cy[,2] cy[,3] cy[,4]  urban income  taxes density
cy[,1]  1.000  0.000  0.000  0.000 -0.618  0.638 -0.474  0.128
cy[,2]  0.000  1.000  0.000  0.000 -0.332 -0.594 -0.467 -0.837
cy[,3]  0.000  0.000  1.000  0.000  0.711  0.487  0.001  0.274
cy[,4]  0.000  0.000  0.000  1.000 -0.041 -0.051 -0.746  0.457
urban  -0.618 -0.332  0.711 -0.041  1.000  0.151  0.480  0.375
income  0.638 -0.594  0.487 -0.051  0.151  1.000  0.014  0.689
taxes  -0.474 -0.467  0.001 -0.746  0.480  0.014  1.000 -0.010
```

```
density 0.128 -0.837  0.274  0.457  0.375  0.689 -0.010  1.000
> # cx = four canonical summaries -- demographic variables
> cx<- x%*%xa
> round(cor(cbind(cx,x)),3)
         cx[,1] cx[,2] cx[,3] cx[,4]    exm    exf births deaths
cx[,1]   1.000  0.000  0.000  0.000 -0.741 -0.205  0.325  0.278
cx[,2]   0.000  1.000  0.000  0.000  0.433  0.734  0.186 -0.672
cx[,3]   0.000  0.000  1.000  0.000 -0.372 -0.481  0.739 -0.660
cx[,4]   0.000  0.000  0.000  1.000  0.354  0.434  0.560 -0.188
exm     -0.741  0.433 -0.372  0.354  1.000  0.802 -0.237 -0.318
exf      0.205  0.734 -0.481  0.434  0.802  1.000 -0.043 -0.314
births   0.325  0.186  0.739  0.560 -0.237 -0.043  1.000 -0.628
deaths   0.278 -0.672 -0.660 -0.188 -0.318 -0.314 -0.628  1.000.
```

Parallel to a principal component summary, the correlations between the individual summaries and the canonical variables can indicate a useful "meaning" for the summarized multivariate observation. However, attributing meaning to the canonical variables is frequently a somewhat subjective process. For the United States data, the first canonical variable Y_1 appears to be most influenced by urbanization and income (correlations of -0.618 and 0.638, respectively) while the second canonical variable Y_2 emphasizes population density (correlation of -0.837). The first canonical variable X_1 appears to be most influenced by expectation of life for males (correlation of -0.741) while the second canonical variable X_2 emphasizes female life expectancy and mortality rates (correlations of 0.734 and -0.672, respectively). Leading to a rough interpretation that the major determinant of the first canonical correlation (0.826) is the association between urban/income status and male expectation of life.

Like all statistical quantities, canonical correlation coefficients are subject to the influence of sampling variation. Significance tests exist to address the question of whether observed canonical correlations are likely due to chance variation or likely a result of systematic relationships between the two compared groups. For the present data, the probability of observing stronger evidence of an association when the x-variables ("health") are unrelated to the y-variables ("demographic") is less than 0.001. This significance test results from a sophisticated manipulation of the correlation array and detailed explanations are found in advanced texts on multivariate analysis (e.g., [9] or [10]). An example of S-code to conduct a significance test (are the observed canonical correlation coefficients likely due entirely to capitalizing on chance variation?) applied to the United States data gives

```
> # number of x-variates
> p<- ncol(x)
> # number of y-variates
> q<- ncol(y)
> total number of observations
> n<- nrow(data)
> mm<- cor(data)
> am<- mm[(1:p),(1:p)]
```

```
> bm<- mm[(p+1):(p+q),(p+1):(p+q)]
> cm<- mm[(1:p),(p+1):(p+q)]
> m<- solve(bm)%*%t(cm)%*%solve(am)%*%cm
> e<- eigen(m)$values
> # transforms e to have a a chi-square distribution
> x2<- -(n-(p+q+1)/2)*sum(log(1-e))
> pvalue<- 1-pchisq(x2,p*q)
> round(cbind(x2,pvalue),3)
          x2 pvalue
[1,] 72.076      0.
```

The S-function *eigen*( ) computes the eigenvalues (latent roots) of the argument matrix and are the key elements in assessing the impact of random variation on the magnitude of a series of canonical correlation coefficients. The large chi-square value (p-value < 0.001) indicates that the correlation between the multivariate measurments of the "health" and the "demographic" characteristics is not at all likely to be a result of random variation.

Problem set VII

1. Use the cholesterol and behavior type data (Table 1.5) to show that a two-sample t-test, a simple linear regression analysis, and an analysis of variance give identical results. That is, all three approaches produce the same significance probability for comparing levels of cholesterol between behavior types A and B.

2. Use the *glm*( ) S-function to reproduce the results found in the chapter using the *aov*( ) S-command for the two-way table of lead level determination data (Table 7.2).

3. Construct and test an S-program to execute a Kruskal–Wallis rank test for independent samples. Compare the results with the S-function *kruskal.test*( ) for a set of simulated data with no identical (tied) values.

   Construct and test an S-program to execute a Friedman rank test for data classified in a two-way table (e.g., the serum lead data—Table 7.2). Compare the results with the S-function *friedman.test*( ) for a set of simulated data with no identical (tied) values.

   Construct and test an S-program to execute a Wilcoxon signed rank test for a set of matched pairs data. Compare the results with the S-function *wilcox.test*( ) for a set of simulated data with no identical (tied) values.

4. Conduct a principal component analysis where $x_1 = \{1, 2, 3, 4, 5, 6, 7\}$ and $x_2 = \{7, 6, 5, 4, 5, 6, 7\}$. Calculate the variance of x_1, the variance of x_2, the variance of the first principal component, and the variance of the second principal component. Why are these variances the same?

5. Using the turtle data (Table 4.4) calculate the first two principal components. To identify differences by gender (clustering), plot the 48 values of each principal component (one against the other).

6. Use the following data to show that a canonical correlation and the multiple correlation coefficient are the same when one group consists of a single variable (y) and the other group (x) has $k = 2$ variables (i.e., compare results from *cancor*( ) with *lm*( ) S-functions).

	y	x_1	x_2
1.	4.8	1	0.2
2.	14.1	2	0.6
3.	10.7	3	0.2
4.	18.3	4	0.8
5.	12.7	5	0.2
6.	17.2	6	1.9
7.	16.0	7	1.3
8.	22.0	8	1.6
9.	22.0	9	1.7
10.	23.6	10	1.1

7. Using the weight gain matched pair data (Table 7.3), assess the association between maternal weight gain and low birth weight ignoring the paired structure (as if the two infants represent samples from separate and unrelated populations). In other words, does the paired pattern of the data collection improve the efficiency of the analysis or not?

8. Write and test an S-program to execute a randomization test for matched pair data. Conduct a matched pair randomization test using the paired data in Table 7.3. Compare the results to the tests used in the chapter to analyze the association between birth weight and maternal weight gain matched for prepregnancy weight.

9. A total of $N = 11$ matched sets of data are collected (one case and two controls). For each infant with a birth defect (case) born in a rural area in France, two infants (controls) were selected who were born at essentially the same time, in the same village and were the same sex. The matched data consist of the distances to electromagnetic radiation exposure (risk factor—measured in meters).

malformation	1150	100	2000	350	400	2700	1200	1800	10	250	350
control 1	300	100	2150	1350	800	1250	450	400	900	1950	1050
control 2	750	650	4050	450	700	2850	50	2300	150	300	1000

Using these 1:2 matched sets assess the association between electromagnetic radiation and birth defects (does the distances among cases differ from distances among controls?).

Ignoring the matched data collection design, again evaluate the association between electromagnetic radiation and birth defects. Does the matched pattern of the data collection improve the efficiency of the analysis?

10. Simulate a data set of $n = 100$ pairs of matched observations.

Demonstrate that the results using the binomial test (without a correction factor) and the Friedman test are identical.

Simulate a data set of $n_1 = 100$ and $n_2 = 100$ observations from two independent populations. Demonstrate that the results using the Wilcoxon two-sample test (*pairs* = F) and the Kruskal–Wallis tests are identical.

REFERENCES

1. Conover, W. J., *Practical Nonparametric Statistics*. John Wiley & Sons, New York, NY, 1971.
2. Tukey, J. W., (1949) One degree of freedom for nonadditivity. *Biometrics*, 5:232–242.
3. Neter, J., Wasserman, W., and Kutner, M. H., *Applied Linear Statistical Models*. Irwin, Homewood, IL, 1990.
4. Miller, A. J., *Subset Selection in Regression*. Chapman and Hall, New York, NY, 1990.
5 Furnival, G. M. and Wilson, R. W. Jr., (1974) Regressions by Leaps and Bounds. *Technometrics*, 16:499–511.
6. Seber, G. A. F., *Linear Regression Analysis*. John Wiley & Sons, New York, NY, 1977.
7. Hosmer, D. W. and Lemeshow S., *Applied Logistic Regression*. John Wiley and Sons, New York, NY, 1989.
8. Hotelling, H., (1936) Relations between two sets of variables. *Biometrics* 28:321–77.
9. Manly, B. F. J., *Multivariate Statistical Methods: a Primer*. Chapman and Hall, New York, NY, 1986.
10. Johnson, R. A., *Applied Multivariate Statistical Analysis*. Prentice-Hall, Englewood, NJ, 1982.

8

Rates, Life Tables, and Survival

RATES

A rate is an instantaneous quantity measuring a change per unit time defined mathematically in terms of the derivative of a function. In fields such as epidemiology and medicine a rate is usually calculated to assess risk and is almost always an approximate average rate. To measure risk, an approximate average rate is defined as

$$approximate\ average\ rate = \frac{number\ of\ events}{total\ person\text{-}years}.$$

A rate is an average because it refers to a period of time and not a single instant; therefore, reflecting the average risk across a period of time. The time period is typically one year, five years, or sometimes ten years. Person-years, in the denominator, is the total time accumulated by the persons at risk over the time considered. A rate is approximate because the person-years is typically estimated by making the assumption that change in the population size is a linear function, or at least, an approximate linear function of time. To define a rate symbolically, notation for three quantities is necessary:

1. the length of the time interval considered: length = δ_x where x denotes a specific interval,
2. the number of persons at risk for the event at the beginning of the interval x: P_x and
3. the number of events such as disease or death that occurred during the interval x to $x + \delta_x$: D_x.

A direct result of this notation is $P_x - P_{x+\delta_x} = D_x$ = number of events.

Using these symbols, the total person-years accumulated in the interval x to $x + \delta_x$ is approximately

$$total\ person\text{-}years = \delta_x P_{x+\delta_x} + \tfrac{1}{2}\delta_x D_x.$$

More precisely, the persons who complete the interval without the event occurring contribute a total of $\delta_x P_{x+\delta_x}$ person-years (when time is measured in years). The persons who experienced the event under consideration contribute a total of approximately $\frac{1}{2}\delta_x D_x$ person-years. The term $\frac{1}{2}\delta_x$ is the approximate average time at risk for each individual up to the time the event occurred. Two equivalent alternative ways to express the total person-years accumulated over a time interval are:

$$total\ person\text{-}years = \delta_x P_x - \tfrac{1}{2}\delta_x D_x = \tfrac{1}{2}\delta_x(P_{x+\delta_x} + P_x).$$

Therefore, an average approximate rate R_x is expressed as

$$approximate\ average\ rate = R_x = \frac{D_x}{\delta_x P_x - \tfrac{1}{2}\delta_x D_x}.$$

Frequently, person-years is estimated using the mid-interval population, then

$$total\ person\text{-}years = \tfrac{1}{2}\delta_x(P_{x+\delta_x} + P_x) = \delta_x(mid\text{-}interval\ population)$$

giving an estimate of a rate as

$$estimated\ rate = R_x = \frac{D_x}{\delta_x(mid\text{-}interval\ population)}.$$

When D_x represents a count of cases of disease or a number of deaths, the quantities D_x and mid-year populations are available from study samples or from government agencies that routinely keep records of disease and mortality. Specifically, for lung cancer (1988–1992—a five-year interval) among males aged 60–64 in the San Francisco Bay area, the number of incident cases $D_{1988} = 1087$ with the corresponding person-years of risk is 351,666 (1990 mid-interval population multiplied by 5) producing an annual rate of 309.1 lung cancer deaths per 100,000 person-years [1]. Rates are usually multiplied by a "base" of 100,000 or some other power of 10 to avoid small fractions.

The probability of an event such as disease or death is related to a rate. The probability of an event is estimated by the ratio of the number of occurrences of the event to the total number of possible occurrences. If D_x represents the number of individuals with a disease or the number of deaths counted between the times x and $x + \delta_x$ and P_x represents the number of individuals at risk at the beginning of interval x, then

$$estimated\ probability = Q_x = \frac{D_x}{P_x}$$

is an estimate of the probability of disease or death during the interval x to $x + \delta_x$ (e.g., the total number of persons who died divided by the number of persons who could have died).

A probability is a unitless quantity that is always between 0 and 1. A rate and a probability, nevertheless, are related. A bit of algebra yields

$$rate = R_x = \frac{Q_x}{\delta_x(1 - \frac{1}{2}Q_x)}.$$

In many situations, particularly for probabilities of disease or death calculated from human populations, Q_x is small (i.e., $1 - \frac{1}{2}Q_x \approx 1$). The approximate relationship of a rate to a probability is then $\delta_x R_x \approx Q_x$. Frequently, δ_x is one (e.g., one year) making a rate and a probability essentially equal, $R_x \approx Q_x$. The two measures of risk are often used, more or less, interchangeably when disease or mortality rates are expressed in terms of one-year intervals or when rate ratios are calculated among groups for equal intervals of time.

Two sets of mortality data are given in Table 8.1. The data are the number of United States cancer deaths among white males and the age-specific population counts for the years 1960 and 1940 (extracted from *Vital Statistics of the United States 1940 and 1960* published by the National Center for Health Statistics).

The populations are the United States census counts (approximate mid-year populations) and, for example, the 1960 age-specific rate of cancer mortality for males aged 65–74 is $R_{65} = 100,000 \times 41,725/4,702,482 = 887.3$ deaths per 100,000 person-years.

When rates refer to disease or death the most important consideration is age. Disease and mortality rates vary considerably depending on the age of the individuals considered. A crude mortality rate ignores age. A crude mortality rate is defined as

$$crude\ mortality\ rate = C = base \times \frac{total\ deaths}{total\ person\text{-}years} = base \times \frac{\sum D_x}{\sum P_{x'}}.$$

The sums are calculated over all age-specific groups (denoted by x and $P_{x'}$ represents the mid-year population). Specifically, the 1960 crude cancer mortality rate is

Table 8.1. United States cancer mortality for the years 1940 and 1960, white males

age	1960 deaths	1960 population	1940 deaths	1940 population
15–24	1 080	10 482 916	670	10 629 526
25–34	1 869	9 939 972	1 126	9 465 330
35–44	4 891	10 563 872	3 160	8 249 558
45–54	14 956	9 114 202	9 723	7 294 330
55–64	30 888	6 850 263	17 935	5 022 499
65–74	41 725	4 702 482	22 179	2 920 220
75–84	26 501	1 874 619	13 461	1 019 504
85+	5 928	330 915	2 238	142 532
total	127 838	53 859 241	70 492	44 743 499

$$C_{1960} = 100{,}000 \times \frac{127{,}838}{53{,}859{,}241} =$$

237.4 cancer deaths per 100,000 person-years.

Similarity, the 1940 crude mortality rate is $C_{1940} = 157.5$ cancer deaths per 100,00 person-years.

Direct comparison of crude rates fails to account for differences in age distributions between the 1960 and 1940 populations. More older and, therefore, higher risk individuals make up the 1960 population. This difference in age distributions is part of the reason for the differences between the two crude mortality rates. To account for the impact of age on the comparison of summary rates, two model-free approaches are popular— direct and indirect rate adjustment.

A direct adjustment uses a single age distribution for all compared groups. Sometimes this single population is an external standard or sometimes the standard population is part of the data under consideration. For the example mortality data, the 1960 population serves as the standard age distribution. Applying the age-specific rates from the 1940 data to the 1960 population age distribution produces the number of estimated "deaths" in each age-specific category that would have occurred if the age distributions were identical in the two groups. The crude rate using the total of these "deaths" is the direct age-adjusted 1940 mortality rate or age-adjusted rate R_{direct} is

$$R_{direct} = base \times \frac{\sum_{x'} \frac{D_x^{comparison}}{P_{x'}^{comparison}} \times P_{x'}^{standard}}{\sum_{x'} P_{x'}^{standard}} = base \times \frac{\sum_{x'} \frac{D_x^{1940}}{P_{x'}^{1940}} \times P_{x'}^{1960}}{\sum_{x'} P_{x'}^{1960}}.$$

Age distributions no longer influence the comparison – they are the same in both groups.

Example S-code to compute a direct age-adjusted rate is

```
> # read data from table 8.1
> # adjust.data is an 8 by 4 file of mortality data
> temp<- scan("adjust.data")
> d<- matrix(temp,8)
> base<- 100000
> # deaths 1960
> d60<- d[1,]
> # population 1960
> pop60<- d[2,]
> # deaths 1940
> d40<- d[3,]
> # population 1960
> pop40<- d[4,]
> # crude rate 1960
> c60<- base*sum(d60)/sum(pop60)
> # crude rate 1940
> c40<- base*sum(d40)/sum(pop40)
```

```
> cat("\n","1960 crude rate/100,000 =",round(c60,1),
    "\n","1940 crude rate/100,000 =",round(c40,1),"\n")
 1960 crude rate/100,000 = 237.4
 1940 crude rate/100,000 = 157.5
> # adjustment
> a40.direct<- base*sum((d40/pop40)*pop60)/sum(pop60)
> cat("\n","direct adjusted 1940 rate/100,000 =",
    round(a40.direct,1),"\n")

 direct adjusted 1940 rate/100,000 = 200.8.
```

An indirect adjusted rate is accomplished by estimating the number of deaths that would have occurred in a comparison population if the age-specific rates were identical to those of a standard population. Again, the single standard may be an external population or derived from the data on hand. For the United States cancer mortality data, the 1960 population again serves as the standard. An indirect adjusted rate is then based on an expected number of deaths calculated as if the 1960 population age-specific rates apply to the 1940 population distribution or

$$expected\ number\ deaths = D_{expected} = \sum \frac{D_x^{standard}}{P_x^{standard}} \times P_{x'}^{comparison}$$

$$= \sum \frac{D_x^{1960}}{P_{x'}^{1960}} \times P_{x'}^{1940}.$$

For the illustrative data, the expected number of deaths in 1940 would be $D_{expected} = 84,187.4$, if the age-specific mortality rates were identical to those in 1960. The observed number of is $D_{observed} = 70,492$. The ratio of observed number of deaths to the expected number is called the standard mortality ratio (*smr*) or

$$standard\ mortality\ ratio = smr = \frac{D_{observed}}{D_{expected}} = \frac{70,492}{84,187.4} = 0.837.$$

An indirect adjusted rate is the crude rate from the standard population multiplied by the standard mortality ratio or

$$R_{indirect} = C_{1960} \times smr = 237.356 \times 0.837 = 198.7$$

and continuing the example S-code gives

```
> smr<- sum(d40)/sum((d60/pop60)*pop40)
> smr
[1] 0.8373225
> a40.indirect<- c60*smr
> cat("\n","indirect adjusted 1940 rate/100,000 =",
     round(a40.indirect,1),"\n")

 indirect adjusted 1940 rate/100,000 = 198.7.
```

The comparison of the crude rate (C_{1940} = 157.5) to the age-adjusted rates (≈ 200 deaths per 100,000 person-years) shows the impact of age on the comparison of the crude mortality rates. The remaining difference (237/100,000—1960 rate versus 200/100,000—1940 adjusted rate) is due to causes other than differences in age distributions; perhaps part of the increase is related to the increase in tobacco-related cancers over the period 1940 to 1960.

An alternative to calculating model-free adjusted rates is to use a model to represent the relationship between age and mortality. Such a model provides a statistical tool to estimate the impact of age and produce an "age-adjusted" rate reflecting non-age-related differences between groups. As in Chapter 4, the logarithm of a rate can be represented by a linear model or

$$log\text{-}rate = \log(R_{ij}) = a + bg_i + c_1 z_{j1} + c_2 z_{j2} + \cdots + c_k z_{j,k-1}$$

where g_i indicates group membership (g_1 = 0 and g_2 = 1; i = 1, 2 = groups) and the z_j-values represent k design variables to account for the influence of age (j = 1, 2, 3, $\cdots$, k = number of age-specific categories). The focus of the "adjusted" comparison is on the coefficient b. The magnitude of b reflects the differences between the compared groups for identical levels of age (age held constant). Specifically, $\log(R_{2j}) - \log(R_{1j}) = b$ or $R_{2j}/R_{1j} = e^b$ is a model defined "standard mortality ratio" measuring the difference between two groups "adjusted" for age. To illustrate, the cancer mortality data in Table 8.1 are again used. Applying the S-function $glm(\ )$ and assuming that the number of deaths in the 16 year/age categories (Table 8.1) are described by Poisson distributions, then

```
> # poisson regression estimated smr and adjusted rate
> g0<- c(rep(0,length(d60)),rep(1,length(d40)))
> d0<- c(d60,d40)
> pop0<- c(pop60,pop40)
> age<- seq(20,90,10)
> a0<- factor(c(age,age))
> otemp<- glm(d0~g0+a0+offset(log(pop0)),family=poisson)
> b<- otemp$coefficient[2]
> b
         g0
-0.1737038
> smr0<- exp(b)
> cat("\n","model smr =",round(smr0,3),"\n")

 model smr = 0.841
> cat("\n","model adjusted rate =",round(c60*smr0,2),"\n")

 model adjusted rate = 199.51.
```

An approximate 95% confidence interval for the estimated "standard mortality ratio" is

```
> sd<- summary(otemp)$coefficients[2,2]
> upper<- exp(b+1.96*sd)
```

```
> lower<- exp(b-1.96*sd)
> smr0<- exp(b)
> cbind(lower,smr0,upper)
        lower       smr0      upper
[1,] 0.832828 0.8405458 0.8483351.
```

The small confidence interval is due to the large number of observations. It could be argued that national data represent population values (not samples), such as the illustrative mortality data, and statistical assessment of calculated values is unnecessary.

The observed rates (dotted lines) and the modeled relationship between age, year (1980 versus 1960), and risk (solid lines) are displayed in Figure 8.1. The right-hand plot was created by the S-code

```
> par(pty="s")
> par(cex=0.75)
> # calculate log-rates
> l40<- log(d40/pop40)
> l60<- log(d60/pop60)
> plot(age,l60,ylim=c(-11,-4),type="n",xlab="age",
    ylab="log-rate")
> points(age,l40,lty=2,type="b",pch="*")
> points(age,l60,lty=2,type="b",pch="o")
> lines(age,predict(otemp)[g0==0])
> lines(age,predict(otemp)[g0==1])
> title("Log-rates by age for 1940 and 1960")
> legend(40,-9,c("estimated","observed"),lty=1:2).
```

The geometric distance between the two estimated log-rate curves (solid lines) is $\hat{b} = -0.174$ for all ages.

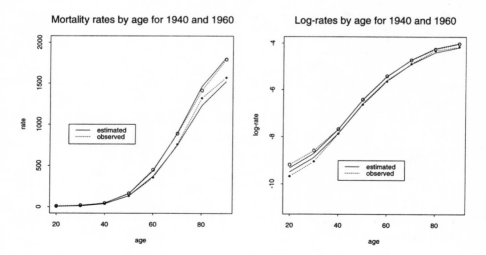

Figure 8.1

A model approach based on a statistical structure allows an assessment of the estimated quantities (e.g., confidence intervals), an evaluation of the fit, and, most important, an assessment of the interaction between group status and age categories. A standard mortality ratio, model based or not, requires the ratio of age-specific rates between the two groups compared to be constant and, therefore, differ among the age categories only because of chance variation. A standard mortality ratio (*smr*) is an estimate of this constant ratio and is useful only if a single value reasonably summarizes the differences between two groups at all ages. If the ratio is not constant (interaction), a single summary does not reflect accurately differences between compared groups, regardless of the age-adjustment method used.

LIFE TABLES

A life table describes the mortality pattern of a stationary population. In general terms, a stationary population results when the number of births each year equals the number of deaths and the age-specific mortality rates remain constant over time. Furthermore, no immigration or emigration occurs. A consequence of a stationary population is that a person whose current age is 60 has the same risk of death a newborn experiences 60 years later. Clearly, postulating a stationary population for human populations is not totally realistic. However, when changes in the human mortality rates are slow, life table summaries can be an approximation of future patterns. Additionally, the requirements of a stationary population are less important when populations or samples are compared, making a life table a useful tool for describing and contrasting mortality patterns among current populations.

Two kinds of life tables exist —a complete and an abridged life table. The difference depends on the age intervals chosen to classify the mortality data. A complete life table consists of age intervals equal to one year ($\delta_x = 1$) for all but the last age category. An abridged life table contains age intervals that are not equal to one year ($\delta_x \neq 1$ for some categories). The construction and interpretation of these two types of life table are essentially the same.

The fundamental feature of a life table is the conversion of current mortality rates into a cohort picture of mortality. The assumption of a stationary population structure translates into

life table cohort mortality rates = observed current mortality rates.

Specifically, for the observed, current age-specific mortality rate R_x

$$\text{life table probability of death} = q_x = \frac{\delta_x R_x}{1 + \frac{1}{2}\delta_x R_x}$$

where q_x represents the life table probability of death before the time δ_x elapses among persons alive at age x and R_x represents a current observed age-specific mortality rate for the same age interval, x to $x + \delta_x$.

Table 8.2 contains age-specific mid-year population counts $P_{x'}$ and the numbers of deaths D_x of California males in 1980. Average age-specific mortality rates calculated from Table 8.2 are, as before, $R_x = D_x/P_{x'}$ for each age interval. Translating these current mortality rates into life table cohort probabilities of death allows the construction of a life table. The current mortality rate for infants less than one year is $R_0 = 2,513/193,310 = 0.0130$ producing $q_0 = 0.0129$; $R_1 = 437/515,150 = 0.008$ producing $q_1 = 0.003$, $\cdots$ etc. Conditional probabilities of death are calculated (one from each age interval) producing the series of life table probabilities $\{q_0, q_1, q_5, q_{10}, \cdots, q_{x+}\}$ from the current age-specific rates $\{R_0, R_1, R_5, R_{10}, \cdots, R_{x+}\}$. The notation x^+ indicates the last age interval, which is open-ended (e.g., 85^+) and, therefore, requires special treatment. For example, $q_{85+} = 1.0$ since all individuals who live to age 85 die at an older age.

Table 8.2. Mid-year populations, deaths (all causes), and mortality rates: California males 1980

age	P_x' population	D_x deaths	R_x rates
0–1	193 310	2 513	0.0130
1–4	515 150	437	0.0008
5–9	843 750	287	0.0003
10–14	915 240	329	0.0004
15–19	1 091 684	1 689	0.0015
20–24	1 213 068	2 482	0.0020
25–29	1 132 811	2 308	0.0020
30–34	1 008 606	2 059	0.0020
35–39	776 545	1 820	0.0023
40–44	629 452	2 102	0.0033
45–49	578 420	3 104	0.0054
50–54	578 795	4 808	0.0083
55–59	573 119	7 403	0.0129
60–64	467 607	9 319	0.0199
65–69	378 259	11 736	0.0310
70–74	269 849	12 593	0.0467
75–79	175 580	12 341	0.0703
80–84	95 767	10 255	0.1071
85+	78 832	13 962	0.1771
total	11 515 844	101 547	0.0088

A life table requires a starting point. An arbitrary population size is chosen such as $l_0 = 100{,}000$. The notation l_x represents the number of individuals alive at the beginning of the life table age interval denoted x. Values of l_x follow directly from the probabilities q_x or

number alive at the start of interval $x + \delta_x = l_{x+\delta_x} = (1 - q_x)l_x = p_x l_x$

where $p_x = 1 - q_x$ is the conditional probability of surviving from x to $x + \delta_x$. Conditional probability in a life table context means that the probability p_x or q_x applies only to those individuals alive at the start of the interval x. The difference equation produces $\{l_1, l_5, l_{10}, \cdots, l_{x+}\}$ starting with l_0. An equivalent expression for l_x is

$$l_{x+\delta_x} = l_0 \times p_0 \times p_5 \times p_{10} \times \cdots \times p_x \qquad x = 1, 5, 10, \cdots, 85^+.$$

The life table number of deaths for each age interval is then

$$\text{deaths} = d_x = l_x - l_{x+\delta_x}.$$

For example, $l_0 = 100{,}000$ and $l_1 = l_0 p_0 = 100{,}000(0.987) = 98{,}708$ making $d_0 = l_0 - l_1 = 1292$ the number of deaths in the first age interval. The life table deaths for each age interval $\{d_0, d_1, d_5, d_{10}, \cdots, d_{x+}\}$ are directly calculated from the l_x-values.

The total person-years lived within the age interval x to $x + \delta_x$ is an important element of a life table. The life table person-years (L_x) calculated from l_x and d_x is

total time lived from x *to* $x + \delta_x = L_x = \delta_x l_x - \frac{1}{2}\delta_x d_x = \delta_x l_{x+\delta_x} + \frac{1}{2}\delta_x d_x.$

The factor $\frac{1}{2}\delta_x$ is again the approximate average time lived by an individual who died during the age interval x. This approximation works well for ages greater than 5 years old. Deaths occur within these age intervals, more or less, uniformly throughout the interval. For the younger ages, mortality is less uniformly distributed, particularly for children under the age of one year where most deaths occur in the first month of life. However, the consequences from assuming that deaths are uniformly distributed in all age intervals are not great. Empirically determined values that can replace $\frac{1}{2}\delta_x$ have been calculated [2] and are used to fine-tune life table estimates. The life table age-specific mortality rate is $r_x = d_x/L_x$ since L_x is the total person-years lived by the l_x persons at risk. As previously noted, the cohort life-table rate equals the current observed age-specific rate, $r_x = R_x$.

The person-years calculation for the last age interval presents a unique problem. The interval length δ_{x+} is not known since the interval is open-ended. However, equating a life table rate to a current observed rate gives an expression for the total person-years lived for the last age interval or

$$R_{x^+} = r_{x^+}, \quad \text{then} \quad R_{x^+} = \frac{d_{x^+}}{L_{x^+}} = \frac{l_{x^+}}{L_{x^+}}$$

since $d_{x^+} = l_{x^+}$ for the last interval. The person-years for the interval x^+ is then

$$\text{total person-years for the last interval} = L_{x^+} = \frac{l_{x^+}}{R_{x^+}}.$$

For example, $R_{85^+} = 13,962/78,832 = 0.177$ making $L_{85^+} = 19,926/0.177 = 112,508$. Therefore, the series of life table person-years $\{L_0, L_1, L_5, L_{10}, \cdots, L_{x^+}\}$ is created from the l_x, d_x, and R_{x^+} values.

The total number of years lived beyond age x (T_x) is the sum of the L_x-values. Therefore,

$$\text{total time lived beyond age } x = T_x = L_x + L_{x+\delta_x} + \cdots + L_{x^+}$$

again creating a series of life table values $\{T_0, T_1, T_5, T_{10}, \cdots, T_{x^+}\}$. The total time lived by all l_0 members of the life table cohort is T_0 person-years.

Perhaps the most important summary of a mortality pattern is the average remaining years of life. Like all averages,

$$\text{average time lived beyond age } x = e_x = \frac{\text{total time lived beyond age } x}{\text{number of individuals alive at age } x} = \frac{T_x}{l_x}.$$

Values $\{e_0, e_1, e_5, e_{10}, \cdots, e_{x^+}\}$ summarize the mortality risk at each life table age interval. A principal single summary from an entire cohort the number of years of life expected to be lived by a newborn (e_0) and, from the California mortality data, males born in 1980 are expected to live

$$e_0 = \frac{T_0}{l_0} = \frac{7,092,448}{100,000} = 70.9 \text{ years.}$$

To repeat, the value e_0 is the expected length of life of a newborn if the population remains stationary.

Example S-code that produces a life table from the current California 1980 mortality data (Table 8.2—contained in the exterior file *life.data*) is

```
> # life table computations
> delta<- c(1,4,rep(5,17))
> # read mortality and population data
> temp<- scan("life.data")
> pop<- temp[seq(1,length(temp),2)]
> deaths<- temp[seq(2,length(temp),2)]
> n<- length(pop)
> R<- deaths/pop
> qx<- delta*R/(1+0.5*delta*R)
> qx[n]<- 1
> lx<- 100000*c(1,cumprod(1-qx))
> d<- -diff(lx)
> lx<- lx[-(n+1)]
> L<- delta*(lx-0.5*d)
> L[n]<- lx[n]/R[n]
> Tx<- rev(cumsum(rev(L)))
```

```
> e<- Tx/lx
> out<- cbind(round(qx,4),round(lx,0),round(L,0),round(Tx,0),
  round(e,1))
> ages<- c("0-1","1-4","5-9","10-14","15-19","20-24","25-29",
  "30-34","35-39","40-44","45-49","50-54","55-59","60-64",
  "65-69","70-74","75-79","80-84","85+")
> matrix(out,n,5,dimnames=list(ages,c("qx","lx","Lx","Tx","ex")))
```

	qx	lx	Lx	Tx	ex
0-1	0.0129	100000	99354	7092448	70.9
1-4	0.0034	98708	394165	6993094	70.8
5-9	0.0017	98374	491452	6598929	67.1
10-14	0.0018	98207	490593	6107477	62.2
15-19	0.0077	98031	488264	5616883	57.3
20-24	0.0102	97275	483900	5128619	52.7
25-29	0.0101	96285	478985	4644719	48.2
30-34	0.0102	95309	474126	4165734	43.7
35-39	0.0117	94341	468958	3691608	39.1
40-44	0.0166	93242	462351	3222649	34.6
45-49	0.0265	91698	452421	2760299	30.1
50-54	0.0407	89270	437271	2307878	25.9
55-59	0.0626	85638	414795	1870607	21.8
60-64	0.0949	80280	382350	1455812	18.1
65-69	0.1440	72660	337149	1073462	14.8
70-74	0.2090	62200	278506	736313	11.8
75-79	0.2989	49203	209245	457807	9.3
80-84	0.4223	34495	136054	248562	7.2
85+	1.0000	19926	112508	112508	5.6.

The S-function *matrix( )* allows the rows and the columns of the argument array to be labeled. The option *dimnames = list(row.names, column.names)* produces labels according to the contents of the S-vectors *row.names* and *column.names*. Chosen labels replace the "default" values of $[i,]$ and $[,j]$.

The life table survival probabilities (l_x/l_0—solid line) and the life table probabilities of death within an interval (q_x—dotted line) are two ways to display the mortality pattern. For the California male life table population based on 1980 mortality rates these values are displayed in Figure 8.2.

The life table crude mortality rate is

$$life\ table\ crude\ mortality\ rate = \frac{total\ deaths}{total\ person\text{-}years}$$

$$= \frac{d_0 + d_1 + d_5 + \cdots + d_{x^+}}{T_0} = \frac{l_0}{T_0} = \frac{1}{e_0}$$

and, specifically, for the California data

$$life\ table\ crude\ mortality\ rate = \frac{100,000}{7,092,448} = 0.014 = \frac{1}{70.924}.$$

Risk (measured by a rate) is inversely related to survival time (measured by the expected amount of life time from birth). This inverse relationship is not surprising but life table summaries give a formal expression for the relationship between risk and survival time. The same inverse relationship is seen in several other contexts as part of the study of survival data (next sections).

Life table -- Mortality pattern California males, 1980

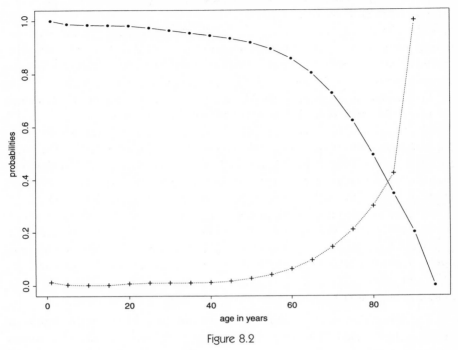

Figure 8.2

Table 8.3. United States mortality rates for the years 1940 and 1960

	1940			1960		
age	population	deaths	rates/1000	population	deaths	rates/1000
0–1	2 020 174	110 908	54.9	4 111 949	111 023	27.0
1–4	8 521 350	24 712	2.9	16 208 952	17 830	1.1
5–9	10 684 622	11 753	1.1	18 691 780	9 346	0.5
10–14	11 745 935	11 746	1.0	16 773 492	6 709	0.4
15–19	12 333 523	20 967	1.7	13 219 243	11 897	0.9
20–24	11 587 835	27 811	2.4	10 800 761	12 961	1.2
25–29	11 096 638	31 071	2.8	10 869 124	14 130	1.3
30–34	10 242 388	34 824	3.4	11 949 186	19 119	1.6
35–39	9 545 377	42 000	4.4	12 481 109	28 707	2.3
40–44	8 787 843	53 606	6.1	11 600 243	42 921	3.7
45–49	8 255 225	71 820	8.7	10 879 485	64 189	5.9
50–54	7 256 846	92 888	12.8	9 605 954	90 296	9.4
55–59	5 867 119	108 542	18.5	8 429 865	116 332	13.8
60–64	4 756 217	126 991	26.7	7 142 452	153 563	21.5
65–69	3 755 526	149 094	39.7	6 257 910	196 498	31.4
70–74	2 569 532	156 998	61.1	4 738 932	224 151	47.3
75–79	1 503 982	142 577	94.8	3 053 559	219 856	72.0
80–84	774 391	112 751	145.6	1 579 927	185 167	117.2
85+	364 752	85 972	235.7	929 252	182 691	196.6

The average number of years of life expected for a "life-table newborn" (e_0) has a straightforward geometric interpretation. The area under the curve described by the life table survival probabilities l_x/l_0 is related to the expectation of life at birth e_0. Specifically, $area \approx e_0 + 2.5$ years. For the California mortality data (Table 8.2), the area enclosed by the estimated survival curve is approximately $e_0 + 2.5$ years ≈ 73.42 years (solid line; Figure 8.2).

To compare patterns of survival based on United States mortality between the years 1940 and 1960 the rates in Table 8.3 are necessary.

Life table survival curves (Figure 8.3) are constructed from the 1940 and the 1960 mortality rates (Table 8.3) with the previous S-code. The area enclosed by the 1940 curve directly reflects $e_0 = 63.028$ years and the area enclosed by the 1960 curve directly reflects $e_0 = 69.796$ years. The difference in areas, shown in the combined plot, is approximately $69.796 - 63.028 = 6.786$ years (shaded area) with the most gain evident in the middle years of life (30–70 years of age). Mortality patterns over the 20 years between 1940 and 1960 have changed to the extent that the expected length of life has increased by nearly seven years. The example illustrates the ease of summarizing and comparing survival experience among groups employing life table measures such as the expectation of life at birth e_0.

SURVIVAL ANALYSIS—AN INTRODUCTION

Data, particularly data from the study of human disease, frequently involve observing an individual until the study ends or a change in status occurs, usually some sort of failure. For example, data might consist of patients followed after experimental surgery and observed until the treatment fails or the study period ends. The variable of primary interest is the time until failure called survival time. Failure can be defined in a number of ways—healthy people can become ill, sick individuals can die or individuals in relapse of a disease can once again show symptoms. The specialized nature of survival time data requires specialized analytic tools. The development and the application of these statistical tools constitute important topics in the analysis of survival data.

A fundamental measure of risk is a survival probability. A survival probability is defined as

$$survival\ probability = S(t) = P(surviving\ from\ time\ 0\ to\ time\ t)$$

or, equivalently,

$$survival\ probability = S(t) = P(surviving\ beyond\ time\ t).$$

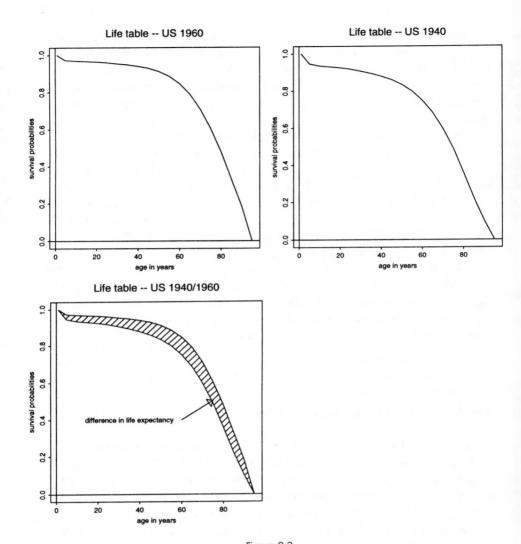

Figure 8.3

For example, the probability a California born female lives to age 90 is about 0.2, which is the same as the probability of living beyond age 90; in both case $S(90) = 0.2$.

Another basic measure of survival is a hazard rate defined as

$$hazard\ rate = \lambda(t) = \frac{-\frac{d}{dt}S(t)}{S(t)}$$

and is an instantaneous measure of risk. A hazard rate is related to a survival probability $S(t)$—large hazard rates imply small survival probabilities and, conversely. A formal relationship is

$$S(t) = e^{-\int_0^t \lambda(x)dx}.$$

Another occasionally used measure of risk that relates survival probabilities and hazard rates is the cumulative hazard function defined as

$$cumulative\ hazard = H(t) = \int_0^t \lambda(x)dx = -log[S(t)].$$

A simple and frequently effective approach to analyzing survival data is based on postulating a parametric model to generate survival probabilities. One choice is the exponential function where

$$survival\ probability = S(t) = e^{-\lambda t}$$

models the probability of surviving beyond a specific time t. For example, if λ = 0.03, then the probability of surviving beyond 50 weeks is $S(50) = e^{-(0.03)50}$ = 0.223. Large values of the parameter λ dictate small survival probabilities and vice versa. The hazard function and cumulative hazard function directly follow as

$$\lambda(t) = \lambda = 0.03 \quad and \quad H(t) = \lambda t = 0.03t,$$

showing that the choice of an exponential function to represent survival probabilities is identical to requiring a constant hazard rate or a linearly increasing cumulative hazard function. The three related measures of survival for the exponential model are displayed in Figure 8.4, created by (λ = 0.03; labeled *lam*)

```
> t<- seq(0,60,0.1)
> lam<- 0.03
> s<- exp(-lam*t)
> plot(t,s,type="l",ylim=c(0,1),xlab="time",ylab="",
      main="Survival data -- three measures")
> abline(h=lam,lty=2)
> lines(t,-log(s),lty=3)
```

Survival data -- three measures

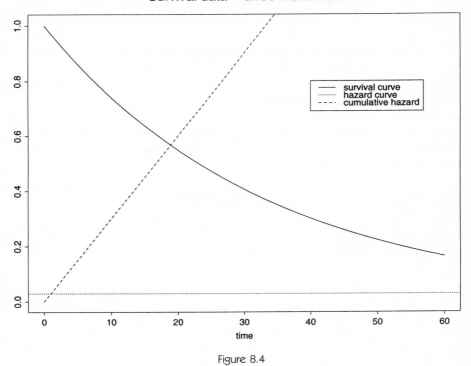

Figure 8.4

```
> legend(40,0.8,c("survival curve","hazard curve",
    "cumulative hazard"),lty=1:3)
```

Estimation of these three quantities is straightforward when the data are complete. By complete it is meant that the n sampled individuals are observed until all observations end in a failure, making the values of all n survival times $\{t_1, t_2, t_3, \cdots, t_n\}$ known. For the exponential distribution, the estimate of λ from complete data was discussed (Chapter 5). The cumulative probability function is $F(x) = 1 - S(x) = 1 - e^{-\lambda t}$ making the probability density function $f(t) = \lambda e^{-\lambda t}$. The maximum likelihood estimate of the hazard rate λ is then $\hat{\lambda} = 1/\bar{t}$ where $\bar{t} = \sum t_i/n$ is the usual mean of n independent observations. The estimated variance of this estimator is $variance(\hat{\lambda}) = \hat{\lambda}^2/n$. Also, the survival function is estimated by $\hat{S}(t) = e^{-\hat{\lambda} t}$ and the estimated cumulative hazard function by $\hat{H}(t) = -log[\hat{S}(t)] = \hat{\lambda} t$. Since these estimates are functions of maximum likelihood estimates, they are themselves maximum likelihood estimates. The mean survival time is also directly calculated as $\bar{t}$ and has an estimated variance given by $variance(\bar{t}) = \bar{t}^2/n$.

In many situations, follow-up data are not complete. Ideally, a study starts with a sample of individuals and continues until all individuals reach the defined end point (disease, death, recurrence, cure,···). However, complete follow-up is frequently not practical. For example, following all patients who received a new cancer treatment until death could involve many years of observation. Most follow-up studies end at a specific time and, typically, some subjects have not yet reached their end point. These incomplete survival times are said to be censored. It is known that followed individuals with censored survival times have not failed before the close of the study but the actual amount of time survived beyond this end point is not known.

Hypothetical survival times recorded in months are

$$8^+, 18^+, 60, 52, 48, 4, 13, 40, 20, 28^+.$$

The "+" indicates data values that have not failed before the close of the study. These data are displayed in Figure 8.5. If the study had continued, the three censored observations would have added more survival time to the total survival time observed. Calculations from censored survival times are therefore biased without the use of special techniques to compensate for the incomplete nature of the data.

n = 10 observation -- three censored

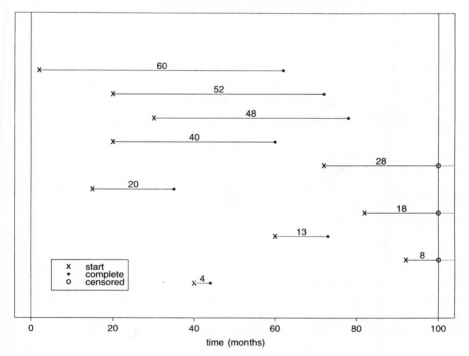

Figure 8.5

When exponentially distributed data are censored, directly calculating the survival rate as $1/\bar{t}$ produces a biased estimate because $\sum t_i$ is an underestimate of the total survival time. Without accounting for the presence of censored data, estimates of the failure rate $\hat{\lambda}$ will tend to be too large. The maximum likelihood estimate of the rate (parameter) λ from a sample of exponentially distributed survival times is

$$estimated\ rate = \hat{\lambda} = \frac{d}{\sum t_i}$$

whether the data is complete or not. The symbol t_i represents the recorded survival time whether the observation is censored or complete, making $\sum t_i$ the total observed survival time, and the numerator is the number of events d not the total sample size n. When the data are complete $d = n$. This estimate of λ is the number of events divided by the total observed person-time at risk, producing the usual estimate of a rate. For the hypothetical data, the estimated failure rate is $\hat{\lambda} = 7/291 = 0.024$. The variance of $\hat{\lambda}$ is $variance(\hat{\lambda}) = \hat{\lambda}^2/d = 0.00058/7 = 0.000083$. The parallel maximum likelihood estimator of the estimated mean survival time when censored data are present is

$$estimated\ mean\ survival\ time = \hat{\mu} = \frac{\sum t_i}{d}$$

where the total observed survival time is not divided by the total number of observations n but rather by the number of events d. Dividing by the smaller value ($d \leq n$) compensates for the reduction in $\sum t_i$ due to including censored observations. Therefore, a rate based on a sample of exponential survival times is again estimated by the reciprocal of the mean survival time but the mean $\hat{\mu}$ is specially adjusted for the presence of censored observations. Again, risk is inversely related to survival, $\hat{\lambda} = 1/\hat{\mu}$. Applied to the hypothetical data, $\hat{\mu} = 291/7 = 41.571$ months and, to repeat, $\hat{\lambda} = 1/41.571 = 0.024$.

The exponential distribution has a property that makes it an unrealistic model for many types of survival data. The exponential survival function yields the probability of surviving to time t_2 given survival to t_1 as

$$S(T > t_2 | T > t_1) = e^{-\lambda(t_2 - t_1)} \qquad t_1 < t_2,$$

which is itself an exponential distribution. The exponential function has "no memory." If a person survives 5 years, then the probability of living 10 more years is $e^{-\lambda 10}$ and for a person who survives 80 years, the probability of living 10 more years is also $e^{-\lambda 10}$. The fact that these two probabilities are identical is not a realistic property for many data sets where past experience influences the likelihood of future outcomes.

NONPARAMETRIC ESTIMATION OF A SURVIVAL CURVE

Estimates of the survival probabilities or an estimate of a survival curve (a series of survival probabilities) is possible without making assumptions about the distribution underlying the sampled survival times. The product-limit or Kaplan–Meier approach produces distribution-free estimated survival probabilities from complete and, more importantly, censored data. To start, a series of intervals is constructed based on the complete survival times. Ideally, these intervals are defined so that they contain only a single failure, which is possible when no identical survival times occur in the collected data. For the illustrative data, the intervals are: 0–4, 4–13, 13–20, 20–40, 40–48, 48–52, and 52–60. When no failure times are identical, the number of intervals is equal to the number of complete survival times ($d \leq n$). For the hypothetical data, the total number of observations is $n = 10$ and the number of complete survival times is $d = 7$. The probability of failure within a specific interval is then estimated by one divided by the number of individuals who died within the interval plus those who completed the interval. That is, all persons alive up to the moment before a specific failure (end point of an interval) form a risk set for the calculation of the probability of failure in that interval. In symbols, the conditional probability of failure in the ith interval is $\hat{q}_i = 1/n_i$ where n_i represents the number of individuals in the risk set. Individuals with censored survival times are members of the ith risk set if they survive the entire i^{th} interval. Only then are they used in the calculation of the interval-specific probabilities of failure. If the data contain identical survival times, the probability $\hat{q}_i$ is the number of individuals who failed in the ith interval divided by the number in the corresponding risk set.

Kaplan–Meier survival probabilities are estimated with the S-function

$$surv.fit(survival.times, censored.status, group.membership).$$

The vector *survival.times* contains the survival times for both complete and censored observations. The *censored.status* vector contains zeros and ones indicating whether an observation is complete (coded as 1) or censored (coded as 0). The *group.membership* vector communicates the possibility that the observed survival times were recorded for members of different groups. If all observations belong to the same group, the *group.membership* option is unnecessary. All three vectors are length n where n is the total number of observations (censored plus complete survival times). For the hypothetical data,

```
> # Kaplan-Meier estimated survival probabilities
> # single group with no tied survival times
> t0<- c(4,8,13,18,20,28,40,48,52,60)
> c0<- c(1,0,1,0,1,0,1,1,1,1)
> surv.fit(t0,c0)
```

```
> 95 percent confidence interval is of type "log"
> time n.risk n.event survival   std.dev lower 95% upper 95%
     4     10       1  0.90000   0.09487   0.73201   1.00000
    13      8       1  0.78750   0.13403   0.56412   1.00000
    20      6       1  0.65625   0.16380   0.40235   1.00000
    40      4       1  0.49218   0.18783   0.23297   1.00000
    48      3       1  0.32812   0.18337   0.10974   0.98113
    52      2       1  0.16406   0.14787   0.02804   0.95979
    60      1       1  0.00000        NA        NA        NA.
```

The column labeled "time" contains the complete survival times, which are the end points of the intervals (e.g., 40 means 20 to 40). The column labeled "n.risk" contains the number of members of the original n observations that form the risk set for a specific interval. The interval-specific probability of failure is the number of failures ("n.event") divided by the number at risk ("n.risk"). For the fourth interval (20–40), there are four individuals in the risk set making the conditional probability of failure in that interval $\hat{q}_4 = 1/4 = 0.25$. The column labeled "survival" contains the survival probabilities (denoted $\hat{P}_i$) that are estimates of the probability of surviving beyond the end point of the interval. For example, $\hat{P}_4 = (1 - 1/10)(1 - 1/8)(1 - 1/6)(1 - 1/4) = 0.492$ is the estimated probability of surviving beyond 40 months. In general, the product

$$\hat{P}_k = (1 - \hat{q}_1)(1 - \hat{q}_2)(1 - \hat{q}_3) \cdots (1 - \hat{q}_k)$$

is the Kaplan–Meier estimate of the probability of surviving beyond the kth interval. Figure 8.6 displays the Kaplan–Meier estimated survival curve and its associated 95% confidence interval based on the 10 hypothetical survival times. The plot is created by the S-function,

```
> plot(surv.fit(t0,c0),xlab="time",
    ylab="survival probability",conf.int=T,
    main= "Kaplan-Meier estimated survival curve")
> abline(h=0)
```

There is one underlying requirement to produce a valid Kaplan–Meier estimated survival curve. It is necessary that the censoring be "noninformative." The censoring of a follow-up observation is "noninformative" when it is censored at random which means that no relationship exists between the reason an observation is censored and the observed outcome.

HAZARD RATE—ESTIMATION

Life table or Kaplan–Meier survival probabilities provide an estimated hazard rate from failure data without a specified model. From a life table, the age-specific life table mortality rate is estimated by

Kaplan-Meier estimated survival curve

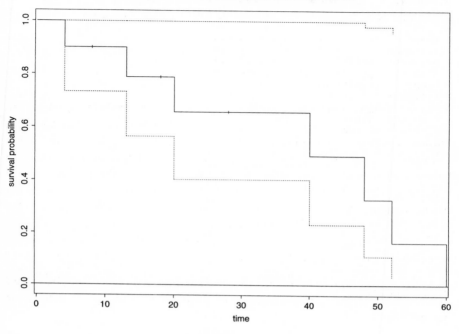

Figure 8.6

$$mortality\ rate\ at\ age\ x = r_x = \frac{d_x}{\delta_x(l_x - \frac{1}{2}d_x)} \approx \frac{q_x}{\delta_x}.$$

This age-specific rate is an estimate of the life table hazard function ($\hat{\lambda}(x) \approx r_x$) at age x when q_x is small ($q_x < 0.1$). Therefore, the life table conditional probabilities q_x reflect the hazard rates associated with the mortality data used to construct the life table. The shorter the age interval (δ_x), the more accurate the estimate of the specific hazard rate $\lambda(x)$. Figure 8.2 displays an approximate hazard curve (dotted lines) reflecting the mortality risk associated with California, white males (1980).

Similarly the $\hat{q}_i$ probabilities from a Kaplan–Meier survival table reflect the hazard rate associated with each time interval. These estimated hazard rates are

$$estimated\ hazard\ rate = \hat{\lambda}_i = \frac{\hat{q}_i}{\delta_i} = \frac{d_i}{\delta_i n_i}$$

where d_i represents the number of failures (usually one) in the ith interval, δ_i represents the length of the ith interval, and n_i represents the number of individuals in the risk set associated with the ith interval. Example S-code applying this definition to the illustrative hypothetical data gives

```
> # Kaplan-Meier hazard rate estimate
> # single group with no tied survival times
> n.event<- surv.fit(t0,c0)$n.event[c0==1]
> n.risk<- surv.fit(t0,c0)$n.risk[c0==1]
> time<- surv.fit(t0,c0)$time[c0==1]
> d.time<- diff(time)
> k<- length(n.risk)
> n.event<- n.event[-k]
> n.risk<- n.risk[-k]
> time<- time[-k]
> h.rate<- n.event/(d.time*n.risk)
> round(cbind(time,d.time,n.risk,n.event,h.rate),4)
       time d.time n.risk n.event   h.rate
[1,]      4      9     10       1   0.0111
[2,]     13      7      8       1   0.0179
[3,]     20     20      6       1   0.0083
[4,]     40      8      4       1   0.0312
[5,]     48      4      3       1   0.0833
[6,]     52      8      2       1   0.0625.
```

The column labeled "d.time" contains the lengths of the time intervals (δ_i) and the column "h.rate" contains the estimated hazard rates ($\hat{\lambda}_i$). The hazard rate is again estimated by the number of events divided by an estimate of the person-time at risk.

MEAN/MEDIAN SURVIVAL TIME

Mean survival time summarizes the survival experience of a group much like any sample mean and is geometrically the area under the survival curve or, in symbols,

$$mean\ survival\ time = \mu = \int_0^\infty S(x)dx.$$

For exponentially distributed survival times, the mean survival time is

$$\mu = \int_0^\infty e^{-\lambda x}dx = \frac{1}{\lambda}.$$

Again, survival time is inversely related to risk.

Estimating the mean survival time from a Kaplan–Meier estimated survival curve translates into a simple geometric argument. The area enclosed by the Kaplan–Meier curve is an estimate of the mean survival time. The area under the Kaplan-Meier curve is the sum of the areas of a series of rectangles formed by the heights of the survival curve and the width of the intervals. Therefore, the mean survival time (total area) is

$$\text{estimated mean survival time} = \hat{\mu} = \sum \hat{P}_{i-1}(t_i - t_{i-1}) \qquad i = 1, 2, 3, \cdots, d$$

where $\hat{P}_i$ (height) represents the estimated survival probability ($\hat{P}_0 = 1$) and t_i represents the interval bounds ($t_0 = 0$) for the d intervals (width $= t_i - t_{i-1}$). The variance of the estimated mean survival time is

$$\text{variance}(\hat{\mu}) = \sum_{i=1}^{d-1} \frac{\hat{q}_i}{n_i(1 - \hat{q}_i)} A_i^2 \qquad \text{where} \qquad A_i = \hat{\mu} - \sum_{j=1}^{i} \hat{P}_{j-1}(t_j - t_{j-1}).$$

If no censoring occurs ($n = d$), then

$$\text{estimated mean survival time} = \hat{\mu} = \sum \hat{P}_{i-1}(t_i - t_{i-1}) = \bar{t}$$

and

$$\text{variance}(\hat{\mu}) = \frac{1}{n^2} \sum (t_i - \bar{t})^2.$$

The mean survival time and its variance based on the estimates $\hat{P}_i$ are computed from the hypothetical data (assuming no identical survival times) by

```
> # mean survival time calculation
> # single group with no tied survival times
> surv<- surv.fit(t0,c0)$>surv
> time<- surv.fit(t0,c0)$time
> n.risk<- surv.fit(t0,c0)$n.risk
> P<- c(1,surv[c0==1])
> t<- c(0,time[c0==1],0)
> tbar<- sum(P*diff(t))
> # standard error calculation
> n<- n.risk[c0==1]
> fact<- 1/(n*(n-1))
> fact<- c(ifelse(fact<Inf,fact,0),0)
> a<- tbar-cumsum(P*diff(t))
> se<- sqrt(sum(fact*a^2))
> cat("mean survival time",round(tbar,3),
      "standard error =",round(se,3),"\n"
mean survival time 37.3 standard error = 6.495.
```

The parametric estimates from the same data based on assuming a constant hazard rate (exponential survival probabilities) are

```
> d<- sum(c0)
> tbar<- sum(t0)/d
> rate<- 1/tbar
> round(rate,3)
[1] 0.024
> se<- sqrt(tbar^2/d)
> cat("mean survival time",round(tbar,3),"standard error =",
      round(se,3),"\n")
mean survival time 41.571 standard error = 15.713.
```

Another summary of the survival time distribution is the median. The median survival time is estimated by the end point of the interval containing the survival probability $P = 0.5$ [3]. More formally, the estimated median survival time is defined to be the smallest observed survival time for which the value of the estimated survival probabilities is less than or equal to 0.5. For the hypothetical data,

```
> # t0 = survival times, c0 = censored(0) or not(1)
> md<- function(t0,c0){min(t0[surv.fit(t0,c0)$surv<=0.5])}
> cat("estimated median =",md(t0,c0),"\n")
estimated median = 40.
```

The median value of 40 months represents an estimate of the expected time where 50% of the sampled population will have failed or, alternatively, 50% would be expected to survive beyond 40 months. A geometric description of a median follows directly from the Kaplan–Meier plot. The median is found by extending a line from the survival probability 0.5 horizontally until it intersects the survival curve. The point on the x-axis directly below the intersection is the estimated median survival time.

Another way to estimate the median is by linear interpolation. The survival time t_{md} corresponding to $S(t_{md}) = 0.5$ is interpolated from the survival probabilities. The S-function

$$approx(x, y, xout = c(< x - values >), \cdots)$$

interpolates for the values identified by *xout* using the x and y values given by the first two vector arguments. The output consists of interpolated values from the curve described by input values x and y calculated at each value given in *xout*. For example,

```
> x<- 1:10
> y<- x^2
> xout<- x+0.5
> yout<- approx(x,y,xout)$y
> cbind(x,y,xout,yout)
          x    y xout yout
 [1,]    1    1  1.5  2.5
 [2,]    2    4  2.5  6.5
 [3,]    3    9  3.5 12.5
 [4,]    4   16  4.5 20.5
 [5,]    5   25  5.5 30.5
 [6,]    6   36  6.5 42.5
 [7,]    7   49  7.5 56.5
 [8,]    8   64  8.5 72.5
 [9,]    9   81  9.5 90.5
[10,]   10  100 10.5   NA.
```

An S-function using interpolation to estimate the median t_{md} is

```
> # estimates the median by interpolation
> # single group with no tied survival times
> md.linear<- function(t0,c0) {
    time<- surv.fit(t0,c0)$time[c0==1]
    p<- surv.fit(t0,c0)$surv[c0==1]
    approx(p,time,xout=0.5)$y
  }
```

The example survival data yield

```
> md.linear(t0,c0)
[1] 39.04762.
```

An estimated median from the illustrative data is then $\hat{t}_{md} = 39.048$ months.

The failure times from a clinical trial [4] conducted to compare two treatments for patients who suffer from acute myelogenous leukemia (AML) are:

nonmaintained (control group)

$$5,\ 5,\ 8,\ 8,\ 12,\ 16^+,\ 23,\ 27,\ 30,\ 33,\ 43,\ 45 \quad (n_1 = 12)$$

and maintained (treatment group)

$$9,\ 13,\ 13^+,\ 18,\ 23,\ 28^+,\ 31,\ 34,\ 45^+,\ 48,\ 161^+ \quad (n_2 = 11).$$

The data are times (weeks) from treatment to relapse for patients who also received the usual treatment (nonmaintained) and patients who additionally received special chemotherapy (maintained). The S-function *surv.fit( )* allows comparison of two or more samples of follow-up data. The comparison of the "survival" probabilities associated with these groups is accomplished with

```
> time<- c(9,13,13,18,23,28,31,34,45,48,161,5,5,8,8,12,16,
     23,27,30,33,43,45)
> c0<- c(1,1,0,1,1,0,1,1,0,1,0,1,1,1,1,1,0,1,1,1,1,1,1)
> g0<- rep(c(1,0),c(11,12))
> surv.fit(time,c0,g0)
 95 percent confidence interval is of type "log"
      Strata:    s = 0
time n.risk n.event  survival  std.dev  lower 95%  upper 95%
    5     12      2    0.8333   0.10758   0.64704    1.00000
    8     10      2    0.6667   0.13608   0.44685    0.99463
   12      8      1    0.5833   0.14232   0.36161    0.94100
   23      6      1    0.4861   0.14813   0.26753    0.88332
   27      5      1    0.3889   0.14699   0.18540    0.81574
   30      4      1    0.2917   0.13871   0.11483    0.74082
   33      3      1    0.1944   0.12187   0.05692    0.66422
   43      2      1    0.0972   0.09187   0.01526    0.61955
   45      1      1    0.0000      NA        NA         NA

      Strata:    s = 1
time n.risk n.event  survival  std.dev  lower 95%  upper 95%
    9     11      1    0.9091   0.08668   0.75413    1.00000
   13     10      1    0.8182   0.11629   0.61925    1.00000
   18      8      1    0.7159   0.13967   0.48842    1.00000
   23      7      1    0.6136   0.15263   0.37687    0.99916
   31      5      1    0.4909   0.16419   0.25486    0.94558
   34      4      1    0.3682   0.16267   0.15488    0.87526
   48      2      1    0.1841   0.15349   0.03593    0.94353.
```

An S-plot of the estimated survival curves for the two treatment groups (Figure 8.7) is created by

```
> plot(surv.fit(time,c0,g0),xlab="time(weeks)",ylab=
     "survival probability",conf.int=F,lty=1:2,
     main="Kaplan-Meier estimated survival curve -- two groups")
> legend(70,0.9,c("maintained","nonmaintained"),lty=1:2)
```

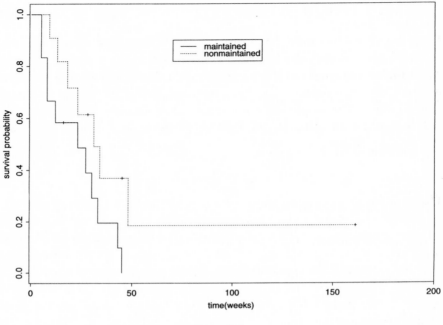

Figure 8.7

The S-plot produces a comparison of Kaplan-Meier survival curves from the maintained and non-maintained groups. The mean survival times are 22.708 with standard error 4.181 for the nonmaintained group and 52.645 with standard error 19.828 for the maintained group. The median survival times are 23 (nonmaintained) and 31 weeks (maintained).

An S-function

$$surv.diff \, (survival.time, censored.status, group.membership)$$

provides a formal test to evaluate observed differences between distributions of survival probabilities (is the survival experience of the maintained group better than the nonmaintained group?). The input arguments are identical to the previous S-function, *surv.fit*( ). This S-function applies a nonparametric technique called the log-rank test, which is one of several approaches to comparing survival experience among groups ([5] or [6] for complete descriptions). The S-function *surv.diff*( ) applied to the AML data yields

```
> surv.diff(time,c0,g0)
```

```
     N Observed   Expected   (O-E)^2/E
  0 12       11      7.311       1.862
  1 11        7     10.689       1.273
```

```
  Chisq= 3.4  on 1 degrees of freedom, p= 0.06534.
```

The log-rank chi-square statistic shows some evidence (p-value = 0.065) of different time to relapse distributions between the maintain and nonmaintained groups. The log-rank test is a special case of a more general approach used to analyze survival data called the proportional hazards model, which is the topic of the next section.

PROPORTIONAL HAZARDS MODEL

If two hazard functions $\lambda_1(t)$ and $\lambda_2(t)$ are proportional, then

$$\frac{\lambda_1(t)}{\lambda_2(t)} = c \quad \text{or, alternatively,} \quad S_1(t) = [S_2(t)]^c$$

where $S_1(t)$ and $S_2(t)$ denote the corresponding survival functions. Proportionality in this context means that the ratio of hazard functions does not depend on the survival time t. Surprisingly, it is possible to estimate the constant of proportionality c without specifying the form of the hazard functions.

Comparison of proportional hazard rates between two groups is a special case of the general proportional hazards model, sometimes called the Cox model after D.R. Cox who originated this analytic approach to survival data. Assuming the hazard functions for the treatment and control (maintained and nonmaintained) groups from the AML data are proportional, the S-function *coxreg*( ) produces an estimate of the proportionality constant c for these two groups where

```
> coxreg(time,c0,g0)
 Alive Dead Deleted
     5   18       0
```

```
        coef exp(coef) se(coef)      z        p
[1,] -0.904     0.405    0.512  -1.77  0.0775
```

```
      exp(coef) exp(-coef) lower .95 upper .95
[1,]      0.405       2.47     0.148       1.1
```

```
Likelihood ratio test = 3.3   on 1 df,   p=0.0694
Efficient score test = 3.32  on 1 df,   p=0.0683.
```

The three S-input arguments are the same as those used to estimate the survival probabilities, to plot the Kaplan–Meier survival curves or to conduct the log-rank test. The output S-term "Alive" denotes the number of censored survival times (coded = 0) and the S-term "Dead" denotes the number of complete observations (coded = 1). The estimated proportionality ratio is $\hat{c}$ = 0.405 ("exp(coef)") indicating that the hazard function associated with the maintained group is 1/0.405 = 2.470 ("exp(-coef)") times smaller than the hazard function associated with the nonmaintained group. The estimate $\hat{c}$ contrasts the risk experience of the two groups and, like all estimates from data, is subject to sampling variation.

The apparent superiority of the maintained treatment can be evaluated statistically in two ways. First by comparing log-likelihood values associated, again, with two nested models. The comparison is accomplished with S-functions by

```
> like<- coxreg(time,c0,g0)$loglik
> like
[1] -42.89812 -41.25011
> x2<- -2*(like[1]-like[2])
> pvalue<- 1-pchisq(x2,1)
> cbind(x2,pvalue)
          x2    pvalue
[1,] 3.296019 0.069448.
```

This same log-likelihood test is part of the *coxreg( )* output (labeled "Likelihood ratio test"). As before, a difference between two log-likelihood statistics multiplied by -2 has an approximate chi-square distribution. In symbols, $X^2 = -2[(log\text{-}likelihood_0) - (log\text{-}likelihood_1)]$ has an approximate chi-square distribution when the model producing $log\text{-}likelihood_0$ is special case of the model producing $log\text{-}likelihood_1$ (i.e., nested models) and the models compared only differ because of random variation. The degrees of freedom are equal to the difference between the degrees of freedom associated with each of the two models. In the AML case, the model with $c \neq 1$ or $\lambda_1(t) \neq \lambda_2(t)$ generates a log-likelihood value of $log\text{-}likelihood_0$ = -41.250. The model where c is constrained or $\lambda_1(t) / \lambda_2(t) = 1$ generates a log-likelihood value of $log\text{-}likelihood_1 = -42.898$. The degrees of freedom for contrasting these two nested models is one. The difference $X^2 = 3.296$ yields a significance probability of 0.069.

A second approach involves calculating the test-statistic

$$z^2 = \left[\frac{estimate - estimate_0}{standard \ of \ the \ estimate}\right]^2 = \left[\frac{\log(\hat{c}) - 0}{S_{\log(\hat{c})}}\right]^2$$

sometimes called the Wald statistic, where $estimate_0$ is a postulated value. For the AML data, $z^2 = (-0.904/0.512)^2 = 3.117$ with a p value of 0.078. Using the logarithm of the estimate of c instead of the estimate $\hat{c}$ itself improves the chi-square distribution approximation. The result from applying *surv.diff( )* to the AML data is also similar ($X^2 = 3.396$ with a p-value = 0.065) since the log-rank test under certain conditions is the same analytic process as the proportional hazards model used to compare risk between two groups. All three tests address the same issue with chi-square statistics and will usually be similar, particularly when the number of failure times in the data set is large.

A formal expression for a k-variate proportional hazards model is

$$\lambda_i(t|x_{i1}, x_{i2}, x_{i3}, \cdots, x_{ik}) = \lambda_0(t) \times c = \lambda_0(t) \times e^{\Sigma b_j(x_{ij}-\bar{x}_j)}.$$

The hazard function $\lambda_i(t|x_{i1}, x_{i2}, x_{i3}, \cdots, x_{ik})$ represents the hazard rate for the ith individual or group and equals a baseline hazard function $\lambda_0(t)$ multiplied by a constant c (constant with respect to time). The x_{ij}-values represent additional measures potentially relevant to a more complete understanding of the hazard functions (i.e., independent variables). The constant of proportionality c is a function of these k independent variables x_{ij}. For this version of the model, these variables do not depend on survival time. The proportional hazards model (Cox model) is a semi-parametric model. It is nonparametric since hazard functions do not need to be specified to estimate c. However, it is parametric in the sense that the role of each independent variable x_{ij} is measured by the parameter b_j. The "baseline" hazard function $\lambda_0(t)$ represents the "average" hazard function since $\lambda_i(t) = \lambda_0(t)$ when all the independent variables equal their mean levels (i.e., $x_{ij} = \bar{x}_j$ for $j = 1, 2, 3, \cdots, k$).

When two hazard functions are compared, the ratio is

$$\frac{\lambda_i(t|x_{i1}, x_{i2}, x_{i3}, \cdots, x_{ik})}{\lambda_j(t|x_{j1}, x_{j2}, x_{j3}, \cdots, x_{jk})} = e^{b_1(x_{i1}-x_{j1})} \times e^{b_2(x_{i2}-x_{j2})} \times e^{b_3(x_{i3}-x_{j3})} \times \cdots \times e^{b_k(x_{ik}-x_{jk})}.$$

The ratio of two proportional hazard functions (called the relative hazard) shows that the Cox model has the three basic properties of the previous additive linear models. The ratio of two hazard rates does not depend on the magnitude of the x_{ij}-values but only on the differences between independent variables. The ratio of hazard functions is the product of a series of individual contributions each associated with a single independent variable. The impact of each of these variables on the hazard ratio is unaffected by the levels of the other independent variables. The interpretation of the hazard model coefficients b_j is also analogous to the general linear model case. A one unit increase in the specific variable x_m causes an expected multiplicative change of e^{b_m} in the relative hazard when the other $k - 1$ variables are held constant (i.e., $x_{il} = x_{jl}$ for all $l \neq m$).

Survival times of lung cancer patients recorded for two groups based on evaluating the vital capacity of their lungs are given in Table 8.4. The 131 cancer patients are classified as "high" vital capacity and as "low" vital capacity on the basis of lung function. Also recorded is their age, which is likely important in understanding the role of vital capacity in the survival from lung cancer, since age is related to both survival and lung function.

Tabulation of the patients classified by lung vital capacity and age as well as censored and complete status gives the following summary table:

		total	censored	complete
high capacity	age ≤ 65	68	41	27
low capacity	age ≤ 65	27	13	14
high capacity	age > 65	27	9	18
low capacity	age > 65	9	3	6
total		131	66	65

Table 8.4. Lung cancer data: "high" vital capacity—survival time and age

complete							
time	age	time	age	time	age	time	age
0	74	1	74	1	63	3	78
4	66	5	40	9	65	19	51
21	73	30	62	36	68	39	50
40	56	48	64	51	72	61	58
89	64	90	41	90	69	92	76
113	73	127	64	131	51	138	75
139	56	143	50	159	60	168	74
170	71	180	69	189	56	192	68
201	64	212	58	223	70	229	76
238	63	265	65	275	63	292	55
317	65	322	55	350	54	357	73
380	51						

censored							
time	age	time	age	time	age	time	age
62	66	75	44	77	60	81	38
83	59	83	42	84	67	86	62
88	53	92	59	98	55	104	62
116	62	129	35	131	43	162	45
167	56	173	54	178	63	179	69
184	69	184	67	194	58	256	57
263	46	269	63	338	47	344	52
347	59	349	61	350	66	362	56
362	60	364	63	364	58	364	58
365	66	368	70	368	39	372	58
388	59	388	68	400	64	524	59
528	63	545	63	546	55	552	52
555	57	558	63				

Note: the first 45 survival times are complete (died within the study period) and the following 50 are censored.

Table 8.4. Lung cancer data (continued): "low" vital capacity—survival time and age

complete							
time	age	time	age	time	age	time	age
0	55	2	75	2	73	2	65
6	61	17	74	22	51	23	66
54	67	56	51	61	36	63	54
64	54	69	70	146	53	155	47
161	46	233	41	248	61	283	53

censored							
time	age	time	age	time	age	time	age
47	56	73	55	86	48	89	65
91	58	169	58	172	62	177	53
183	48	188	52	194	67	266	53
266	53	267	52	351	71	372	71

Note: the first 20 survival times are complete (died within the study period) and the following 16 are censored.

Survival and vital capacity

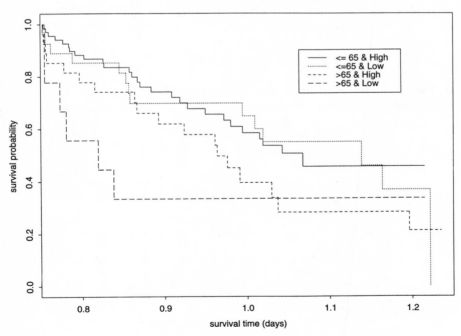

Figure 8.8

441

A plot of these data gives strong indications that both age and vital capacity play a role in the survival of these patients. A plot (Figure 8.8) of the four survival curves is produced by

```
> # time is a vector of 131 survival times
> # c0 is a vector: censored (0) or complete (1)
> # g0 is a vector: high (0) or low (1) vital capacity
> # age is a vector of 131 reported ages
> cplot<- function(id1,id2,id0) {
    ttmp<- time[age0==id1 & g0==id2]
    ctmp<- c0[age0==id1 & g0==id2]
    stmp<- g0[age0==id1 & g0==id2]
    par(new=T)
    plot(surv.fit(ttmp,ctmp,stmp),conf.int=F,xlab="",
        ylab="",yaxt="n",mark.time=F,xaxt="n",lty=id0)
    }
> plot(time,time,ylim=c(0,1),type="n",xlab="survival time (days)",
        mark.time=F,ylab="survival probability",
        main="Survival and vital capacity")
> age0<- ifelse(age<66,1,2)
> cplot(1,1,1)
> cplot(1,2,2)
> cplot(2,1,3)
> cplot(2,2,4)
> legend(250,.9,c("<= 65 & High","<=65 & Low",">65 & High",
        ">65 & Low"),lty=1:4)
```

To analyze the joint influences of both vital capacity ($x_{i1} = 0$ [high] and $x_{i1} = 1$ [low]) and age ($x_{i2} =$ age in years, as reported), a bivariate proportional hazards model is postulated where

$$\lambda_i(t|x_{i1}, x_{i2}) = \lambda_0(t) \times e^{b_1 x_{i1} + b_2(x_{i2} - \bar{x}_2)}.$$

The estimation of the model coefficients b_1 and b_2 as well as the other elements of the analysis employing this bivariate model are generated by the S-function $coxreg()$. For the 131 lung cancer patients,

```
> coxreg(time,c0,cbind(age,g0))
 Alive Dead Deleted
    66   65       0

        coef exp(coef) se(coef)    z      p
age 0.0383      1.04   0.0154  2.49 0.0128
g0  0.6350      1.89   0.2742  2.32 0.0206

      exp(coef) exp(-coef) lower .95 upper .95
age      1.04      0.962      1.01      1.07
g0       1.89      0.530      1.10      3.23

Likelihood ratio test= 10   on 2 df,     p=0.00667
Efficient score test = 10.3  on 2 df,    p=0.00572.
```

The estimated model is

$$\hat{\lambda}_i(t|x_{i1}, x_{i2}) = \lambda_0(t) \times e^{0.635 x_{i1} + 0.038(x_{i2} - 59.450)}.$$

where $\hat{b}_1 = 0.635$ (*vital capacity group*) and $\hat{b}_2 = 0.038$ (*age*) and the mean age of the study participants is $\bar{x}_2 = 59.450$ years. A few selected estimated hazard ratios (i.e., $\hat{\lambda}_i/\lambda_0$) are:

age $x_2 = 55$ high vital capacity ($x_1 = 0$)   estimated hazard ratio = 0.843
age $x_2 = 65$ high vital capacity ($x_1 = 0$)   estimated hazard ratio = 1.237
age $x_2 = 75$ high vital capacity ($x_1 = 0$)   estimated hazard ratio = 1.814

age $x_2 = 55$ low vital capacity ($x_1 = 1$)   estimated hazard ratio = 1.591
age $x_2 = 65$ low vital capacity ($x_1 = 1$)   estimated hazard ratio = 2.334
age $x_2 = 75$ low vital capacity ($x_1 = 1$)   estimated hazard ratio = 3.423.

A person 59.450 years old belonging to the high vital capacity group has a hazard ratio of exactly 1.0. Furthermore, the hazard ratio comparing low vital capacity group to the high vital capacity group is $\lambda_{low}(t)/\lambda_{high}(t) = e^{0.635} = 1.887$, accounting for the influence of age.

To evaluate the influence of a specific variable, the proportional hazards model with the variable included is once again compared to the model with the variable excluded in terms of -2 times the increase in log-likelihood values. For example, to assess the influence of age, the model with age included is compared to the model with the age variable excluded. The model depending on vital capacity status alone (age excluded) is

```
> coxreg(time,c0,g0)
 Alive Dead Deleted
    66    65       0

       coef exp(coef)  se(coef)     z       p
[1,] 0.539      1.71     0.274  1.97 0.0491

       exp(coef) exp(-coef) lower .95 upper .95
[1,]        1.71      0.583         1      2.93

Likelihood ratio test= 3.61  on 1 df,   p=0.0574
Efficient score test = 3.96  on 1 df,   p=0.0465.
```

The log-likelihood values are extracted from the S-objects for these two nested models. To evaluate the role of age, then

```
> # additive model -- age  and vital capacity
> like1<- coxreg(time,c0,cbind(age,g0))$loglik
> # age excluded (vital capacity only)
> like0<- coxreg(time,c0,g0)$loglik
> x2<- -2*(like0[2]-like1[2])
> pvalue<- 1-pchisq(x2,1)
> cbind(x2,pvalue)
           x2      pvalue
[1,] 6.40924 0.0113528.
```

The comparison is not affected by vital capacity status since both models contain a term that accounts for any influence. The same analytic process yields an assessment of the vital capacity variable or

```
> # vital capacity excluded (age only)
> like0<- coxreg(time,c0,age)$loglik
> x2<- -2*(like0[2]-like1[2])
> pvalue<- 1-pchisq(x2,1)
> cbind(x2,pvalue)
           x2      pvalue
[1,] 4.922531 0.02650866.
```

Age, as expected, has a substantial influence on the survival time (p-value = 0.011). The vital capacity classification has a somewhat less but also important impact (p-value = 0.027).

Another example of using a proportional hazards model is provided by the analysis of predictors of AIDs onset. Two indications of the extent of HIV infection are β_2-microglobulin levels and CD4 counts. To assess these prognostic indicators and their relation to the time (in months) to onset of AIDs, a proportional hazard model is applied to the data in Table 8.5. The recorded variables are: the time to AIDs ("survival") for a group of $n = 89$ men with HIV infection reported in weeks, the status of the observation (0 = censored and 1 = complete), measured β_2-microglobulin levels, and CD4 counts [7].

The baseline Kaplan–Meier survival curve (ignoring the independent variables) estimated from these data (Figure 8.9) is created by

```
> # read and define input variables (Table 8.5)
> temp<- scan("aids.data")
> time<- temp[seq(1,length(temp),4)]
> c0<- temp[seq(2,length(temp),4)]
> plot(surv.fit(time,c0),xlab="time (months)",
    ylab="survival probability",conf.int=T,
    main="Kaplan-Meier estimated survival curve -- time to aids")
```

As before, the S-vector *time* contains all "survival" times (censored and complete = $n = 89$) and the S-vector $c0$ indicates their censored status.

A bivariate model assuming proportional hazard rates is

$$\lambda_i(t|x_{i1}, x_{i2}) = \lambda_0(t) \times e^{b_1(x_{i1}-\bar{x}_1)+b_2(x_{i2}-\bar{x}_2)+b_3(x_{i1}-\bar{x}_1)(x_{i2}-\bar{x}_2)}$$

where x_1 represents the β_2-microglobulin levels and x_2 represents the CD4 counts. Unlike the baseline survival function (Figure 8.9), the hazard rates are influenced by two independent variables. Example S-code that reads the HIV data from the exterior file named *aids.data* and implements the estimation of the Cox model parameters is

```
> # read and define input variables
> temp<- scan("aids.data")
> time<- temp[seq(1,length(temp),4)]
> c0<- temp[seq(2,length(temp),4)]
> beta<- temp[seq(3,length(temp),4)]
> cd4<- temp[seq(4,length(temp),4)]
> cd4bybeta<- beta*cd4
> x<- cbind(beta,cd4,cd4bybeta)
> # model estimation
> coxreg(time,c0,x)
```

Table 8.5. Survival times (weeks to AIDs) for $n = 89$ men with recorded serum β_2-microglobulin and CD4 counts

time	status*	β_2	CD4	time	status*	β_2	CD4	time	status*	β_2	CD4
5	1	5.51	263	97	0	1.79	648	46	1	2.67	643
96	0	2.17	681	54	1	1.94	1359	95	0	1.68	788
45	1	3.95	261	26	1	3.62	373	37	1	3.15	830
96	0	2.97	493	13	1	3.70	346	21	1	2.58	918
77	1	2.71	536	25	0	2.61	341	101	1	2.35	800
97	0	1.66	970	22	0	2.62	528	98	0	3.00	534
1	1	2.79	485	100	0	1.97	1468	98	0	2.02	742
50	1	1.86	738	100	0	3.95	598	102	1	2.67	1199
18	1	4.13	389	85	1	1.97	356	98	0	2.53	922
59	1	4.22	981	49	0	1.79	764	102	0	1.98	1137
45	1	2.40	533	97	0	1.52	872	98	0	3.22	928
76	1	1.84	568	22	1	3.19	451	101	0	2.46	774
95	0	2.52	342	18	1	4.73	431	98	0	2.55	1140
20	1	2.12	581	97	0	2.40	825	48	1	2.45	297
100	0	1.60	592	25	1	3.22	389	101	0	1.95	543
37	0	1.81	937	20	1	0.79	417	101	0	4.86	685
22	1	3.03	296	63	1	2.12	625	101	0	1.71	897
19	1	2.21	570	101	0	1.15	782	70	0	2.06	410
85	1	4.02	640	42	1	1.96	544	57	1	3.39	906
47	1	2.39	805	102	0	1.78	467	61	1	2.66	562
101	0	2.98	406	74	1	2.20	827	3	1	3.90	49
45	1	2.77	439	76	1	2.08	692	16	1	4.67	341
80	0	2.61	724	62	1	2.83	677	100	0	1.61	654
101	0	2.34	799	102	0	2.46	413	69	1	2.79	615
6	0	2.18	908	75	1	2.55	598	49	1	1.76	558
2	1	2.74	74	60	1	1.69	476	16	1	2.59	567
100	0	1.95	745	90	1	2.03	676	65	1	2.94	646
84	0	1.81	1013	98	1	1.60	873	42	1	1.74	996
97	0	1.64	597	56	0	2.11	478	12	1	3.36	1020
84	1	1.49	747	47	1	2.57	719				

* status = 1 = complete observation and status = 0 = censored observation
Note: the first 52 observations are patients less than 30 years old and the remaining 37 patients have ages greater than or equal to 30.

```
Alive Dead Deleted
  37    52      0
                  coef exp(coef) se(coef)        z         p
     beta  1.26055        3.527 0.459063    2.746  0.00603
      cd4  0.00152        1.002 0.002041    0.747  0.45533
cd4bybeta -0.00133        0.999 0.000741   -1.787  0.07387

          exp(coef) exp(-coef) lower .95 upper .95
     beta     3.527      0.283     1.434      8.67
      cd4     1.002      0.998     0.998      1.01
cd4bybeta     0.999      1.001     0.997      1.00

Likelihood ratio test= 23.8   on 3 df,    p=2.76e-05
Efficient score test = 33.4   on 3 df,    p=2.65e-07.
```

Kaplan-Meier estimated survival curve -- time to aids

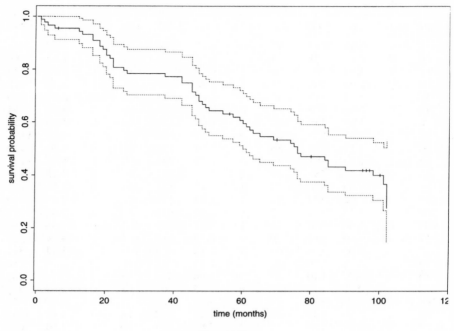

Figure 8.9

This version of a proportional hazards model includes an interaction term. Specifically, the association between the time to AIDs ("survival" time) and CD4 counts may be influenced by the level of β_2-microglobulin. The magnitude of the b_3 coefficient measures the impact of the joint influence of these two independent variables on "survival" time.

To assess statistically the influence from this interaction, an additive model is purposed and the respective log-likelihood values compared. The additive model (no interaction—$b_3 = 0$) is

$$\lambda_i(t|x_{i1}, x_{i2}) = \lambda_0(t) \times e^{b_1(x_{i1}-\bar{x}_1)+b_2(x_{i2}-\bar{x}_2)}$$

and the estimates of b_1 and b_2 are given by

```
> coxreg(time,c0,x[,-3])
 Alive Dead Deleted
    37   52       0

          coef exp(coef) se(coef)     z       p
beta   0.46908     1.599 0.153611  3.05 0.00226
 cd4  -0.00198     0.998 0.000691 -2.87 0.00410
```

```
      exp(coef) exp(-coef) lower .95 upper .95
beta    1.599      0.626    1.183     2.160
 cd4    0.998      1.002    0.997     0.999

Likelihood ratio test= 20.8  on 2 df,   p=3.11e-05
Efficient score test = 21.5  on 2 df,   p=2.13e-05.
```

The contrast of log-likelihood summaries (interaction term included and excluded)

```
> # interaction present
> like<- coxreg(time,c0,x)$loglik
> # interaction absent
> like0<- coxreg(time,c0,x[,-3])$loglik
> x2<- -2*(like0[2]-like[2])
> pvalue<- 1-pchisq(x2,1)
> cbind(x2,pvalue)
            x2       pvalue
[1,] 3.035368 0.08146807
```

indicates marginal evidence of an interaction influence. That is, the impact of CD4 counts on the time to AIDs may depend on the level of the β_2-micro-globulin. Note the expected similarity to the Wald test ("p" in the output corresponding to the "cd4bybeta" term) produced as part of the first *coxreg*( ) analysis where the p-value associated with the interaction coefficient $(\hat{b}_3 - 0.00133)$ is 0.074.

Based on the additive model, the separate influences of each of the two prognostic variables are once again evaluated by contrasting log-likelihood values from nested models. The impact of β_2-microglobulin is evaluated from the following:

```
> # additive model -- cd4 and beta included
> like1<- coxreg(time,c0,x[,-3])$loglik
> # beta variable excluded (CD4 only)
> like0<- coxreg(time,c0,cd4)$loglik
> x2<- -2*(like0[2]-like1[2])
> pvalue<- 1-pchisq(x2,1)
> cbind(x2,pvalue)
          x2       pvalue
[1,] 8.25851 0.004056141.
```

Similarly, the impact of CD4-counts is evaluated from

```
> # CD4 variable excluded (beta only)
> like0<- coxreg(time,c0,beta)$loglik
> x2<- -2*(like0[2]-like1[2])
> pvalue<- 1-pchisq(x2,1)
> cbind(x2,pvalue)
            x2       pvalue
[1,] 9.143166 0.002496487.
```

Both variables appear to have substantial influence on "survival" time. Again the log-likelihood tests are similar to the Wald's z-statistic from *coxreg*( ) output based on the additive, bivariate model (p-values 0.002 (β) and 0.004 (*CD4*), respectively).

Much like a linear model, analysis of residual values can indicate failures of a proportional hazards model to adequately represent the structure underlying the data. A simple start are plots of the residual values associated with each independent variable. If the data conform to the requirements of a proportional hazards analysis, then the residual values, as before, are expected to be randomly distributed about a horizontal line = 0. Visual assessment of residual value plots can indicate the presence of outlier observations, non-proportionality, trends or other problems associated with a specific variable. For the AIDs data, the residual value plots associated with the β_2-microglobulin levels and the CD4 counts using the additive model ($b_3 = 0$) are created by

```
> otemp<- coxreg(time,c0,x[,-3],resid="schoen")
> rcox<- otemp$resid
> tcox<- otemp$time
> par(mfrow=c(2,1))
> labels<- c("beta level","cd4 count")
> for(i in 1:2){
   plot(tcox,rcox[,i],xlab="time",ylab="Schoenfeld residuals",
   pch=i,main=paste("Residual values -- ",labels[i]))
   abline(h=0)
   lines(tcox,smooth(rcox[,i]),lty=2)
   abline(lsfit(tcox,rcox[,i]))}
```

Figure 8.10 displays these two plots along with a smoothed line (dotted line) and a least squares estimated straight line (solid line) summarizing the residual values ("+") to help identify non-random patterns. The same residual plots based on the interaction model can be created by replacing the input data array $x[, -3]$ with x. Both plots of residual values from the additive model show indications of non-random trends. The β_2-microglobulin residual values slope downward while the CD4 residual values slope upward, or in terms of correlation coefficients between the residual values and the "survival" times,

```
> round(cor(rcox,tcox),3)
        beta    cd4
  [1,] -0.307 0.359.
```

Ideally, the correlations should be close to zero. Based on the plots of the residual values (Figure 8.10), a model restricted to "survival" times between 30 and 85 weeks removes much of the observed pattern among the residual values. The correlation between residual values and the "survival" times decreases where

```
> # rcox1 and tcox1 -- output from truncated analysis
> round(cor(rcox1,tcox1),3)
        beta    cd4
  [1,] 0.028 0.105.
```

The truncated data appears to conform somewhat better to the requirements of the proportional hazards model.

Residual values -- beta level

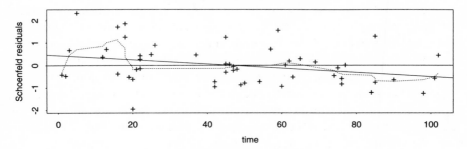

Residual values -- cd4 count

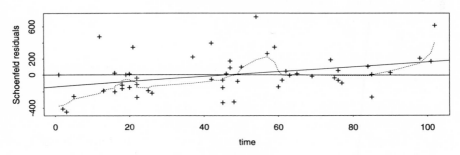

Figure 8.10

The S-function *coxreg( )* allows a stratified analysis of survival data. Strata can be combined where the hazard functions are proportional within each stratum but differ among strata. That is, the "baseline" hazard functions differ among specified strata. The analysis is made under a "no-interaction" assumption producing one set of estimated model coefficient based on combining estimates from each stratum. Applied to the AIDs data, an additive model stratified by age (< 30 and ≥ 30 years of age) gives

```
> age0<- rep(c(0,1),c(52,37))
> coxreg(time,c0,x[,-3],strata=age0)
  Alive Dead Deleted
0    22   30       0
1    15   22       0

          coef exp(coef) se(coef)     z       p
beta   0.44017     1.553 0.155447  2.83 0.00463
 cd4  -0.00189     0.998 0.000697 -2.71 0.00670

       exp(coef) exp(-coef) lower .95 upper .95
beta       1.553      0.644     1.145     2.106
 cd4       0.998      1.002     0.997     0.999

Likelihood ratio test= 19.1  on 2 df,  p=7.19e-05
Efficient score test = 19.6  on 2 df,  p=5.63e-05.
```

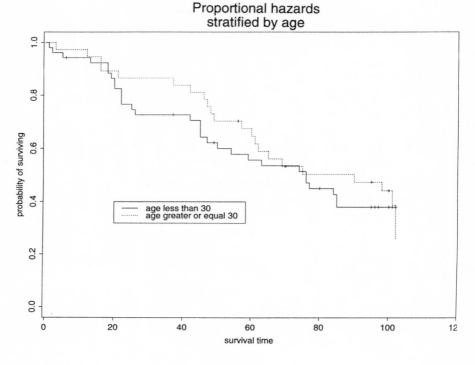

Figure 8.11

No important differences appear to exist between the AIDs prognostic variables and time to AIDs using an analysis stratified by age. The values of the estimates and the statistical tests are essentially the same as the previous additive model ignoring age. The baseline Kaplan–Meier survival curves for each age group are plotted (Figure 8.11) showing the younger group with a slightly better "survival" experience.

Problem set VIII

1. Show* the equivalence of the three expressions:

$$\text{person-years} = \delta_x P_{x+\delta_x} + \tfrac{1}{2}\delta_x D_x,$$
$$\text{person-years} = \delta_x P_x - \tfrac{1}{2}\delta_x D_x,$$
$$\text{person-years} = \tfrac{1}{2}\delta_x (P_{x+\delta_x} + P_x).$$

Show* that for an exponential survival model

$$S(T > t_2 | T > t_1) = e^{-\lambda(t_2 - t_1)}.$$

Show* that when $\lambda_1(t)/\lambda_2(t) = c$, then $S_1(t) = [S_2(t)]^c$.

2. If the survival times from one group are $\{7.5, 12, 18, 33^+, 55.5, 61.5\}$ and for another group are $\{34.5, 60, 64.5, 76.5^+, 79.5^+, 93\}$, show that the log-rank test (i.e., *surv.diff*( ) function) gives essentially the same results as the proportional hazards model (i.e., *coxreg*( ) function). The "+" indicates a censored survival time.

3. If d observations are complete (not censored) in a sample of n distinct survival times from exponentially distributed data, the likelihood function is

$$L = \prod_i \lambda e^{-\lambda t_i} \times \prod_j e^{-\lambda t_j'} \qquad i = 1, 2, 3, \cdots, d \quad \text{and} \quad j = 1, 2, 3, \cdots, n - d$$

where t_i represents complete observations and t_j' represents censored observations. Find the maximum likelihood estimate* of λ. Verify this estimator using the survival data from problem 2 and the S-function *ms*( ).

4. If the survival function is $S(t) = 1 - t/b$ where $0 \le t \le b = constant$, find the hazard function $\lambda(t)$ and the cumulative hazard function $H(t)$. Plot these three curves on a single page. Derive an expression for the average rate (R_t = deaths/person-years). Show* that $R_t \approx \lambda(t)$ for small time intervals.

5. Consider the $n = 11$ complete survival times $t = \{1, 4, 6, 8, 2, 12, 24, 23, 25, 27, 31\}$.

Use an S-program to demonstrate that the Kaplan–Meier estimated mean survival time is the same as the usual mean value $\bar{t} = \sum t_i/n$ and the variance is $(n - 1)variance(t)/n^2$.

Show* algebraically that for complete survival data

$$\bar{t} = \frac{1}{n}\sum t_i = \sum P_{i-1}(t_i - t_{i-1})$$

where $i = 1, 2, 3, \cdots, n$.

*Solve theoretically and not with a computer program.

REFERENCES

1. Cancer in California: Cancer Incidence and Morality California, 1988, California Tumor Registry, Cancer Surveillance Section, Department of Health Services, 1991.
2. Chiang, C. L., *The Life Table and Its Application*. Robert E. Krieger Publishing Company, Malabar, FL, 1984.
3. Collett, D., *Modeling Survival Data in Medical Research*. Chapman-Hill, New York, NY, 1994.
4. Miller, R. G., *Survival Analysis*. John Wiley and Sons, New York, NY, 1981.
5. Johnson, R. C. and Johnson, N. L., *Survival Models and Data Analysis*. John Wiley & Sons, New York, NY, 1980.
6. Kalbfleisch, D. J. and Prentice, R. L., *The Statistical Analysis of Failure Time Data*. John Wiley & Sons, New York, NY, 1980.

7. Anderson, R.E., Lang, W., Shiboski, S., *et al.* (1990) Use of β_2-microglobulin level and CD4 lymphocyte count to predict development of acquired immunodeficiency in persons with human immunodeficiency virus infection. *Archives of Internal Medicine* 150:73–77.

Index

Note: The parentheses following an index entry indicate an S-function. For example, $q(\ )$ indicates the S-function q for quit.

abline 92
ABO blood type 348–9
abridged life table 417
abs( ) 17
acceptance region 159
acceptance/rejection procedure 158, 189
acceptance/rejection sampling 157, 181, 188
accurate 267
acf( ) 152
acute myelogenous leukemia 435
additive data 127, 129
additive effect 127
additive linear model 206
additive logistic model 238, 243
additive model 238, 243, 254, 359, 370–1, 375, 381, 383, 446, 449
additive relationship 126, 129
additive structure 126, 132
additivity 127, 255, 260, 384
adj 400
adjusted 207
adjusted odds ratio 238, 245
adjusted R-squared 385
age-adjusted rate 415
age-specific mortality 417
age-specific rate 413–14, 419, 431
AIC criteria 386, 389
AIDs 445
Akaike Information Criterion 386
alpha-particles 170
analysis of matched pair data 379
analysis of variance 192, 361, 364–5, 369–70
anova( ) 246, 372, 383
aov( ) 364, 371, 381
apply( ) 33–5
approx( ) 434
approximate average rate 410
arithmetic operation 19

array( ) 38–9
array of values 7
arrow( ) 6
arrow 47
as.numeric( ) 60
atomic bomb 250
attach( ) 203
.Audit-file 57–8
autocorrelation coefficient 150
autocovariance 151
  function 152
axes 95

backwards stepwise procedure 386
bandwidth 73, 75, 95, 115
barplot( ) 70
behavior type 50
benign breast disease 323
benzene exposure 81, 316
Bernoulli variable 162
bias 300, 358
  estimate 300
binary data 270
binary design variable 342, 344
binary outcome 237, 239
binary variable 326
binom.test( ) 329
binomial coefficient 46, 163
binomial distribution 162, 171, 268, 329
binomial probability 163
birth weight 65–6, 76, 99
  distribution 92
  of newborn infants 202
  study 363
bivariate density function 115
bivariate model 447
bivariate normal contours 102
bivariate normal distribution 101, 114
bivariate random uniform value 188
Bode's rule 176

bootstrap bias estimator 300
bootstrap distribution 297
bootstrap estimate 283–6, 288–90,
    292–6, 299–302
    of the standard error 285
    of the statistical summary 285
bootstrap estimated mean 302
bootstrap replicate 284–6, 290, 295, 297
bootstrapping the residual 295
Box-Muller transformation 181
boxplot( ) 80, 82–3
breakfast cereals 120
Butler's method 186

c( ) 6
California lottery 76, 155
cancer mortality rate 310, 312
cancer prevention study 111
cancor( ) 403
canonical correlation 401, 403, 405–7
canonical summary 393, 401
    variable 403
canonical variable 392, 402, 405–6
capture/recapture strategy 167
carapace dimensions 229
case sensitive 6
case/control 239
    data 333
    status 240
cat( ) 48
categorical variable 37, 349, 364
cbind( ) 7
CD4 count 445
ceiling( ) 21
censored 274–5, 317, 428–9, 430, 437
cex 98
chi-square distribution 49, 183, 245,
    247, 249, 332, 344, 346, 357, 362,
    367, 376, 438
chi-square statistic 145, 242, 246,
    248–50, 260, 333, 335–6, 347
chi-square test 324–5
chisq.test( ) 49, 324, 344
chol( ) 190
Choleski decomposition 190–1
cholesterol 50
classification 228, 233
    error 233
clinical trial 326, 435
clustering 115
coefficient of contingency 335
coffee consumption 239
colon cancer cases 111
column effect 372
column percentages 128

column sum of squares 370
complementary log-log
    transformation 225
complete 429
complete life table 417
complete survival time 429
computer simulation 154
concatenate 48
concordant 328
confidence interval 48, 222, 271, 288–9,
    296, 302, 415–16
confidence limits 286
confounding 328, 378
consistency 266–7
consistent estimator 266
continuous distribution 178, 182, 188
continuous random variable 177
contour( ) 101, 103, 115
contour plot 103, 115
convex hull 135–6
cor( ) 26–7, 204
cor.test( ) 196
coronary heart disease 55
    data 130–1
coronary risk factors 244
correction factor 329
correlation 196, 214, 397, 401–2
counts of coronary events 289
covariance 46
Cox model 437, 439, 444
coxreg( ) 437, 442, 449
Cramer's *C* 336
Cramer's *V* 336
crude mortality rate 412
crude rate 413
cumsum( ) 20
cumulative binomial probability 163
cumulative hazard function 425–6
cumulative probability 174
    distribution 84, 87, 89, 146–7, 162,
    177–9, 185
cumulative standard normal
    distribution 179
cumulative sum 20
cut( ) 34, 36–7

.Data 57
.Data-directory 57
data frame 203, 204, 221, 368
data.frame( ) 221, 316
data.matrix( ) 306
deciles of risk 248–9
dendrogram 116
density( ) 70, 87
density estimate 72–3, 94

density function 73, 113, 174, 176
density plot 70, 75, 87
depth of a fourth 80–1
derivative( ) 276
derivative of a function 272–3
describe( ) 67–8
descriptive statistics 65
design variable 349, 415
deviance-table 247
diag( ) 40
diagnostic 365
diastolic blood pressure 195
diff( ) 20
differences 20
dim( ) 39
dimnames 421
direct adjustment 413
direct age-adjusted rate 413
discr( ) 230
discrete probability distribution 157,
    161–2, 166
discriminant analysis 228, 230
discriminant coefficient 229
discriminant function 232
discriminant score 228–30, 232–4, 392
dispersion parameter 207
dist( ) 118–19
distribution-free 429
dnorm( ) 174, 186
dose-response 331
dot notation 337
double arrow convention 48

editors 60
efficient 377
eigen( ) 407
eigenvalue 407
electromagnetic radiation 101
emacs 60
empirical cumulative probability
    distribution 84–5
error term 206, 292
Esterase D, 164
estimated logistic probabilities 241
estimated regression coefficient 292
estimated standard error 358
estimation 200
Euclidean distance 118, 120
exp( ) 17
expectation 157, 173
expected length of life 420
expected value 163, 167–9
exponential distribution 179, 272, 315,
    426, 432
exponential function 425, 428

exponential model 425
exponential probability distribution 178
exponential survival time 428
extreme value 65
eye 99

F-distribution 183–4, 211, 235, 296, 363
F-statistic 56, 211, 216, 236, 363–4, 372,
    377, 380, 384
F-test 212, 245
F-to-remove 212, 235
faces( ) 123, 126
factor( ) 351, 364
factor 349
failure rate 428
family 201
Fibonacci series 44
finite population correction factor 167–8
Fisher's exact test 324–5
five-dimensional model 355
follow-up study 427
for( ) 43
for-loop 43–4, 282
forward stepwise procedure 386
fourth-spread 82–3
Friedman rank test 376
full period 143
full regression equation 386

gamma( ) 17
gamma function 18
Gauss-Markov theorem 305, 307
Gaussian 201
general linear model 199, 236, 361, 439
geographic calculations 133
geometric distance 118
geometric distribution 173
geometric mean 184
geometric probability 173
    distribution 172
geometric standard deviation 184
glm( ) 199, 201, 203–4, 206, 216, 236,
    342, 357, 361, 415
goodness-of-fit 207, 248–9, 346, 386
graphic display 133, 365
graphic technique 95
graphics window 70, 97

harmonic mean 287
Hasting's approximation 180–1
hat matrix 218
hazard function 437–9, 449
hazard rate 425–6, 431–2, 439, 443–4
hclust( ) 118–19

health and demographic
    characteristics 404
help( ) 3, 109
hierarchical cluster 120
hierarchical grouping 116
hist( ) 68, 87
histogram 68, 70, 72, 78, 87, 95, 145
history 60
homemade function 45
homogeneity 325, 330, 347–8
homogeneous loglinear model 351
homogeneous model 352
Hotelling's T^2 test 54, 236
hypergeometric distributed variable 166
hypergeometric probability 167, 325
    distribution 165, 168

identify( ) 197
if( ) 45
ifelse( ) 16
independent variable 200–1, 207
indirect adjusted rate 414
integral 176
inter-quartile range 26
interaction 127, 132, 257, 259, 262, 373,
    384, 446
    effect 371
    sum of squares 381
    term 222
interpolation 434
interquartile range 75
inverse function 31, 178, 180, 185
inverse transformation 160, 171, 178–9
    method 160, 162, 177

jack( ) 298
jackknife estimate 298
jackknife estimated mean 299
jackknife estimation 297
jackknife replicate 297–9
jackknife residual 220

k-dimensional table 354
Kaplan-Meier estimate 430
Kaplan-Meier plot 434
Kaplan-Meier survival curve 431–2,
    436–7, 444, 450
Kaplan-Meier survival probability 429
Kendall's τ-measure 340
Kendall's τ-statistic 339
kernel 73
    function 75, 113–14
Kolmogorov 148
    procedure 85
    statistic 148

Kruskal-Wallis test 367
kruskal.test( ) 367

labex 103
lag 151
lambda measure 338
    of association 337
latent root 407
leaps( ) 387, 390–1
least squares analysis 306
least squares diagnostic 54
least squares estimate 198, 229, 294,
    305, 308, 311
least squares estimation 310
least squares fit 52
least trimmed squares 198
leaves 76
legend( ) 98
length( ) 16, 206
less.smooth( ) 112
leukemia incidence rates 109
leverage 197–9, 218–19
life table 417–19, 421
    hazard function 431
    person-years 419
    probabilities 418
    survival curves 423
likelihood 303
    function 268, 274, 277, 279–80,
        317–18
    ratio test 438
line type 95
linear combination 405
linear congruential sequence 142
linear discriminant analysis 192
linear equation 42
linear logistic model 236, 238, 240
linear model 200, 204, 206–8, 212, 222,
    250, 257–8, 372, 403, 448
linear regression 292
    analysis 192, 200, 203
    model 52, 216, 218, 234
lines( ) 107
link function 237, 254
list 314
lm( ) 204, 206, 211
location 65
log( ) 17
log-likelihood 275, 317, 319, 438, 443,
    446–7
    function 270–1, 276, 282
log-odds 240
log-rank test 436–8
logarithm of the odds 237
logarithmic transformation 310

logical condition 13, 16
logical operators 14
logistic analysis 237, 391
logistic function 237
logistic model 242, 318
logistic probability 248–9, 318
logit 237
loglinear model 341, 344, 348, 352, 354
lognormal distribution 183–4
lower fourth observation 80
ls.diag( ) 54
lsfit( ) 52–3, 98, 195, 198
ltsreg( ) 198
lty 95
lung cancer data 440
lung cancer deaths 250
lung cancer mortality 260
lung cancer patients 439

Mahalanobis distance 231
main 71
Mallow's *Cp* criteria 385, 387, 389
Mantel-Haenszel estimate 327
Mantel-Haenszel odds ratio 327
Mantel-Haenszel test 326
matched pair data 328, 378–9, 381
matched pair design 380
matched pairs 379
maternal/paternal variables 394
mathematical function 17
matplot( ) 261
matrix( ) 9, 11, 38, 40, 421
matrix algebra 39
max( ) 25
maximum 68, 185–6, 188, 277
maximum likelihood estimate 267,
    271–2, 277–8, 280, 282, 315, 317,
    318–19, 426
maximum likelihood estimation 281,
    283, 308
maximum likelihood estimator 268–9,
    270, 272, 428
McNemar chi-square analysis 378
McNemar matched pair test 328
McNemar test 329
mean( ) 25
mean 130, 144
mean squared error 375
mean survival time 428, 432–3
mean weight gain 310
measure of association 334, 336, 340
median( ) 25
median 80–2, 130, 144, 290–1, 433
median smoothed 109, 111
median survival time 433, 436

median/average smoothing 111
mid-square process 142
mid-year population 411
min( ) 25
minimum 68, 185–6, 188
minimum sum 314–15
minimum variance 267, 305
mod-function 23
model selection 387
    criteria 389, 391
model-free adjusted rate 415
modern cowboy 49
modulo arithmetic 142
modulo operator 23
mortality rate 418
motif( ) 70, 97
moving average 111
ms( ) 314–15, 318
multiple correlation coefficient 208–9,
    216, 403
multiplicative relationship 132
multiplicative structure 131–2
multiplicative terms 257
multivariable linear model 199, 204, 229
multivariable regression 385, 400
multivariate classification scheme 123
multivariate data 200
multivariate distance 231, 235
multivariate function 29
multivariate measurement 392, 395,
    401–2, 407
multivariate normal data 192
multivariate normal distribution 56, 190,
    232
multivariate normal random
    observation 191
multivariate observation 231, 236, 393,
    400, 405–6

NA 16, 27, 205–6
NA-values 27
na.omit( ) 205
ncol( ) 39
Neanderthal man 49
nearest neighbor distance 116
negative triangular distribution 188
nested design 367
nested model 245–6, 352, 438
nls( ) 309
non-additivity 373, 383–4
noninformative 430
nonlinear least squares 313
    estimate 308, 313
nonlinear model 311
non-monotonic criterion 387

nonparametric 367, 376–7, 439
nonparametric matched pair 380
nonparametric technique 436
normal cumulative distribution 87
normal distribution 29, 31, 72–3, 75, 83,
    174, 180, 186, 200, 214, 267, 278,
    285–6, 294, 317
normal probability function 176
normalized residual value 219
nrow( ) 39, 206
NULL 44
null deviance 208, 247, 307
null distribution 304
null hypothesis 329
nutritional contents 121

object 53
odds ratio 238, 327, 334–5, 342, 345–8
offset( ) 258–9
one observation per cell 381
one-way analysis 377
    of variance 364, 372–3
one-way design 361
order( ) 22–3
ordinal variable 338
ordinary least squares 205
ordinate 174
orthogonal polynomial 223
outer( ) 43, 47, 99
outlier 78, 82
    cut-off 81
    value 65
Oxford Childhood Cancer Study 330

p-value 79
paired observations 378
pairs( ) 104–5, 398
pairwise association 347–8
pairwise product term 345, 347
pairwise relationship 403
par( ) 94, 107, 214
partition 333
paste( ) 109
pch 97
pclust( ) 118
perimeter 134
perinatal mortality 224
permissible parameter 269
permutation 155
person-years 410–11, 419
persp( ) 98–9, 101, 103, 115
perspective plot 115
petroleum workers 368
pie( ) 71
pie chart 71

plclust( ) 119
plot( ) 97
plot character 97
plot type 101
pnorm( ) 29, 31, 84, 174
points( ) 97
pointwise( ) 222
pointwise confidence interval 222
Poisson distribution 168, 170–1, 254,
    271, 274, 342, 415
Poisson model 250, 254–5, 258–60, 342
Poisson parameter 276
Poisson probability distribution 169
Poisson regression 258, 341
poly( ) 223
Polya 180
polygon( ) 133, 134–6, 189
polynomial function 223
polynomial model 225
polynomial regression 223
positive triangular distribution 174, 178,
    188
postscript( ) 97
prcomp( ) 395
precise 267
precision 283
predict( ) 208, 221, 227, 230, 241, 248,
    260, 347
predicted sum of squares 385
prediction 385
PRESS 385
principal component 391–3, 395–40
    analysis 393, 399, 403
    coefficient 398–9
    plot 400
    summary 396, 398–9, 406
prior probabilities 232
probability 411–12
    density 101, 186
    density function 174
    distribution 72, 157, 159
    of failure 429
    of misclassification 232
prod( ) 20, 46
product-limit 429
product-moment correlation 26, 204,
    403, 405
projection 104
prop.test( ) 324
proportional hazards analysis 448
proportional hazards model 442–4
proportional hazards rate 437
pseudo-random number 141–2
pty 101

q( ) 3
qchisq( ) 179
qnorm( ) 31, 87, 179
qqline( ) 85
qqnorm( ) 85, 87, 92, 146, 214, 216
qqnorm plot 365
qqplot( ) 87, 91–2
quadratic function 197
quantile( ) 26, 81, 288
quit 5

R-squared adjusted 387
random binomial 164
random maximum value 185
random minimum value 185
random normal value 180
random number 141
    generator 143
random permutation 155
random statistical value 141
random.seed( ) 144
randomization test 302, 304
range( ) 25, 74
rank( ) 21
rank 367, 376
rate 410–16, 425
rbind( ) 8
rbinom( ) 164
rchisq( ) 183
read.table( ) 201, 203
regression analysis 205, 220, 399
regression coefficient 206–7, 210, 223,
    229, 245, 254, 293, 295–6
regression equation 247
regression model 385, 387
regression parameter 295
relative risk 289–90
remove( ) 57
rep( ) 11
residual( ) 132
residual deviance 207, 211, 234–5,
    245–8, 255–6, 260, 307, 343, 346,
    352, 357–8
residual plot 213
residual standard error 213
residual sum of squares 307, 370, 372,
    377, 381–3, 385
residual value 198, 207, 211–14, 217,
    219–20, 371, 373, 448
    plot 448
rev( ) 21
rexp( ) 178
rf( ) 184
rgeom( ) 173
rhyper( ) 168

risk set 430
rlnorm( ) 184
rnorm( ) 21, 32, 180, 191
row effects 372
row percentages 128
row sum of squares 370
rpois( ) 172
rt( ) 183
runif( ) 33, 143–5, 148, 150, 286

S-geometry 136
S-object 53–4, 199, 201, 246, 314
sample( ) 155, 286
sample mean 267
sampled with replacement 156, 284
sampling without replacement 155
saturated model 343–5, 354–5, 357–8
scale( ) 217, 393
scan( ) 10
scoring process 274
second partial derivative 277
seed value 144
segments( ) 135
semi-parametric model 439
seq( ) 12
serial correlation coefficient 150–1
serum lead level 369
set.seed( ) 144
sign( ) 17
significance probability 79, 260, 325,
    364, 384
simple linear regression model 291
simulation technique 141
single value 6–7
slope 272
smoking data 336
smoking status 334, 336
smooth( ) 290–1
smooth.spline( ) 112
smoothing parameter 73
smoothing techniques 109
smoothness 291
solve( ) 42
source( ) 59
spatial clustering 152
spatial data 113
spatial pattern 155
spin( ) 105, 107
Splus BATCH, 59
sqrt( ) 17
square brackets 9, 12–13, 15, 40
square root 190
squared multiple correlation
    coefficient 236, 296–7, 385
standard deviation 67, 395

standard error 67, 217, 219, 221, 285–6, 289–90
standard mortality ratio 414–15, 417
standard normal distribution 31–2, 36, 83, 85, 146, 175, 179, 181–2, 184–6, 188, 301, 316, 333, 347, 380
standard normal value 180, 191
standard normal variates 190
standard random normal value 214
standardization 393
standardized coefficient 210, 234, 355
standardized difference 353
standardized discriminant score 230–1
standardized residual value 219–20
stars( ) 126
stationary population 417
statistical distribution 29, 201
statistical independence 343
statistical test 28, 271
stem( ) 76
stem-and-leaf display 76, 78
stems 76
step( ) 289, 386
step-function 147
stepfun( ) 147
stepwise selection process 386–7
Student *t*-test 50
Student's *t*-distribution 308
Studentized residual value 220
subscript 13
sum( ) 24
sum of squares 362
summary( ) 67
summary 67, 204–5, 210, 245, 314, 344, 346, 354
  technique 65
super smooth 198
supsmu( ) 112, 198–9
surv.diff( ) 429, 435–6
survival curves 435, 442
survival data 428, 449
survival function 444
survival probability 421, 423, 425, 430, 433, 434–5
survival time 427, 430, 432, 448
sweep( ) 127–9, 397
symbolic name 6
systolic blood pressure 197, 292

t( ) 41
t-distribution 183, 220
t-statistic 197
t-test 79–80, 196, 302
T^2 statistic 236
T^2 test 54

table( ) 34–5, 37, 68, 145
tabulations 34
tapply( ) 37, 364
test of randomness 146, 214
tests of homogeneity 346
text( ) 107, 400
three-dimensional plot 98
three methods of determining serum lead level 370
total sum of squares 307, 362–3
transformation 106, 217, 225, 237, 393
transpose 41
tree( ) 126
triangular distribution 175
trigonometric function 18
trunc( ) 21
TRUNC_AUDIT 58
Tschuprow's *T* 336
turtle's carapace 228
twin data 280
twins 279
two by two table 323
two-dimensional array 8
two-dimensional distribution 136
two-dimensional plot 104, 135
two-dimensional table 126
two-sample test 301
two-way analysis of variance 381–2
two-way classification 369–70, 377, 384
two-way data 381
two-way table 127, 382
twoway( ) 130

unbiased 267, 300, 345
unif( ) 32
uniform distribution 32, 145–6, 148, 177–8, 190
uniform random variable 144, 181, 185, 188
uniroot( ) 273
United States cancer deaths 412
United States cancer mortality 412
United States mortality rates 422
UNIX 97
UNIX command 59
unix( ) 59–60
unordered categorical variable 349, 351
upper fourth 81
upper triangular matrix 190

var( ) 25, 27
variability 65
variance 67, 157, 163, 167–9, 173
  of a continuous probability distribution 175

of the maximum likelihood
  estimate 270
variance/covariance array 54, 56, 190–2,
  277, 280, 282, 307–8
vector variable 7
vi 60

waiting time distribution 172
Wald statistic 438
Wald test 447
Wald z-statistic 447
width 75
wilcox.test( ) 380
Wilcoxon signed rank test 380
Wilcoxon two-sample test 50
Wilk's lambda 231
win.graph 70

within pair differences 379
within sum of squares 362
wrong model bias 358

*X*11( ) 70, 97
xlab 71, 74, 95
xlim 74
xy-coordinate system 118
xy-plot 95

yaxt 214
ylab 74, 82, 95
ylim 74
Yule's measure 335

z-statistic 159